AIDS
and the
Allied Health
Professions

AIDS

and the
Allied Health Professions

Joyce W. Hopp, Ph.D., M.P.H.

Dean, School of Allied Health Professions
Professor, Health Education
School of Public Health
Loma Linda University
Loma Linda, California

Elizabeth A. Rogers, Ed.D., PT

Professor and Associate Chairperson
Department of Physical Therapy
School of Allied Health Professions
Loma Linda University
Loma Linda, California

 F.A. DAVIS COMPANY • Philadelphia

Printed in the United States of America

Last digit indicates print number: 10 9 8 7 6 5 4 3 2 1

Library of Congress Cataloging-in-Publication Data

AIDS and the allied health professions / [edited by] Joyce W. Hopp, Elizabeth A. Rogers.
    p.   cm.
   Includes bibliographies and index.
   ISBN 0-8036-4677-1
   1. AIDS (Disease) 2. Allied health personnel.   I. Hopp, Joyce W., 1927–   . II. Rogers, Elizabeth A.
   [DNLM: 1. Acquired Immunodeficiency Syndrome. 2. Allied Health
   Personnel.   WD 308 A287796]
   RC607.A26A345556   1989
   362.1′969792—dc20
   DNLM/DLC
   for Library of Congress   89-11934
                                                                                        CIP

Preface

"Allied health professionals play a major role in the care of people with AIDS," states Dr. Thomas Freeland, President of the American Society of Allied Health Professions.[1] We wholeheartedly agree. This text has been written to help allied health professionals fill that role as the worldwide epidemic rages unchecked. Effective treatment for sexually transmitted diseases has not always led to their control; penicillin, although potent against syphilis, has not kept the rate of syphilis cases from rising. Education targeted at personal behavior and societal change is necessary. With an estimated 10 million persons infected worldwide, the number of individuals who will develop AIDS will continue to increase, even if both a vaccine and effective therapeutic drugs are developed.

Every health professional will be touched by the tragedy of this epidemic. AIDS has many faces: a young child who will know no mother other than the nurse on his hospital unit, the expectant mother who has just learned that the virus she carries will probably infect her baby, or the successful businessman who has the early signs of AIDS dementia. How a health care worker responds to their needs depends on the values held, the education gained, and the service he or she is willing and able to render.

The Institute of Medicine's 1988 report states that the health professions have a compact with society to treat patients with all forms of illness, including human immunodeficiency virus (HIV) infection and AIDS.[2] To deny or compromise treatment to any patient on the grounds that a medical risk is posed to the provider breaks the fundamental trust between patient and caregiver. Health care personnel, however, also deserve to know the occupational risks they face in caring for infected patients. This text provides an assessment of the risks of occupational transmission, along with techniques to further reduce the risks of occupational HIV transmission.

The care of AIDS patients is sufficiently complex that it requires personnel of many different skills, all trained in the context of HIV-caused disease. It is the responsibility of each of the allied health professions to provide adequate training in HIV infection and AIDS. The Institute of Medicine urges that every health professional curriculum be modified to ensure adequate training in the diagnosis, prevention, and treatment of HIV infection and AIDS, as well as in infection control measures.[3]

- We have written this book with the needs of a variegated audience in mind. Although the chapters unfold in a logical manner, we have made sure that each chapter stands on its own so that the use of this book can be adapted to individual needs.

- Each chapter begins with an outline—"a road map" of the material to be covered—and a list of the chapter's objectives. Discussion questions at the end of each chapter help reinforce newly acquired learning.

- Because caring for persons with AIDS (PWAs) is a team effort, in Chapter 10 we identify the contributions of 12 Allied Health professions in the treatment and prevention of HIV infection and AIDS. This chapter strongly emphasizes the health care worker's (HCW's) role in limiting the spread of HIV and in self-protection.

- In the last chapter, we provide 2 case studies to help the readers explore their attitudes toward caring for PWAs. One health professional and a volunteer for an AIDS project relate their experience with HIV infection and the health care system and, quietly but forcefully, make the case for professionalism and compassion on the part of the HCW.

- Finally, a glossary of AIDS-specific terms is provided at the back of the book for quick review along with 3 appendices: one on AIDS resources, one on HIV testing, and one on safer sex guidelines.

- A Teacher's Guide is available, upon adoption, to facilitate the use of the book in a variety of settings. In it, instructors will find an extensive list of additional sources (print as well as audio-visual), specific information for use in different disciplines, as well as sample examinations.

Terminology in the field of AIDS continues to change. In the early days of the epidemic, both AIDS (a disease definition limited to those diagnosed with Kaposi's sarcoma or *Pneumocystis carinii* pneumonia) and ARC (AIDS-related complex, representing other symptomatology related to HIV infection) were used. Since that time, the term ARC has been discarded in recognition of the fact that infection by HIV is a continuum of conditions associated with immune dysfunction.

Writing this textbook on AIDS was like trying to paddle up a whitewater stream; no matter how fast we stroked, the flood of information pushed us downstream. Hundreds of scientific articles are appearing yearly on AIDS. Laboratories in educational institutions, research institutes, and pharmaceutical companies around the world pour forth information. To keep up to date, the reader must go beyond this text to current scientific and professional journals.

AIDS is the most widely researched disease in history. The fruits of that research may eventually conquer the disease. Until such a time, the care and commitment of dedicated health care workers can provide quality of life for those afflicted with the virus that causes AIDS.

J.W.H.
E.A.R.

1. Allied Health Professions Seen Playing Major Role in AIDS Crises. Trends, newsletter of the Amer Soc of Allied Health Professions, June 1988, p. 3.

2. Confronting AIDS: Update 1988, Institute of Medicine. Washington DC: Academic Press. 1988, p. 15.

3. Confronting AIDS: Update 1988, Ibid.

Acknowledgments

We heartily thank our contributors who generously worked under tight time constraints. We thank our students who challenged us to give them material they could use. We thank the PWAs with whom we have worked and who helped us understand the urgent need for education and caring. Finally, we thank our valiant reviewers who read and re-read the manuscript under the "impossible" schedule set by Jean François Vilain, our editor: Mary F. Belmont, Ed.D., R.N., AIDS Consultant, New York City Department of Health, and Director of Program, National Student Nurses' Association; Linda D. Crane, M.M.Sc., PT, CCS, Instructor, Division of Physical Therapy, University of Miami School of Medicine; Brenda M. Foster, B.S., CMA, Instructor, Medical Assisting, School of Public and Allied Health, East Tennessee State University; Robert J. Kus, R.N., Ph.D., Associate Professor, College of Nursing, The University of Iowa; Sharan L. Schartzberg, Ed.D., OTR, FAOTA, Professor and Chairperson, Tufts University-Boston School of Occupational Therapy; Walter A. Stein, M.A. in HCA, PA-C, Assistant Professor of Health Care Sciences, George Washington University; Mary Louise Turgeon, Ed.D., MT (ASCP), Assistant Director of Medical Education, Guthrie Medical Center, Robert Packer Hospital, Sayre, PA, and Clinical Assistant Professor, University of North Dakota School of Medicine; and Frances K. Widmann, M.D., Associate Professor of Pathology, Duke University Medical Center.

Contributors

Leif Kristian Bakland, D.D.S.
Associate Dean and Professor of Endodontics
School of Dentistry
Loma Linda University
Loma Linda, California

Sylvia A. Burlew, M.P.H., RRA
Assistant Professor
Department of Health Information Administration
School of Allied Health Professions
Loma Linda University
Loma Linda, California

Mark J. Clements, M.A., RT(R)
Assistant Professor and Associate Chairman
Department of Radiologic Technology
School of Allied Health Professions
Loma Linda University
Loma Linda, California

Eunice Diaz, M.S., M.P.H.
Member, National AIDS Commission
Cerritos, California

Harvey A. Elder, M.D.
Professor of Medicine
School of Medicine
Loma Linda University
Chief, Infectious Disease Control
Jerry L. Pettis Memorial Veterans Hospital
Loma Linda, California

Mary Ann Frew, M.S., R.N., CMA-C
Director, Medical Assistant Program
Gannon University
Erie, Pennsylvania

Kathleen R. Guindon, R.N.
Case Manager, Inland AIDS Project
Riverside, California

Delia Gutierrez, M.P.H., PT
Assistant Professor
Program Director, Physical Therapist Assistant Program
Department of Physical Therapy
School of Allied Health Professions
Loma Linda University
Loma Linda, California

Fritz Guy, Ph.D.
Lecturer in Ethics
School of Religion
Loma Linda University
Loma Linda, California

Marianne Hart, M.S.W., L.C.S.W.
Social Work Consultant and Private Practitioner
Victorville, California

Joyce W. Hopp, Ph.D., M.P.H.
Dean, School of Allied Health Professions
Professor, Health Education
School of Public Health
Loma Linda University
Loma Linda, California

Marguerite McMillan Jackson, R.N., M.S., CIC
Director, Epidemiology Unit
Assistant Professor of Community and Family Medicine
University of California Medical Center
San Diego, California

George Edward Johnston, Ph.D.
Associate Dean
Program Director and Associate Professor of Environmental Health
School of Public Health
Loma Linda University
Loma Linda, California

Cindy L. Kosch, M.S.
Assistant Professor
Department of Nutrition and Dietetics
School of Allied Health Professions
Loma Linda University
Loma Linda, California

John Edwin Lewis, Ph.D.
Associate Professor
Chairman, Department of Clinical Laboratory Science
School of Allied Health Professions
Associate Professor of Pathology and Medicine
School of Medicine
Loma Linda University
Loma Linda, California

Edwinna May Marshall, M.A., OTR
Associate Professor and Chairperson
Department of Occupational Therapy
School of Allied Health Professions
Loma Linda University
Loma Linda, California

David Pauley
Volunteer with Inland AIDS Project
Riverside, California

Ann Elizabeth Ratcliff, Ph.D.
Assistant Professor
Department of Speech-Language Pathology and Audiology
School of Allied Health Professions
Loma Linda University
Loma Linda, California

Elizabeth A. Rogers, Ed.D., PT
Professor and Associate Chairperson
Department of Physical Therapy
School of Allied Health Professions
Loma Linda University
Loma Linda, California

Roland T. Sedillos, B.S., PT
Physical Therapist and Artist
Long Beach, California

Juliette Monique So'Brien van Putten, M.P.H., M.S.
Assistant Professor
Department of Health Promotion and Education
School of Public Health
Loma Linda University
Loma Linda, California

Robert L. Wilkins, M.A., R.R.T.
Assistant Professor
Co-ordinator of Clinical Education
Department of Respiratory Therapy
School of Allied Health Professions
Loma Linda University
Loma Linda, California

Contents

ONE

HISTORY OF THE ACQUIRED IMMUNODEFICIENCY SYNDROME (AIDS) EPIDEMIC

John Edwin Lewis

OUTLINE

OBJECTIVES

After reading this chapter, the reader will be able to:
1. Describe the worldwide character of the AIDS epidemic.

1

2. List 5 major events in the history of the AIDS epidemic.
3. Describe the role of the Centers for Disease Control in the AIDS epidemic.
4. Identify the first known high-risk groups.
5. Trace the way in which the means of transmission were identified.
6. Describe the contributions of scientists worldwide to knowledge of the viral cause of AIDS.
7. Identify the serologic tests for HIV.
8. Distinguish among the 3 patterns of HIV distribution.
9. Analyze why different patterns exist among various racial and ethnic groups in the United States.
10. Summarize the primary challenge posed by the AIDS epidemic.

HISTORY OF THE AIDS EPIDEMIC

Scientists worldwide have embarked on a mission to understand and arrest the epidemic of the human immunodeficiency virus (HIV) and acquired immunodeficiency syndrome (AIDS). The ravages of this modern affliction know no boundaries. AIDS has been reported in 138 countries.[1]

This century has witnessed and benefitted from the scientific development of antibiotics and vaccines—the faithful and widely used standbys against the onslaught of infectious agents. There are at present no magic bullets to render people infected with the HIV noninfectious, no vaccines that will stimulate the human immune system and augment its ability to fend off this enemy. The introduction of penicillin in 1941 revolutionized and transformed medicine. Forty years later an elusive and subtle virus has become a medical and scientific obsession. AIDS has the distinction of being the first great pandemic of the second half of the 20th century.

The syndrome has become a global calamity. It is a physical and emotional calamity for people who have AIDS and know that there is no cure; a social calamity for groups and families whose members have been affected by the virus; a psychosocial calamity for people frightened by the disease—the worried well who are seropositive, that is, whose blood has tested positive for the virus but who have no clinical symptoms, and the general population who are afraid of contracting the HIV and who do not understand the modes of transmission of the virus; and a financial calamity for all—the person with AIDS (PWA), the family, the health care facilities, and communities attempting to deal with the economic impact of the epidemic.

AIDS First Identified (1981)

The clinical observation of AIDS burst upon the American scientific community in the spring of 1981.[2] Five young gay men were seen by Dr. Gottleib at the

University of Los Angeles School of Medicine, and by Dr. Pozalski at Cedars of Sinai Hospital, both in Los Angeles, California. The red flag that triggered profound interest was that all 5 men were hospitalized with *Pneumocystis carinii* pneumonia (PCP), a rare infection seldom seen in healthy young persons. In addition, all 5 men developed other opportunistic infections (OI) generally affecting only patients whose immune systems have been purposefully depressed to enable them to accept tissue and organ transplants. These findings were promptly reported in the United States Centers for Disease Control weekly publication, The Morbidity and Mortality Weekly Report (MMWR).

One month later, the MMWR carried another alarming report from Dr. Friedman and his colleagues at New York University.[3] They noted a high number of gay men presenting clinically with Kaposi's sarcoma (KS). In the 30 months from January 1979 to July 1981, 20 cases of KS had been discovered in New York and 6 in California. All 26 patients were sexually active, and 4 had both KS and PCP. Within 2 years of the diagnosis of KS, 8 had died.[4]

Kaposi's sarcoma was first described by a Hungarian named Moricz Kaposi in 1872.[5] This form of cancer causes pink, brown, or purplish skin blotches; the cause is unknown. Before the onset of AIDS, the disease seldom affected North American men under age 50. It was most prevalent in men over age 50 of Jewish, Italian, or Greek lineage. Little wonder, then, that when 26 young men suddenly developed these unusual skin colorations, the medical community took notice.[6]

CDC Task Force Mobilizes

The federal agency responsible for controlling, monitoring, and preventing disease in the United States is the Centers for Disease Control (CDC). A task force headed by Dr. James Curran of the CDC started a systematic search for cases of this new disease and for its possible cause. The task force's early conclusion was that this was indeed a new disease.[7]

A rapid plan of attack was quickly initiated. Interviews were conducted and questionnaires about patients' medical histories and lifestyles, including homosexual sexual activity and drug use, were distributed to private physicians and sexually transmitted disease (STD) clinics in New York, San Francisco, and Los Angeles.[8] Biological specimens for laboratory analysis were obtained, and after a year of interpretation, the results supported the original hypothesis: a new and deadly disease was spreading within certain identified groups.

Groups Displaying High-Risk Behaviors Identified

The puzzle became even more complex when physicians at Jackson Memorial Hospital in Miami, Florida reported to the CDC that immigrants from Haiti were being treated for PCP and KS. Some of those patients had died.[9] By July 1982, only 10 months after the first report of the disease, there were 216 cases in the United

States. Of these, 84% were gay men, 9% were intravenous drug users, and 5% were women. This new disease claimed the lives of 88 of the 216 persons affected.[10]

The medical mystery continued to unfold. In that same month, July of 1982, the CDC[11] reported that "the occurrence among 3 hemophiliac cases suggests the possible transmission of an agent through blood products." Hemophiliacs require infusions of a blood-clotting protein component called Factor VIII. Factor VIII is derived from processing blood from donors. Dr. Curran and other investigators were already strongly considering the theory that a virus was a probable cause of the disease. Evidence that people had contracted the disease from transfused blood products (Factor VIII) confirmed their suspicions.

In 1982, soon after the first cases of AIDS were reported in the United States, similar cases were described in a number of European countries.[12] In Europe, this new disease was confined initially to gay men; early in its course it did not affect intravenous drug users. In 1983, AIDS was observed in Africans who had immigrated to Europe (particularly Belgium).[13]

AIDS did not discriminate. Children were not immune. By 1983, cases of pediatric AIDS (or as it was then called, PAIDS) were reported in the literature.[14,15] PAIDS was observed in places where there were significant numbers of AIDS cases, such as New York City, San Francisco, Los Angeles, and Miami. The majority of pediatric cases involved children born to drug-addicted mothers who were prostitutes.[16] Other infants developed PAIDS after a blood transfusion from a donor with AIDS, as did a small number of adults.[17] A laboratory test to screen the blood supply had not yet been developed.

The cumulative data then clearly showed that whatever the nature of this new agent, it could be transmitted in several ways: sexually, by men having sex with men; by transfusion of blood and blood products, as cases involving hemophiliacs, blood transfusion recipients, and drug addicts who shared hypodermic needles demonstrated; and by transplacental or perinatal passage to newborns. Furthermore, it became apparent that the incubation period—the period from infection with this new agent to the clinical manifestation of AIDS—could be months or maybe years. This new piece of evidence emerged when a 20-month-old baby developed fatal PCP after receiving a blood-platelet transfusion at birth from a man who subsequently died of AIDS.[18]

The complacency of the heterosexual population was shattered in January 1983, when 2 well-documented cases of AIDS in female partners of male intravenous drug abusers were reported.[19] Clearly, the AIDS virus could be transmitted to a man's female partners as well as to his male partners. Male–female sex was added to the list of modes of transmission.

A general hysteria began to develop in the United States as scientific journals, newspapers, popular magazines, and periodicals published a plethora of information, some excellent and informative, but some misleading. Some of the fear and panic pervasive in 1983 still exist today. Talk of quarantine and isolation of persons diagnosed with AIDS was reminiscent of the segregation and ostracism of lepers in the early years of this century. Isolation of lepers was found to be epide-miologically unjustified, but only after countless lives had been disrupted or ruined.

The public's perception that scientists knew little about AIDs fueled the hysteria. In reality, the syndrome had been remarkably well characterized clinically, epidemiologically, and immunologically in the brief span of 2 years. As scientific researchers churned out volumes of information much of it too detailed and complex for the public, the goal of educating the layperson unfortunately fell through the cracks. Dr. Curran of the CDC wrote:

> We must do what we can to put the problem in perspective by educating others about AIDS and preventing the misuse or misinterpretation of medical data about the syndrome.[20]

By 1983, scientists had collected enough data to determine that AIDS was the manifestation of an immunosuppressive disease that allowed life-threatening infections to develop. These infections were caused by opportunistic organisms or neoplasms or both and usually led to death. In the search for the cause of AIDS, the single factor observed in all patients was the peculiar breakdown of the immune system, caused by no apparent genetic predisposition. Most AIDS investigators had come to the conclusion that AIDS was caused by a virus.

The Transatlantic Research Duel

Intensive research efforts paid off when 3 groups of scientists independently isolated a virus transmitted by body fluids, especially blood, semen, and vaginal secretions. The retrovirus they isolated (See Chap. 2 for a full description) causes death to a specific population of white blood cells, the T-helper lymphocytes. When these cells are decreased in number, the immune system fails to function properly and ceases to defend the body, and renders the person susceptible to strange and unusual microorganisms in the environment. *Pneumocystis carinii* pneumonia is an example of such an opportunistic disease; by 1983, it had been the cause of death in hundreds of AIDS patients.

In January of that year, a specimen from the swollen lymph nodes (a condition called lymphadenopathy) of a young gay man in France was sent to the laboratory of Dr. Luc Montagnier and his colleagues Francois Barre-Sinoussi and Jean-Claude Chermann at the Pasteur Institute in Paris. They processed the tissue and isolated a virus from the preparation. They called this new retrovirus lymphadenopathy-associated virus (LAV) because of its origin in the patient's enlarged lymph node.[21]

Meanwhile, in the United States, Dr. Robert Gallo at the National Cancer Institute in Bethesda, Maryland continued his relentless search for the AIDS agent. Gallo[22] had already described 2 human retroviruses, HTLV-1 and HTLV-2, the human T-lymphotropic virus type 1 and type 2. HTLV-1 infects T lymphocytes and causes a highly malignant but rare form of cancer called adult T-cell

TABLE 1-1. **Development of AIDS Virus Nomenclature**

LAV: Lymphadenopathy-associated virus, 1983, Montagnier, France
HTLV-3: Human T-lymphotropic virus type 3, 1984, Gallo, United States
ARV: AIDS-related virus, 1984, Levy, United States
HIV-1: Human immunodeficiency virus type 1, 1986, International committee consensus
HIV-2: Human immunodeficiency virus type 2, 1987, West Africa

leukemia (ATL), which tends to occur in Africa, the Caribbean and Japan. The HTLV-2 causes a disease called hairy-cell leukemia. Gallo noted a common denominator linking the 2 viral types, the fact that both could be spread by blood, by sexual intercourse, or from a mother to her unborn child. Both caused disease after a long period of latency or incubation. In addition, both viruses infected T-helper lymphocytes.[23]

To Gallo and his colleagues, it seemed reasonable to call the new virus found in AIDs patients HTLV-3, the human T-lymphocyte virus type 3. In the same year that Gallo published his findings, a third group, led by Dr. J. A. Levy[24] at the University of California, San Francisco, isolated and named a retrovirus from the blood of patients with AIDS, calling it ARV (AIDS-associated retrovirus).

When all the accumulated data were critically reviewed and interpreted, the results showed that HTLV-3, LAV, and ARV were the same virus, with small but expected genetic differences. Regrettably, heated debates erupted between the French and American investigators. Who should get credit for first identifying the virus? What should it be named? Who would rightfully acquire the patent rights on any vaccines that might be developed? In 1986, an international commission[25] settled the debate by naming the virus human immunodeficiency virus (HIV). Table 1-1 outlines the sequence of events in the naming of the AIDS virus.

The scientific bridges between the French and American researchers have since been mended. Gallo and Montagnier[26] recently published their first collaborative article, entitled "AIDS in 1988." They recount their discoveries of the virus and offer prospects for a vaccine, for therapy, and for the epidemic itself. The HIV causes AIDS (Table 1-2). This fact has now been firmly and unequivocally established; Gallo and Montagnier's article[27] documents the accumulated evidence.

The HIV is considered a new pathogen because it fulfills the required original (Koch's) postulates: new disease, new agent. With the isolation, characterization, and identification of the HIV came laboratory tests to detect its presence in patients' blood. The first laboratory tests showed evidence of the HIV in only a fraction of patients with AIDS. Researchers did not despair, however, but perfected the tests and made them more sensitive. When patients with AIDS were tested using more refined and exacting test methods, the blood of almost all of the patients was positive for the HIV (HIV+).[28]

TABLE 1–2. **Evidence That HIV Causes Aids**

Type of Evidence	Description
Animal systems	Several types of retroviruses can cause severe immune deficiencies in animals. For example, the feline leukemia (FeLV) can cause immune deficiency or cancer, depending on slight genetic variations in the virus. A virus related to the HIV, the simian immunodeficiency virus (SIV), can cause AIDS in macaque monkeys. The second AIDS virus, HIV-2, may also cause AIDS in macaques.
Epidemiology	In every country studied so far, AIDS has appeared only after the appearance of the HIV. Using the most recent technology, the HIV can be isolated in the blood of the majority of people with AIDS. Earlier in the epidemic, the virus was present in the groups at risk for the disease but in almost no healthy heterosexuals.
Blood transfusion data	A study of people who received blood transfusions in 1982-1983 (when the fraction of blood donors infected with the HIV was about 1 in 2,000) showed that of 28 people who contracted AIDS, the virus could be found in all 28. Furthermore, for each recipient who contracted AIDS an infected donor could be found. Today most of those infected donors have also developed AIDS. Elimination by antibody screening of the HIV in blood for transfusion has drastically reduced the number of AIDS cases resulting from transfusions.
Test tube studies	In the laboratory the virus kills the very T-4 cells whose depletion is the hallmark of AIDS. It also infects and alters the function of cells of the monocyte–macrophage lineage, which may serve as a reservoir of infection in AIDS patients.

Serologic Tests Developed

New tests for HIV, called serologic tests because the specimen tested is blood serum, opened up new epidemiological vistas. It was now possible to ascertain if antibodies to the virus were present in populations at risk long before AIDS became clinically apparent. Serologic tests for the HIV were licensed by the Food and Drug Administration (FDA) in 1985. Preliminary reports to the FDA showed that results of a laboratory testing method called enzyme-linked immunosorbent assay (ELISA) were reproducible and acceptably accurate. Initially, the test was used exclusively to screen blood and plasma donations in an urgent effort to protect the American blood supply from transfusion-transmitted HIV. Since 1985, millions of HIV antibody tests have been performed in laboratories of blood and plasma collection centers, in clinical facilities, and in public health laboratories. The tests have also been used to screen the blood of active duty military personnel and of applicants for military service.[29]

Because of the medical and social implications of a positive test result for the HIV antibody, it is important that test results be accurate and their interpretation correct. The stigma attached to HIV+ serology knows no bounds.

The amount of knowledge we have about the HIV, one of the most complex viruses, is a testimony to the stamina and persistence of scientists. Never before in medical history has so much energy, time, and money been directed to a single purpose. This knowledge also reflects the fact that 1980s' technology was not available in the 1960s and 1970s. Had the HIV appeared 20 years earlier, before the tools of molecular biology and recombinant DNA were developed and perfected, the story would be much different. Our knowledge today about the molecular complexity, life cycle, and target cell affinity of the HIV outstrips our knowledge about any other virus.

EPIDEMIOLOGY OF AIDS

Origins

Armed with a serologic test for HIV, researchers in dozens of countries anxiously investigated where and how far the virus had spread. Their discoveries were alarming: the virus had been around for years before it surfaced in the United States in 1981. Blood stored as early as 1959 in Zaire (central Africa) was found to contain antibodies to the HIV.[30] Seventy-five serum samples collected in the west Nile district of Uganda between August 1972 and July 1973 revealed 50 HIV+ tests results.[31] The serum had been collected, frozen, and stored for studies of Burkitt's lymphoma, a totally different clinical entity. This new information gave credence to the suspicion that the HIV might have originated in Africa.

The AIDS Epidemic in Central Africa

A collaborative study involving Zaire, the CDC and the National Institutes of Health (NIH) in the United States, and the Institute of Tropical Medicine in Belgium[32] revealed a different pattern of infection in central Africa from the pattern in the Western hemisphere. In the United States, the AIDS male:female patient ratio is 14:1; in Africa it is 1:1. The high incidence of infection in that society enables the virus to spread evenly between the sexes by male–female sex. Estimates of infection in the general population of Central Africa range from 10%–18%, as compared with 0.03% in the United States.

Fauci and colleagues[33] estimate that 10%–20% of all infants born in central Africa will be born to HIV-infected mothers. Additionally, because blood for transfusions is seldom screened, between 10%–20% of transfusions are HIV-contaminated. The alarm may have sounded too late. Heroic and dramatic public health measures will take years to stop the spread of AIDS in areas already ravaged by tropical diseases, malnutrition, and poverty.

The actual origin of the HIV is still not known; it may never be known. In 1987 the World Health Assembly[34] stated that the HIV is a "naturally occurring retrovirus of *undetermined* geographic origin" (italics supplied).

The epidemiology of AIDS in Africa differs from the epidemiology of AIDS in the United States. Sex between men and the use of shared, contaminated needles and syringes (called parenteral transmission) are the major modes by which the HIV is transmitted in the United States; sex between men and women is the major mode of transmission in Africa. One study revealed that prostitutes in Nairobi, Kenya, were sexually transmitting the HIV to men from other parts of central Africa; this study suggests the continental spread of the epidemic.[35] Infection rates in some prostitute groups range from 27%–88%. Sexual activity with multiple partners, not sexual orientation, appears to be the overwhelming risk factor in the African AIDS epidemic. Available studies strongly suggest that vaginal intercourse is the dominant mode of HIV transmission on that continent.

In 1986, the World Health Organization's Global AIDS Program (GPA) was formed as a collaborative effort to keep track of the AIDS pandemic. Director Mann and colleagues[36] estimate that there are over 250,000 cases of AIDS worldwide, and between 5 and 10 million persons infected with the HIV.

There is little question that the continent hardest hit is Africa, particularly central and east Africa. Currently, approximately half of all patients in the medical wards of hospitals in such cities as Kinshasa, Nairobi, and Butare are infected with the HIV.[37]

The health care systems in developing African countries are often not capable of coping with their current patient loads. How will these systems manage the additional 400,000 cases projected for the next 5 years? The Harvard Institute of International Development[38] estimates that by 1995 the annual loss due to AIDS deaths in the country of Zaire alone will be $350 million, 8% of the country's gross national product. The same study estimates that economic losses in central Africa will be $980 million by 1995. There is no easy solution. The control and ultimate prevention of AIDS internationally require an immediate and substantial long-term national and global commitment.

To compound the complexity of the problem, a new retrovirus, HIV-2, has emerged. The HIV-2 is related to the HIV-1 in overall structure, and both cause AIDS. Initially isolated in West Africa,[39] it was later identified in New Jersey in a West African who came to the United States in 1987.[40] The pathogenic potential of the HIV-2 is not yet well established. The HIV-2 is found primarily in West Africa, whereas the HIV-1 is concentrated in central Africa and other regions of the world (Fig. 1–1).

Where did the HIV-2 originate? Some hints come from the discovery that other primate species harbor a closely related virus called simian immunodeficiency virus (SIV). This virus, found in the macaque monkey, is closely related

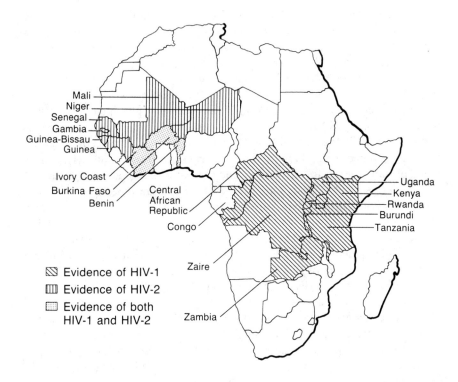

FIGURE 1-1. The African picture. The first AIDS virus, HIV-1, appears mostly in central Africa; HIV-2 occurs in the west. Note that not all African nations have been tested for the AIDS viruses. (Data from *Newsweek*, January 4, 1988, p 60.)

genetically to the HIV-2. This finding raises the obvious question: is there a possibility that the HIV-2 in humans originated in another primate species? The origin of the HIV-1 remains even more questionable than does that of its relative HIV-2. Gallo and Montagnier[41] suspect that the "HIV has infected human beings far more than 20 years but less than 100."

Where was the HIV hiding all those years? Gallo and Montagnier[42] believe that the virus had been present in small isolated groups in central Africa for many years, and that the spread of the virus was limited by the sequestered nature of the groups. Thus the HIV-1 could have been confined and contained for decades.

Because HIV infection precedes the development of symptomatic AIDS by several years, it is necessary to understand the patterns of HIV distribution. Using the HIV serologic tests, epidemiologists have been able to establish the prevalence of HIV infection as measured by the presence of HIV antibodies in the blood (seroprevalence data). Three infection patterns have emerged[43] (Fig. 1–2).

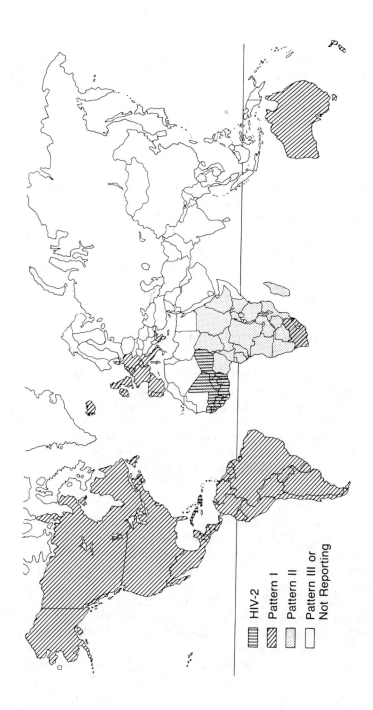

FIGURE 1-2. Worldwide HIV infection patterns. (Data from Mann, JM, et al: The international epidemiology of AIDS. Scientific American, October 1988, p 83.)

Patterns of HIV Distribution

Pattern I typically occurs in industrial countries reporting large numbers of documented AIDS cases: the United States, Mexico, Canada, Australia, New Zealand, parts of Latin America, and many Western European countries. In areas designated pattern I, most AIDS cases occur among gay or bisexual men and urban intravenous drug users. In these areas, the male:female patient ratio ranges from 10:1 to 15:1.[44]

Pattern II is observed in some areas of central, eastern, and southern Africa. This pattern is also developing in some Latin American countries. Like pattern I, pattern II probably is associated with the spread of the HIV beginning in the late 1970s. In pattern II, however, AIDS predominantly affects heterosexuals; the male:female patient ratio is approximately 1:1.[45]

Pattern II involves Eastern Europe, north Africa, the Middle East, Asia, and most of the Pacific, excluding Australia and New Zealand. The HIV probably infiltrated these areas in the early or middle 1980s. This pattern accounts for the smallest number of reported AIDS cases. When AIDS is reported in these areas, it generally involves travelers to pattern I and pattern II areas.

Distribution of Cases in the United States

Heyward and Curran[46] have documented the distribution of AIDS in the United States (Fig. 1–3). Much of the information and statistics used in scientific journals, periodicals, and newspapers is provided by their office and their publications. Their article provides the following information. As of March 1989, 86,656 cases of AIDS have been reported in the United States; 49,870 (57.5%) of these patients have died. By 1992, the number of cases is estimated to reach 365,000. Of this number, it is estimated that 72% will have died of AIDS.

Adults

Sixty-two percent of adult AIDS patients are gay or bisexual men with no history of intravenous drug use (Fig. 1–4). An additional 7% are gay or bisexual men who also have a history of intravenous drug use. Twenty percent are heterosexual men and women who acquired the HIV because of intravenous drug habits. Transfusion-contaminated blood that was administered before 1985 caused approximately 3% of AIDS cases. (After 1985, the blood supply for transfusion was protected by HIV testing.) Hemophiliacs who contracted AIDS through administered blood products account for 1%. The cause of 3% of cases is undetermined because of lack of sufficient information. Male-female transmission is responsible for 4% of reported cases. Of these patients, nearly half had a history of sexual contact with a person with documented HIV infection or with a person in another high-risk group, such as intravenous drug users. The other half are persons born

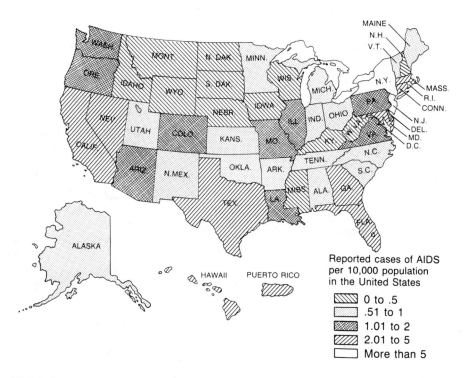

FIGURE 1-3. Geographic distribution of HIV in the United States. (Data from Heyward, WL and Curran, JW: The epidemiology of AIDS in the United States. Scientific American, October 1988, p 75.)

in countries where male–female sexual contact is the major mode of transmission.

Children

The fastest growing group of reported AIDS patients is children. In 1987–1988, there was a 114% increase over the previous year in reported cases among children under age 12 (Fig. 1–5). Seventy-eight percent of pediatric HIV infections were acquired perinatally, that is, before, during, or soon after birth. In most of these cases the infection can be traced directly to an intravenous drug user, either the mother or the mother's sexual partner. Twelve percent of pediatric AIDS cases to date have been associated with blood transfusion, and 6% involve children with hemophilia or other coagulation disorders.

Other Modes of Transmission

Transfusion of a single unit of HIV-contaminated blood has a high risk potential. It is reported that between 89% and 100% of recipients of HIV-contaminated blood become infected.[17] Fortunately, because the blood supply has been

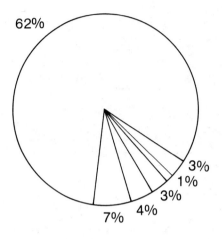

62% Homosexual or Bisexual Men

19% Heterosexual IV drug abusers

7% Homosexual or Bisexual IV Drug Abusers

4% Heterosexual Men and Women

3% Recipients of Blood or Blood-Product Transfusions

1% People with Hemophilia or other Coagulation disorders

3% Other or undetermined

FIGURE 1-4. AIDS cases among adult population groups as of March 1989.

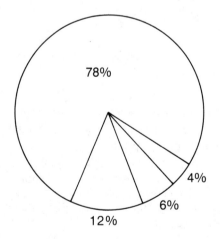

78% Children of mothers with AIDS or at increased risk for AIDS

12% Recipients of Blood or Blood product transfusions

6% Children with hemophilia or other Coagulation disorders

4% Other or undetermined

FIGURE 1-5. AIDS cases among pediatric population groups as of March 1989.

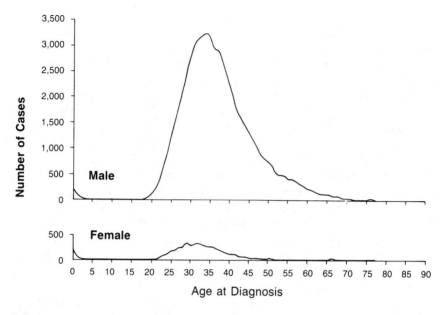

FIGURE 1-6. AIDS distribution for male and female patients in the United States.

screened routinely since 1985, transfusion of HIV-infected blood is extremely rare in the United States today. Contrary to beliefs expressed by many people, there is *no* risk of HIV infection from *donating* blood.

Sharing of needles and other drug paraphernalia provides contaminated blood easy access to the body. In the United States, intravenous drug use is presently the major source of male–female sexually transmitted and perinatal infection. The HIV in contaminated blood poses an occupational risk for health care workers. Four of 870 health care workers who accidentally punctured their skin with contaminated needles while treating HIV-infected patients have developed HIV infection.[48] Precautions for health care workers are discussed in Chapter 4.

Figure 1–6 depicts the age distribution for male and female AIDS patients in the United States. Most patients are men between the ages of 25 and 45. Female AIDS patients tend to cluster between the ages of 25 and 40. The left peaks represent the small but growing numbers of male and female children with AIDS.

Racial and Ethnic Groups

A disproportionate percentage of AIDS cases are reported among black and Hispanic intravenous drug users, their sex partners, and their children. Blacks and

Hispanics living in the northeastern United States have a 2–10 times higher risk of contracting the HIV because of the high incidence of intravenous drug abuse in that region of the country.[49]

Fifty-nine percent of adults with AIDS are white, and 23% of children with AIDS are white. Figure 1–7 shows the disparity between infection rates for racial and ethnic minorities and rates for the white population. Blacks account for 36% of all reported AIDS cases and 53% of pediatric cases, but account for only 12% of the general population. Hispanics account for 16% of all reported AIDS cases and 23% of pediatric cases, but account for only 7% of the general population.

As with black and Hispanic adult AIDS patients, black and Hispanic children with AIDS are more likely than white children with AIDS to reside in New York, New Jersey, or Florida. Ninety percent of children with perinatally acquired AIDS are black or Hispanic.[51] Whether the fetus becomes infected during pregnancy, at birth, or soon afterward, is still unknown. The fact that the HIV has been detected in fetal tissues supports the hypothesis that infection occurs *in utero*. Reports of women who became infected with the HIV immediately after giving birth, and subsequently infected their infants, suggest that the HIV may also be transmitted through breast-feeding.[52]

The incidence of AIDS is rising for all racial and ethnic groups in all geographic regions of the United States, but cumulative incidences of AIDS among blacks and Hispanics are over 3 times the incidence among whites.[53] Seventy-three percent of all women with AIDS are black or Hispanic. Risk factors, not ethnicity, are the underlying reasons.

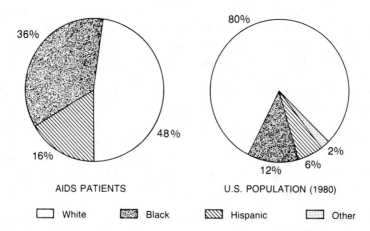

FIGURE 1-7. Racial and ethnic classification of adult AIDS cases.

THE CHALLENGE OF AIDS

In an interview published in American Medical News,[54] Dr. Gallo described his primary mission as follows:

> To develop a vaccine, and before I die, to contribute to the cure of one or two other diseases. We know an awful lot about the AIDS virus, but we do not know enough . . . I do believe that we're going to get a vaccine against AIDS, and in this century. We need a vaccine fast because of two reasons: the drug addicts, they don't learn; and Africa, well, Africa is too big to learn. These are the real issues for the future of the epidemic because the gays have learned.

It would be an error to pretend that the HIV will be easily defeated. Scientists necessarily have not narrowed their vision to the hope of finding a single remedy. Investigators worldwide have as their goal to develop a variety of ways to attack the HIV at different points.

DISCUSSION QUESTIONS

1. Compared with the identification and conquering of viruses causing diseases such as polio, why has the identification of the HIV been more rapid? How does knowing the identity of the virus assist in controlling AIDS?
2. Considering the leading causes of death in the United States, how would you set priorities for the amount of effort that should be put into prevention for these diseases? Where does AIDS fit into the picture?
3. What kinds of questions are still unanswered about the epidemiology of AIDS?
4. How would you prevent the spread of the HIV in areas of the world where there is not yet a high rate of infection (pattern III)?
5. Why do you suppose it has taken at least 2 decades to identify AIDS in Africa?
6. What projections can you make for the year 2000 about (a) number of people with HIV+ blood, (b) number of deaths, (c) number of heterosexuals with AIDS?
7. How likely is it that one or more new HIV viruses (HIV-3 and HIV-4) will appear in the next decade? Why do you think so?
8. If you were a health officer in Africa, where would you start your efforts to arrest the epidemic?

REFERENCES

1. Mann, JM, et al: The international epidemiology of AIDS. Sci Am 259:89, 1988.
2. Centers for Disease Control: Pneumocystis pneumonia: Los Angeles. MMWR 30:250, 1981.
3. Centers for Disease Control: Kaposi's sarcoma and Pneumocystis pneumonia among homosexual men: New York City and California. MMWR 30:305, 1981.
4. Centers for Disease Control (1981): Ibid.
5. Cantwell, AR: Bacteriologic investigation and histologic observations of variably acid-fast bacteria in three cases of cutaneous Kaposi's sarcoma. Growth 45:79, 1981.
6. Shilts, R: And the Band Played On. Viking Penguin, New York, 1987.
7. Curran, JW, et al: The epidemiology of AIDS: Current status and future prospects. Science 229:1352, 1985.
8. Curran, JW: Ibid.
9. Centers for Disease Control: Update on Kaposi's sarcoma among Haitians in the United States. MMWR 31:353, 1982.
10. Centers for Disease Control: Update on Kaposi's sarcoma and opportunistic infections in previously healthy persons: United States. MMWR 31:277, 1982.
11. Centers for Disease Control: Update on acquired immunodeficiency syndrome (AIDS) among patients with hemophilia. MMWR 31:644, 1982.
12. Rozenbaum, W, et al: Multiple opportunistic infections in a male homosexual in France. Lancet 1:572, 1982.
13. Clumeck, N, et al: Acquired immune deficiency syndrome in Black Africans (Letter). Lancet 1:642, 1983.
14. Oleske, J, et al: Immune deficiency syndrome in children. JAMA 249:2345, 1983.
15. Ammann, AJ: Is there any acquired immune deficiency syndrome in infants and children? Pediatrics 72:430, 1983.
16. Oleske, J: Ibid.
17. Ammann, AJ, et al: Acquired immunodeficiency in an infant: Possible transmission by means of blood products. Lancet 1(8331):956, 1983.
18. Heyward, WI and Curran, JW: The epidemiology of AIDS in the U.S. Sci Am 259:72, 1988.
19. Centers for Disease Control: Human immunodeficiency virus infection in the United States: A review of current knowledge. MMWR 36:S6, 1987.
20. Curran, JW: Editorial. N Engl J Med 309:609, 1983.
21. Barre-Sinoussi, F, et al: Isolation of a T-lymphotropic retrovirus from a patient at risk for immune deficiency syndrome (AIDS). Science 220:868, 1983.
22. Gallo, RC: The AIDS virus. Sci Am 256:47, 1987.
23. Gallo, RC and Montagnier, L: AIDS in 1988. Sci Am 259:41, 1988.
24. Levy, JA, et al: Isolation of lymphopathic retroviruses from San Francisco patients with AIDS. Science 225:840, 1984.
25. International Committee on Taxonomy of Viruses: What to call the AIDS virus? Nature 321:10, 1986.
26. Gallo, RC and Montagnier, L: Ibid.
27. Gallo, RC and Montagnier, L: Ibid.
28. Gallo, RC and Montagnier, L: Ibid.
29. Centers for Disease Control: Update: Serologic testing for antibody to Human Im-

munodeficiency Virus. MMWR 36:833, 1988.

30. Mann, JM, et al: The international epidemiology of AIDS. Sci Am 259:82, 1988.
31. Saxinger, WC, et al: Evidence of exposure to HTLV-III in Uganda before 1973. Science 227:1036, 1985.
32. Fauci, AS: AIDS: Pathogenic mechanisms and research strategies. American Society for Microbiology News 53:264, 1987.
33. Fauci, AS: Ibid.
34. Mann, JM: Ibid.
35. Kreiss, JK, et al: AIDS virus infection in Nairobi prostitutes. N Engl J Med 314:414, 1986.
36. Mann, JM: Ibid.
37. Mann, JM: Ibid.
38. Mann, JM: Ibid.
39. Clavel, F, et al: Human immunodeficiency virus type 2 infection associated with AIDS in West Africa. N Engl J Med 316:1180, 1987.
40. Centers for Disease Control: AIDS due to HIV-2 infection: New Jersey. MMWR 37:33, 1988.
41. Gallo, RC and Montagnier, L: Ibid.
42. Gallo, RC and Montagnier, L: Ibid.
43. Mann, JM: Ibid.
44. Mann, JM: Ibid.
45. Mann, JM: Ibid.
46. Heyward, WL and Curran, JW: The epidemiology of AIDS in the United States. Sci Am 259:72, 1988.
47. Heyward, WL and Curran, JW: Ibid.
48. Heyward, WL and Curran, JW: Ibid.
49. Heyward, WL and Curran, JW: Ibid.
50. Centers for Disease Control: Trends in reported cases of AIDS. MMWR 37:552, 1988.
51. Centers for Disease Control: Acquired immunodeficiency syndrome (AIDS) among blacks and Hispanics: United States. MMWR 35:655, 1986.
52. Heyward, WL and Curran, JW: Ibid.
53. Centers for Disease Control (1986): Ibid.
54. Breo, DL (ed): Robert C. Gallo. Am Med News 4:3, 1987.

TWO

BIOLOGY OF HIV INFECTION

John Edwin Lewis

OUTLINE

THE ETIOLOGY OF AIDS
GENERAL CHARACTERISTICS AND
  PROPERTIES OF VIRUSES
Viral Structure
Viral Replication
RETROVIRUSES

Lentiviruses
The Molecular Biology of the HIV
The Life Cycle of the HIV
THE ROLE OF T-HELPER LYMPHOCYTES
  IN THE IMMUNE RESPONSE

OBJECTIVES

After reading this chapter, the reader will be able to:
1. State 2 major characteristics of viruses.
2. List and describe the 2 basic components of all viruses.
3. Define *antigen* and *antibody*.
4. Define the role of antigenic spikes.
5. Describe the stages of viral replication.
6. Explain why the HIV is termed a retrovirus.
7. Describe the role of reverse transcriptase in viral replication.
8. List the characteristics of diseases caused by lentiviruses.
9. Distinguish between the HIV-1 and the HIV-2.
10. Label components of a drawing of HIV.
11. List and describe 3 genes common to retroviruses.
12. State the importance of the CD_4 receptor to the HIV.

13. Identify the human cells that possess CD_4 receptors.
14. Explain the importance of being able to identify cofactors.
15. Describe the function of T_H cells and T_S cells in the immune response.
16. Analyze the potential effect on the body of damage to the T_H cells.

THE ETIOLOGY OF AIDS

The etiologic or causative agent of acquired immunodeficiency syndrome (AIDS) is a retrovirus, the human immunodeficiency virus (HIV).[1] Of all the body's enemies, the greatest in number and the most primitive in form are the viruses.

Viral diseases have caused some of the major scourges of humanity and include such historical disorders as smallpox, yellow fever, rabies, and poliomyelitis. Science has accomplished wonders with vaccines for the prevention and virtual elimination of many of the more lethal viral diseases humans suffer, but even today viruses are the most common cause of human ailments. The common acute respiratory and gastrointestinal infections, as well as chronic infections such as hepatitis, genital herpes, and AIDS, are caused by viruses.

Viruses are not unique to humans. Viruses have been isolated from a wide variety of animals, plants, and even bacteria. A great deal of our knowledge about the structure and life cycle of viruses has been gained from the study of bacteriophages, the viruses that infect bacteria.

GENERAL CHARACTERISTICS AND PROPERTIES OF VIRUSES

Viruses are the smallest agents that cause disease in living organisms. They are obligate intracellular parasites, capable of multiplying only in a living cell. Once inside a host cell they use the host cell's organelles for their own reproduction. Viruses have a host cell preference, or specificity. The common cold viruses attack cells of the respiratory tract, the hepatitis virus attacks liver cells, and the rabies virus uses nerve cells for growth and reproduction. The HIV has a preference for invading the cells that play a major role in defending the body against infection, the white blood cells.

All cells contain both deoxyribonucleic acid (DNA) and ribonucleic acid (RNA). Viruses contain only one of the nucleic acids, either DNA or RNA. It is on the basis of their genetic composition that human viruses are generally classified. For example, the herpes virus that causes chickenpox, cold sores, and infectious mononucleosis is a DNA virus. The HIV is one of many viruses whose genetic information (*genome*) is RNA. Others include the common cold viruses, measles, and mumps.

Viral Structure

Routine study of the structure and size of viruses was not possible until the electron microscope was perfected in the early 1930s. The structure of a virus is relatively simple compared with that of other disease-causing microscopic agents. All viruses consist of 2 basic components: nucleic acid (DNA or RNA), and a surrounding layer of protein known as the *capsid,* which gives shape to the virus particle (Fig. 2–1). The capsid is composed of protein subunits called *capsomeres.* Because of its protein composition, the capsid is *antigenic*; it is the structural component of the virus to which the body actively responds with the production of antibodies during immune processes. An *antigen* is a molecule that can be recognized by an antibody. *Antibodies* are protein molecules produced by certain lymphocytes in response to a foreign agent or antigen. The term *nucleocapsid* refers to the genome and the capsid together.

Many viruses are surrounded by a flexible outer membrane known as the *envelope.* The envelope, acquired from the host cell during viral replication and escape, is composed of lipid and protein, or *lipoprotein.* It is similar to the host's cell membrane except that it contains viral-specific components, that is, proteins produced by the host cell in response to virus genetic dictation.

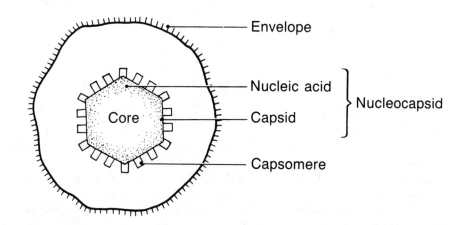

All viruses possess a protein capsid surrounding the genome.
The capsid is composed of protein subunits called capsomeres.

Genome + capsid = nucleocapsid

Some viruses — the enveloped viruses — possess a lipoprotein outer envelope in addition to the capsid.

FIGURE 2-1. Basic structure of a virus.

Certain viruses contain functional projections of the envelope called *spikes,* which are *glycoprotein* (carbohydrate and protein) in chemical composition. The spikes, which are on the external surface of the virus, are also termed *antigenic spikes* because they, too, induce the production of antibodies.

Viral Replication

Viral replication inside the host cell is a remarkable process. A virus invades a living cell that is 1000 or more times its size, and then uses the metabolic machinery of the cell to efficiently produce copies of itself.

Two distinctly different virus reproductive life cycles are now known. One is referred to as *lytic,* the other as *latent.* The first initiates a series of events that ends in *lysis,* the death of the host cell. The second, which is more elusive, results in the virus lying dormant but viable in the host cell.

The first step in replication is the union of virus and host cell. The presence of molecules called *receptor sites* on the host cell membrane is a major determinant in virus-host cell specificity. Without such an interaction the virus cannot absorb to the cell surface, and without adsorption, infection of the cell is not initiated. The receptor molecule on the virus "matches" and interacts specifically with its counterpart on the host cell surface. Adsorption is the initial step leading to all events of the replication cycle.[2]

RETROVIRUSES

The HIV is a retrovirus whose genetic information (genes) is encoded in RNA. Retroviruses are so named because they *reverse* the normal flow of genetic information. In all cellular organisms the genetic material is DNA. DNA passes its information to RNA, which in turn translates this information into the precise construction of proteins, whose building blocks are amino acids.

Before the genetic information carried by an RNA virus can be expressed, the RNA must first be converted to a DNA copy. The copying enzyme, called *reverse transcriptase* because it transcribes in a reverse fashion, takes an RNA genome and makes a complementary DNA strand. This DNA strand then acts as a template for its proper DNA complement, and a normal double-stranded DNA is formed. This newly formed viral DNA, indistinguishable from host DNA, may then incorporate into the host's DNA and become a permanent part of the host cell genetic material. Once integrated into the host's own DNA, the viral segment of DNA is called a *provirus.* The provirus remains with the host genome until it is activated to make new virus particles.

Lentiviruses

Through morphologic and genetic studies the HIV has been assigned to the *lentivirus* subfamily of retroviruses. Viruses in this subfamily cause a number of diseases in other mammalian species. These diseases are characterized by the following:

a. Long incubation periods
b. Persistent infection
c. Impairment of the immune system

The HIV was the first lentivirus to be described with the capability to profoundly suppress the immune system.[3] A number of related lentiviruses have subsequently been identified. Simian immunodeficiency virus (SIV) has been found in a variety of monkey species.[4,5] Researchers have also identified lentiviruses as potential agents of immunodeficiency in cats (feline immunodeficiency virus)[6] and cows (bovine immunodeficiency virus).[7]

In 1987, Clavel and colleagues[8] isolated and identified a new lentivirus, designated the HIV-2, that is associated with AIDS in West Africa. The HIV-2 has subsequently been found in the United States.[9] Despite a number of similarities with the HIV-1, the HIV-2 has some noteworthy differences.[10] It grows readily not only in humans, but also in several species of monkey and ape. The HIV-1 infects only humans and chimpanzees. In addition, the geographic distribution of HIV-2 infection is different than that of HIV-1 infection. In Africa, HIV-2 infection occurs predominantly in West Africa, namely in Senegal, the Ivory Coast, Guinea, Guinea Bissau, and the Gambia.[11,12] HIV-1 infection predominates in east, central, and southern Africa.

The Molecular Biology of the HIV

The HIV is not an ordinary virus.[13] The genetic information consists of 2 strands of RNA surrounded by 2 protein coats (Fig. 2–2). The 2 protein coats are called protein 18 and 24 (p18 and p24), representing their molecular weight (18,000 and 24,000). These proteins play a major role in the laboratory identification of the HIV. As can be seen in Figure 2–2, the HIV possesses a spiked envelope. The outer portion of the spike is called gp120, because it is a glycoprotein with a molecular weight of 120,000. The stalk that penetrates the envelope is called gp41, because it is a glycoprotein with a molecular weight of 41,000. Glycoproteins 120 and 41 span and extend beyond the virus membrane. Core proteins 24 and 18 cover the viral RNA.

All retroviruses possess 3 common genes that are required for replication and synthesis or manufacturing of new virus proteins.[14] The 3 genes are called *gag, pol,* and *env.*

In the case of HIV, these stand for the following:

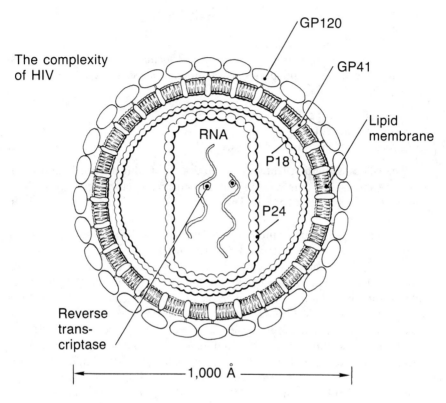

FIGURE 2-2. Structure of the human immunodeficiency virus.

Gag: Group-specific antigens, codes for the synthesis of p24 and p18
Pol: Codes for the synthesis of the enzyme reverse transcriptase, also called
    polymerase
Env: Codes for the synthesis of the *env*elope proteins, gp120 and gp41

In addition to these 3, the HIV genome includes at least 6 other genes that are associated with the regulatory pathways of the virus.[15] Recall that a *gene* is a segment of DNA or RNA that codes for a functional product. The genetic blueprint for the structure and life cycle of the HIV is about 100,000 times smaller than the genetic blueprint contained in a human cell.

The Life Cycle of the HIV

Viruses do not haphazardly attach to host cells. They can only enter a specific host cell membrane receptor, the cell site of attachment and entry. The initial step in any viral infection is the binding of the virus particle to the receptor. In the case of the HIV it has been shown that the gp120 virus projection binds to a specific cell surface protein known as CD_4.[16] CD_4 receptors are abundant on the surface of cells such as the white blood cells called T-helper lymphocytes (T_H). T lymphocytes are so named because they mature and differentiate in the *thymus gland*.

The kinds of cells and tissues to which the HIV binds are a reflection of the distribution and types of host cells possessing CD_4. Cells other than T_H lymphocytes also possess the CD_4 receptor and are capable of hosting the HIV. These include monocytes and macrophages, brain cells (microglial cells), certain epithelial cells, and certain cells that line the intestinal mucosa.[17]

Binding of viral gp120 to cellular CD_4 is the first step in the life cycle of the HIV. Evidence suggests that the HIV enters by fusing directly with the host cell membrane.[18] The virus can do no damage until it enters a target host cell. Once inside the cell, the HIV governs its own life cycle because the 2 identical strands of RNA carry the genetic blueprint not only for the structure of new virus particles, but also for the virus's own life cycle.

As with other lentiviruses, the HIV genetic information now in the form of double-stranded DNA integrates into the host cell's DNA. Permanent infection is established when the provirus (viral DNA) and the cell's own DNA duplicate together every time the cell divides.

The virus exhibits variable courses of interaction with the host cell depending on the kind of cell infected and the cell's own level of activity. In T_H lymphocytes the provirus can remain indefinitely, sequestered from the host's immune defenses, resulting in the so-called latent period. Recent data shows that during the latent period, once thought to be a quiescent stage of the HIV life cycle, the provirus actually expresses some gene messages that gradually kill T_H lymphocytes.[19] If the T_H lymphocytes are stimulated, however, the virus can destroy them in a burst of replication. In other immune system cells, monocytes and macrophages (the phagocytic or debris-collecting cells of the body), the HIV grows continuously but slowly. These cells are altered in their function but are not destroyed as stimulated T_H lymphocytes are destroyed.[20] Thus the monocytes and macrophages may serve not only as a reservoir for the HIV, but also as a major contributor to the viral burden of an infected host.

What triggers the production of new virus particles, which takes place only sporadically and only in some infected cells, is not perfectly known. Speculation abounds, and the term *cofactors* has emerged to encompass a multitude of possible initiating factors. Stress, alcohol, diet, and drugs have been suggested. The activation phase is especially likely to be triggered by antigenic stimulation, as occurs with transfusions and exposure to semen, and by contact with pathogens such as cytomegalovirus (CMV), herpes virus, and the hepatitis B virus (HBV), all of which are common in settings where HIV transmission is especially likely. When lymphocytes are stimulated by an antigen and begin to multiply, proteins within the cell may stimulate viral growth.

Cofactors are known to trigger the rapid reproduction of the HIV virus particles by the host cell. At this stage, the virus is no longer latent, but undergoes reproduction, maturation, and assembly. New viruses literally bud out from the host cell's membrane. The host membrane serves as the outer envelope of the virus. The new virus acquires its host cell's manufactured spikes as it exits.

As mature virus particles bud from an infected cell, the newly formed gp120 spikes on the exiting virus bind to surrounding CD_4 molecules on adjacent cells, tearing holes in their membranes. The punctured cells than swell and die.[21]

The virus envelope gp120 can kill T_H cells in large numbers by yet another method. HIV-infected cells manufacture gp120 and carry it on their own cell membranes. When an infected cell comes in contact with a healthy cell that carries the CD_4 receptor, the gp120 of the infected cell can bind to the CD_4 on the healthy cell and the two cells join, probably by direct fusion.[22] The process can continue until many uninfected cells have combined into a giant cell mass called a *syncytium*. Syncytia die soon after their formation.

THE ROLE OF T-HELPER LYMPHOCYTES IN THE IMMUNE RESPONSE

The immune deficiency caused by the AIDS virus results mainly from the depletion of T_H lymphocytes. These cells are responsible directly and indirectly for the induction and initiation of a wide array of immune defense responses.

Lymphocytes are the central cells involved in the humoral and cell-mediated immune defense mechanisms of the host. Without them the immune system collapses and leaves the host vulnerable to many foreign agents.

The body requires defense against invasion by *pathogens* (disease-producing microorganisms or substances) and against invasion by *opportunistic infections*. Opportunistic infections are caused by microbes commonly present in or on the human body or in the environment. These infections occur only when there is a change from normal, healthy conditions, such as when the immune system becomes depressed.

Two major kinds of lymphocytes defend the body against invasion. The *B lymphocytes* are influenced and programmed in the bone marrow to perform the special defense task of making antibodies. This type of immune response is called *humoral immunity*. The *T lymphocytes* leave the bone marrow and are conditioned in the thymus to perform specialized and complex duties called *cell-mediated immunity*.

Within the thymus, T lymphocytes mature and develop into either T-helper (T_H) cells or T-suppressor (T_s) cells. There are twice as many helper cells as suppressor cells; the ratio is stated as follows:

$$T_H:T_s = 2:1$$

While in the thymus, the lymphocytes destined to be helpers mature and acquire glycoprotein cell membrane markers (62,000 molecular weight) called CD_4. These surface glycoproteins are the receptor sites for HIV adsorption or attachment. The T-suppressor lymphocytes also mature in the thymus and differentiate into cells that are distinguishable from T-helper cells by their surface glycoproteins (76,000 molecular weight), called CD_8.

The membrane markers CD_4 and CD_8 differentiate not only the identity but also the function of the 2 types of lymphocytes.[23] Because these 2 markers are found on T lymphocytes, CD_4 T lymphocytes are also designated T_4, and CD_8 T lymphocytes are designated T_8. Depletion of T_4 cells leads to immunodeficiency and the collapse of a major defense mechanism of the host. Opportunistic microorganisms in the environment may obtain a foothold in the host, who lacks an intact immune system. See Chapter 3 for a listing of opportunistic infections.

DISCUSSION QUESTIONS

1. How does the relationship of a virus and the host cell determine the outcome of a disease?
2. If you were a medical scientist today, where would you direct research to deter the HIV in its attack on the body?
3. How essential is animal research to understanding the action of viruses such as the HIV?
4. If you could select animals for research on the HIV, which animals would be most appropriate?
5. What immunologic interventions might hamper the HIV in its attack on the CD_4 receptor cells?
6. If viruses require specific cell receptors for adsorption, why is the HIV not transmitted casually?
7. Which of the 2 virus life cycles, lytic or lysogenic, is of greatest concern to a person infected with the virus? Why?
8. If you could chemically influence the education of T lymphocytes in the thymus gland, would this arrest the spread of AIDS?

REFERENCES

1. Gallo, RC and Montagnier, L: AIDS in 1988. Sci Am 259:41, 1988.
2. Harrison, S: Principles of virus structure. In Fields, BN and Knipe, DM (eds): Fundamental Virology. Raven Press, New York, 1986, p 27.
3. Gallo, RC: The first human retrovirus. Sci Am 255:88, 1986.
4. Daniel, MD, Letvin, NL, and King, NW: Isolation of a T-cell tropic HTLV-III-like retrovirus from macaques. Science 228:1201, 1985.
5. Kanki, PJ, Alroy, J, and Essex, M: Isolation of T-lymphotropic retrovirus related to

HTLV-III/LAV from wild-caught African green monkeys. Science 230:951, 1985.

6. Pederson, NC, Ho, EW, and Brown, ML: Isolation of a T-lymphotropic virus from domestic cats with immunodeficiency-like syndrome. Science 235:790, 1987.

7. Gonda, MA, Braun, MJ, and Carter, SG: Characterization and molecular cloning of a bovine lentivirus related to Human Immunodeficiency Virus. Nature 330:388, 1987.

8. Clavel, F: Human Immunodeficiency Virus type 2 infection associated with AIDS in West Africa. N Engl J Med 316:1180, 1987.

9. Centers for Disease Control: AIDS due to HIV-2 infection: New Jersey. MMWR 37:33, 1988.

10. Fox, JL: Scrutinizing AIDS from a molecular vantage point. American Society for Microbiology News 53:477, 1987.

11. Bottiger, B, Palme, IB, and da Costa, JL: Prevalence of HIV-1 and HIV-2/HTLV-IV infections in Luanda and Cubinda, Angola. Journal of Acquired Immune Deficiency Syndromes 1:8, 1988.

12. Clavel, F, Guetard, D, and Brun-Vezinet, F: Isolation of a new human retrovirus from West African patients with AIDS. Science 233:343, 1986.

13. Fauci, AS: The Human Immunodeficiency Virus: Infectivity and mechanisms of pathogenesis. Science 239:617, 1988.

14. Lowry, DR: Transformation and oncogenesis: Retroviruses. In Fields, BN and Knipe, DM (eds): Fundamental Virology. Raven Press, New York, 1986, p 235.

15. Haseltine, WA and Wong-Staal, F: The molecular biology of the AIDS virus. Sci Am 259:51, 1988.

16. Redfield, RR and Burke, DS: HIV infection: The clinical picture. Sci Am 259:90, 1988.

17. Haseltine, WA: Replication and pathogenesis of the AIDS virus. Journal of Acquired Immune Deficiency Syndromes 1:217, 1988.

18. Weber, JN and Weiss, RA: HIV infection: The cellular picture. Sci Am 259:101, 1988.

19. Ginsberg, HS (moderator): Scientific forum on AIDS: A summary. Journal of Acquired Immune Deficiency Syndromes 1:165, 1988.

20. Pavza, CD: HIV persistence in monocytes leads to pathogenesis and AIDS. Cell Immunol 112:414, 1988.

21. Haseltine, WA: Ibid.

22. Weber, JN and Weiss, RA: HIV infection: The cellular picture. Sci Am 259:90, 1988.

23. Roitt, IM: Essential Immunology. Blackwell Scientific Publications, Boston, 1988.

THREE

WHAT THE HIV CAUSES: CLINICAL MANIFESTATIONS AND DIAGNOSES

Harvey A. Elder

OUTLINE

31

OBJECTIVES

After reading this chapter, the reader will be able to:

1. State the 2 components necessary for a diagnosis of AIDS.
2. Differentiate between infection and disease.
3. List the 4 possible manifestations of AIDS.
4. List a minimum of 2 major and 4 minor criteria for a diagnosis of AIDS.
5. List, in order, the 4 groups of HIV infection.
6. Analyze why primary HIV infection may go unrecognized.
7. List 3 constitutional symptoms of AIDS.
8. Relate the possible role of HIV infection in neurologic disease.
9. Identify and describe the common opportunistic infections associated with AIDS.
10. Explain why an HIV-infected person remains infectious for the rest of his or her life.
11. Describe the difference in incubation periods for the HIV in newborns and adults.
12. Trace the usual time course of HIV infection.
13. Compare survivor rate with case fatality rate.
14. List and describe the steps in confirmatory antibody testing.
15. Describe the potential of new HIV detection methods.
16. Distinguish between sensitivity and specificity of a test.
17. List and evaluate current treatments for HIV infection.

In order for health care professionals to understand the clinical manifestations and diagnostic schemata associated with human immunodeficiency virus (HIV) infection, they need to know the meaning and use of specialized words that apply to acquired immunodeficiency syndrome (AIDS). Each professional needs to comprehend the magnitude of patients' clinical and personal problems associated with HIV infection, in order to become a cooperative team member who supports and cares for such patients.

When does a person have AIDS? Clinicians diagnose AIDS when there is both evidence of HIV infection and clinical findings typical of AIDS. In general, diagnosis of a specific infectious disease[1] requires specific findings; the diagnosis of upper respiratory infection, for example, requires upper respiratory symptoms and signs and evidence that these symptoms are caused by an infectious agent.

INFECTION AND DISEASE

What is the difference between *infection* and *disease?* To understand the difference, and apply it to the HIV, consider the following definitions.

Colonization occurs when nonviral organisms multiply on the body's surface (skin or mucosa) without immunologic or physiologic evidence that the host responds.[2] Bacteria growing in the axilla is an example of colonization. A colonizing organism does not affect the person, is not infecting, and does not cause disease unless it later invades the person. The HIV infects, it never simply colonizes; no virus ever does.

Infection refers to invasion of the host by a virus or other organism or by an organism's toxin. Infection is manifested by immunologic, physiologic, and/or anatomic changes.[3] To diagnose infection there must be evidence of the presence of the infecting organism and change in the host's body of at least one of the following: (1) function, (2) structure, or (3) immune response. A positive test result for HIV antibody is immunologic evidence of HIV infection.

Infectious disease refers to host symptoms or abnormal physical findings caused by infection.[4] Infection associated with appropriate signs and symptoms is a disease; an infection without appropriate signs and symptoms is not a disease. Subclinical infection is asymptomatic and thus not a disease.

AIDS is a disease caused by HIV infection. Diagnosis of AIDS requires evidence, usually immunologic, of HIV infection *and* signs and symptoms of specific HIV-caused host disease. Four manifestations are possible:[5]

1. The special neuropathy (nervous system abnormalities) of AIDS
2. The special wasting of AIDS
3. The opportunistic infections characteristic of AIDS
4. The special cancers characteristic of AIDS

HIV infection occurs when the HIV invades a person's body. The disease AIDS is the symptomatic phase of HIV infection. Symptoms typical of AIDS may appear years after a person becomes infected with the HIV, although shorter incubation periods do occur.[6,7]

DIAGNOSIS OF AIDS

In principle, the diagnosis of disease is based on identifying abnormalities in a body system or systems, and documenting the disease process and/or the etiologic agent (cause). The same principles apply to diagnosing HIV infection. In the early phase of infection, symptoms are not localized; therefore diagnosis is based on clinical findings and systemic evidence of HIV infection. If infection has reached the phase where clinical signs of AIDS appear, procedures are used to visualize and take specimens from the anatomic area revealing abnormalities, for specific identification of the pathologic process and etiology. If secondary infection or cancer is not identified, the HIV may be the direct cause.

In countries with limited budgets, the diagnosis of AIDS may rest on clinical criteria rather than extensive laboratory procedures. The diagnosis is often made by nurses, medical technologists, and other allied health workers. The World Health Organization[8] has developed a definition requiring that 2 of the following major and 1 of the following minor criteria be present in order to make the diagnosis of AIDS. The major criteria are: fever lasting longer than 1 month, weight loss greater than 10% of body weight, and chronic diarrhea lasting more than 1 month. The minor criteria are general pruritic dermatitis; herpes zoster; oropharyngeal candidiasis; chronic or aggressive ulcerated herpes simplex; and general lymphadenopathy. Aggressive or disseminated Kaposi's sarcoma or cryptococcal disease alone make the diagnosis of AIDS.

DISEASES RELATED TO HIV INFECTION

The clinical classification of HIV infections is found in Table 3–1. This classification reflects the progression of HIV infection from the appearance of initial signs and symptoms through a long asymptomatic period with or without the development of generalized lymphadenopathy,* to the development of AIDS, the final and symptomatic stage of HIV infection. AIDS follows 1 of the 4 courses described above. Each course is progressive, tragic, and dehumanizing. Once AIDS develops, even if opportunistic infections are successfully treated or encephalopathy improves, the diagnosis of AIDS remains.[9] Patients deteriorate; as of this writing there is no cure for HIV infection. Regression of AIDS is not documented.

The National Academy of Science Committee on AIDS[10] states that "HIV infection itself should be viewed as a disease, a continuum of conditions associated with immune dysfunction. The term AIDS-related complex (ARC) is no longer a useful term. All symptoms are part of the same disease.[11]

Group I—Primary HIV Infection Syndrome: Patient Infected, and Possibly Infectious, With Transient Symptoms

Presentation: vague symptoms
Systemic studies: none diagnostic

---

*Generalized lymphadenopathy means that lymph nodes at several sites are enlarged.

TABLE 3-1. **Types of HIV Infection**

Group I. Primary HIV Infection
Group II. Asymptomatic Infection
Group III. Generalized Lymphadenopathy
Group IV. AIDS
  Subgroup A: Constitutional Disease
  Subgroup B: Neurologic Disease
  Subgroup C: Secondary Infectious Diseases
      C-1: Specified Infections from surveillance definition of AIDS
         Pneumocystis carinii pneumonia
         Cryptosporidiosis, chronic
         Isosporiasis
         Strongyloidiasis, extraintestinal
         Candidiasis of esophagus, trachea, or bronchi
         Cryptococcosis, extrapulmonary
         Histoplasmosis, disseminated
         Mycobacterium avium-intracellulare or M. kansasii, disseminated
         Cytomegalovirus infection
         Herpes simplex, chronic mucocutaneous or disseminated
         Progressive multifocal leukoencephalopathy
      C-2: Other specified infectious diseases
         Hairy leukoplakia, oral
         Multidermatomal herpes zoster
         Recurrent *Salmonella* bacteremia
         Nocardiosis
         M. tuberculosis extrapulmonary
         Oral thrush
  Subgroup D: Secondary Cancers
     Kaposi's sarcoma
     Non-Hodgkin's lymphoma
     Primary lymphoma of the brain
  Subgroup E: Other
     Lymphoid interstitial pneumonitis (child less than 13 years old)

From: Revision of the CDC Surveillance Case Definition for Acquired Immunodeficiency Syndrome. MMWR 36:1S, 1987; and from Classification system for Human T-Lymphotropic virus type III/lymphadenopathy-associated virus infections. MMWR 35:334, 1986.

Localizing signs and symptoms: none recognized
Abnormal anatomy: none recognized
Specimen needed: serum
How specimen studied: serotest for HIV

Primary HIV infection syndrome is an infectious mononucleosis-like illness that most HIV-infected patients develop within the first few weeks of acquiring HIV infection.[12] Patients report a history of exposure to the HIV by such means as male–male sex or other high-risk sexual practices, intravenous drug use, or accidental needle stick. Manifestations include fever, generalized aches, lymphadenopathy, rashes of various types, headache, temperature elevation, pharyngitis, and arthralgia (joint pain). Typically, the patient is ill for 2–5 weeks and has an uneventful recovery.

To make this diagnosis, evidence of HIV infection must be present. If the presence of HIV cannot be documented* but HIV infection is suspected, the case should be followed so as to document seroconversion; seroconversion usually within the next few weeks.[13] If the *possibility* of HIV infection is not considered, symptoms may be erroneously attributed to a disease such as infectious mononucleosis (a common infection in young persons, caused by the Epstein-Barr virus, or EBV) or to infection by the cytomegalovirus (CMV).

Nurses, counselors, and health educators are often called upon to counsel patients whose blood is HIV positive to protect others by sexual abstinence or practicing "safe sex" and by absolutely avoiding the donation of blood, sperm, and organs. Experts do not recommend that persons in this group receive therapy with the antiviral agent zidovudine (AZT). Persons whose blood is HIV positive should practice good health habits, be vaccinated once against pneumococcus (Pneumovax) and annually against influenza, and receive regular clinical follow-up care.[14] During these visits, lymph node enlargement and other symptoms should be monitored. Laboratory technicians perform tests measuring sedimentation rate, hemoglobin, white blood count, and platelet count. Patients need support and the opportunity to deal with their physical, emotional, and spiritual needs (see Chapter 5).

Group II—Asymptomatic Infection: Patient Infected and Infectious But Without Symptoms

Presentation: no symptoms or signs
Systemic studies: document HIV infection
Localizing signs and symptoms: none
Abnormal anatomy: none recognized
Specimen needed: none recognized
How specimen studied: none recognized

During convalescence from primary HIV infection, the lymphadenopathy clears and patients return to "good health." Physically, patients feel normal and

---

*In 1989, tests sensitive enough to detect HIV antigen early infection are not available but are under development.

continue their daily activities, often unaware that they have HIV infection.

Diagnosis of asymptomatic HIV infection depends on a positive test result for HIV and the patient reporting no history of AIDS-like symptoms. The nurse or dental hygienist may identify increased skin disorders such as acne and other nonspecific rashes or oral lesions.[15] There is no recommended treatment for this stage, but patients need counseling, support, and regular laboratory testing as indicated under Group I. Patients not yet vaccinated against pneumococcus should receive Pneumovax.

Group III—Persistent Generalized Lymphadenopathy: Patient Infected and Infectious But Without Other Symptoms

Presentation: enlarged lymph nodes
Systemic studies: document HIV infection, no other illness
Localizing signs and symptoms: lymphadenopathy
Abnormal anatomy: studied by physical examination (palpation)
Local specimen needed: lymph node biopsy
How specimen studied: histological and cytological studies to find etiology

Patients unaware of their generalized lymphadenopathy may seek care from nurses or other allied health professionals for other reasons. Though otherwise asymptomatic, such persons may have skin rashes, nonspecific upper respiratory symptoms, or occasional diarrhea not otherwise explained.[16] Health care professionals may find skin lesions; if the lesions are identified as Kaposi's sarcoma, they are diagnostic of AIDS. They may find thrush (oral candidiasis), or perirectal lesions (herpes or condyloma). Dental hygienists may note a finding specific for HIV infection called *hairy leukoplakia*, characterized by white hair-like ridges on the sides of the tongue.[17]

Young adults often have lymphadenopathy; occasional transitory lymphadenopathy does not suggest HIV infection. The diagnosis of persistent generalized lymphadenopathy requires that lymph nodes be more than 1 cm in diameter, with the enlargement not otherwise explained, and bilaterally symmetric, affecting at least 2 extra-inguinal sites for at least 3 months.[18] Persistent generalized lymphadenopathy usually involves the neck and axillae and lasts for several years.

The Food and Drug Administration (FDA) has not approved specific treatment for patients in group III. As of 1989, studies have not shown that the benefits of AZT administered during this stage outweigh risks.

Patients with persistent generalized lymphadenopathy should be counseled, supported, vaccinated annually against influenza and pneumococcus (if not done previously), and their cases medically followed. At this stage, the laboratory technician is often called on to perform counts of the T-helper cells to assess the progress of the HIV.

Group IV—AIDS: Patient Infected and Infectious

Subgroup A: Constitutional Symptoms

Presentation: fever, weight loss, diarrhea, possible lymph node enlargement
Systemic studies: document HIV infection and the absence of any other cause of illness
Localizing signs and symptoms: diarrhea, lymphadenopathy
Abnormal anatomy: colon and small bowel studied by endoscopy and/or radiograms
Local specimen needed: stool, colon or small bowel for biopsy; lymphadenopathy
How specimens obtained: stool stain or culture; biopsy specimen by histology; lymphadenopathy

Constitutional symptoms include unexplained fever lasting longer than 1 month, diarrhea lasting longer than 1 month and not otherwise explained, and involuntary weight loss greater than 10% of baseline weight.[19]

Weight loss is the most common presentation of AIDS in Africa, where it is called the "slim disease." In the United States, fewer than 15% of AIDS patients present with constitutional findings. Constitutional symptoms were previously termed AIDS-related complex (ARC). Because this term became nebulous, it lost its diagnostic value and its use was discontinued.[20]* Constitutional symptoms point to bowel and lymph node disease. Endoscopy and radiographic studies rarely reveal anatomic abnormalities of the bowel. Stool or bowel biopsies are studied using microbiologic and histologic techniques to determine the cause of the diarrhea.

Diarrhea that is a constitutional characteristic of AIDS differs from specific diarrheas (see Subgroup C), which may be evidence of opportunistic infections.

Subgroup B: Neurologic Disease

Presentation: dementia, depression, impairment of fine movements
Systemic studies: document HIV infection
Localizing signs and symptoms: neurologic signs and symptoms

The designation *AIDS-related complex* was excluded from the CDC case definition in 1986. It continues to be absent in the revision of the CDC surveillance case definition of 1987. Most of the elements indicating progressive disease are included in the term "HIV wasting syndrome."

Abnormal anatomy: studied with magnetic resonance imaging (MRI) or computed tomography (CT)

Local specimen needed: cerebral spinal fluid (CSF); occasionally a brain biopsy

How specimen studied: CSF stain, serology, and culture; biopsy specimen by cytology and histology

About 10% of patients with AIDS present with *HIV encephalopathy* and 60% eventually develop this neurologic complication caused by HIV infection (these percentages exclude patients whose neurologic findings are caused by opportunistic agents or malignancies).[21,22] The neurologic diseases of AIDS include 3 syndromes: dementia, myelopathy (disease of the spinal cord), and peripheral neuropathy (disease in the peripheral nerves). See Chapter 6 for further information.

Subgroup C: Secondary Infectious Diseases

Presentation: fever, or some localized manifestation

Systemic studies: document HIV infection

Localizing signs and symptoms: depend on site of infection

Abnormal anatomy: radiologic studies, scans, occasionally direct (endoscopic) visualization

Local specimen needed: specimen from diseased site, secretions, occasionally biopsy required

How specimen studied: fluid stain, cytology, and histology

Certain microorganisms that rarely cause disease in immunologically normal people are the etiologic agents of opportunistic infectious diseases associated with AIDS. These microbes are omnipresent and frequently enter healthy persons' bodies without causing disease. But when opportunistic organisms enter the bodies of people with immune defenses badly damaged by leukemia, chemotherapy, or AIDS, they cause serious diseases. The opportunistic organisms *Pneumocystis carinii* is a common cause of pneumonia (PCP) in patients with AIDS in the United States.

The most common sites for secondary infections in HIV-infected patients are the lungs, throat and esophagus, bowel and colon, blood stream, central nervous system, and the eye. Many of these infections can be effectively treated.

The most common opportunistic organisms affecting AIDS patients are listed in Table 3–2. These present major challenges to the microbiologist, parasitologist, and cytologist. Often the presence of an organism is not adequate to document that it is a pathogen; it is necessary to demonstrate its role in pathogenesis. Laboratory technicians frequently identify additional infectious agents not classified as opportunistic in AIDS patients but commonly affecting them. These agents are listed in Table 3–3.

Respiratory Infections. Respiratory symptoms such as shortness of breath, cough, and sputum production suggest pulmonary disease. In patients with AIDS, or who are suspected of having AIDS, these findings should trigger an urgent and

TABLE 3–2. **Most Common Opportunistic Organisms Affecting AIDS Patients**

Organism	Specific Disease	How Diagnosed	Treatment
Parasites			
Pneumocystis carinii	Pneumonia	Sputum washing Bronchial alveolar lavage	Pentamidine Trimethoprim/ sulfamethoxazole
Toxoplasma gondii	Intracerebral	MRI or CT scan/ brain biopsy	Pyrimethamine + sulfonamide
Cryptosporidium	Diarrhea	Stool/acid-fast stain	None effective
Isospora belli	Diarrhea	Stool/acid-fast stain	Trimethoprim/ sulfamethoxazole
Strongyloides stercoralis	Extra-intestinal	Stool and sputum culture Serology	Thiabendazole
Fungi			
Candida	Esophagitis Tracheitis Bronchitis	Clinical symptoms Bronchoscopy Bronchoscopy	Ketoconazole
Coccidioides	Disseminated	CSF culture, serology	Amphotericin B
Cryptococcus	Extrapulmonary Meningitis	CSF Gram's stain CSF antigen	Amphotericin B Amphotericin B
Histoplasma	Disseminated	Blood culture Bone marrow culture CSF culture	Amphotericin B Amphotericin B
Viruses			
Cytomegalovirus	Retinitis Esophagitis Pneumonitis Colitis	Clinical symptoms Biopsy/CMV Biopsy/CMV Biopsy/CMV	Ganciclovir
Herpes simplex	Disseminated or chronic mucocu- taneous	Biopsy/HSV	Acyclovir
Bacteria			
Mycobacterium avium- intracellulare	Disseminated	Blood culture	No effective therapy

From: Revision of the CDC surveillance case definition for Acquired Immunodeficiency Syndrome. MMWR 36:1S, 1987; and from Classification system for human T-lymphotropic virus type III/lymphadenopathy-associated virus infections. MMWR 35:334, 1986.

TABLE 3–3. **Additional Infectious Agents Commonly Affecting AIDS Patients**

Organism	Specific Disease	How Diagnosed	Treatment
Parasites			
Entamoeba histolytica	Diarrhea	Colon biopsy	Metronidazole
Giardia lamblia	Diarrhea	Small bowel biopsy	Metronidazole
Viruses			
Epstein-Barr virus (EBV)	Hairy leukoplakia	Clinical symptoms	Only
Herpes zoster	Shingles, multiple	Clinical symptoms	Acyclovir
Fungi			
Candida	Stomatitis	Clinical symptoms	Clotrimazole
Bacteria			
Mycobacterium tuberculosis	Extrapulmonary	Biopsy or culture	INH + Rifampin + pyrazina-mide
Nocardia	Disseminated	Acid-fast and Gram's stain Culture	Trimethoprim/ sulfamethox-azole
Streptococcus pneumoniae	Pneumonia and bacteriemia	Sputum culture and blood culture	Penicillin
Hemophilus influenzae	Pneumonia and bacteriemia	Sputum culture and blood culture	According to susceptibility
Branhamella catarrhalis	Pneumonia and bacteriemia	Sputum culture and blood culture	According to susceptibility
Staphylococcus aureus	Pneumonia	Sputum culture	According to susceptibility
Salmonella	Recurrent bacteriemia	Stool Blood culture	Ciprofloxacin

vigorous evaluation of pulmonary anatomy, secretions, and tissues so that diagnosis can be made and treatment begin. A large health care team is needed in order to properly diagnose and treat the patient (Table 3–4).

Pulmonary anatomy is studied by chest x-ray. The cause of infection is usually found by staining and culturing sputum and culturing blood. When common pathogens are found, they are treated. Respiratory disease not easily explained by common pathogens triggers a search for interstitial lung disease (including PCP).[23]

TABLE 3–4. **Contributions of Various Allied Health
Personnel in Evaluation of Secondary
Respiratory Infections**

Profession	Study	Indication	Outcome	Response
Radiologic technologist	Chest x-ray	Respiratory distress	Infiltrate	Find cause
Respiratory therapist	Induce sputum	Cough or respiratory distress	Sputum	Stain and culture
Medical technologist	Stain sputum	Adequate specimen	Pus and few epithelial cells	Culture sputum
	Culture	Adequate specimen	Bacteria susceptibility	Identify and treat
	Culture blood	Septic patient	Bacteria susceptibility	Identify and treat
Radiologic technologist	Chest x-ray	Respiratory distress	Find interstitial disease	Rule out *Pneumocystis carinii*
Respiratory therapist	Diffusion capacity	Suspect interstitial disease	Find interstitial disease	Rule out *Pneumocystis carinii*
Nuclear medicine technician	Gallium scan	Suspect interstitial disease	Find interstitial disease	Rule out *Pneumocystis carinii*
Respiratory therapist	Induce sputum	Interstitial disease	Sputum	Stain for *Pneumocystis carinii*
Cytologist	Stain	Sputum or washings	Etiology	Treatment is agent-specific

Lung structure is studied by chest x-ray. If the roentgenogram reveals nothing, lung diffusion capacity is measured. If the symptoms are still unexplained, many physicians then perform a gallium lung scan.

If any of these tests reveal evidence of interstitial pulmonary disease, specimens are collected to identify the cause.[24] If induced sputum does not produce an adequate specimen for diagnosis, bronchoscopy is performed and specimens are obtained by bronchial alveolar lavage (washing the lungs). Specimens are stained for *P. carinii* and other pathogens and cultured for likely agents, including opportunistic bacteria, fungi, and viruses. Treatment is pathogen-specific. If PCP is diagnosed, it is treated and prophylaxis continues for life.[25]

The laboratory technologist should be able to identify the following pathogens, listed in the approximate order of frequency: *Streptococcus pneumoniae,*

P. carinii, Branhamella influenzae, B. catarrhalis, Myobacterium avium-intracellulare, Staphylococcus aureus, Mycobacterium tuberculosis, nonspecific interstitial pneumonia, CMV, and Kaposi's sarcoma.[26]

Infections of the Upper Gastrointestinal Tract. Pain or other difficulty swallowing suggests esophageal disease. Painful swallowing (dysphagia) identifies the anatomic abnormality in AIDS patients and oral candidiasis (thrush) is adequate evidence of the etiologic agent to diagnose candidal esophagitis.[27,28]

If the patient experiences painful swallowing but oral candidiasis is not present, endoscopy (to identify etiology) may be necessary. Biopsy of the esophageal lesion may be performed. Histologists and microbiologists can determine the cause by evaluating the tissue.

Epigastric Symptoms. Epigastric distress in AIDS patients usually indicates peptic ulcer disease or gastritis. Kaposi's sarcoma, lymphoma, and other complications of HIV infection are infrequent causes.[29] Even with the use of a gastroscope (to diagnose etiology), a biopsy specimen enabling diagnosis of Kaposi's sarcoma or lymphoma may be difficult to obtain.

Biliary Infections. Evaluation of right upper quadrant abdominal distress in AIDS patients requires assistance by allied health professionals (Table 3–5). Stones are the most likely cause of biliary disease in all patients with biliary

TABLE 3–5. **Contribution of Allied Health Professionals to Evaluation of AIDS Patients With Right Upper Quadrant Abdominal Distress**

Profession	Study	Indication	Outcome	Response
Medical technologist	Liver function tests	Signs and symptoms or screening	Other abnormality	Liver biopsy
	Alkaline phosphatase test	Signs and symptoms	Very high alkaline phosphatase level	Ultrasound
Sonographer	Ultrasound	Very high alkaline phosphatase level	Ducts dilated or ducts not dilated	ERCP* Liver biopsy
Radiologic technologist	ERCP*	Dilated ducts	Cause of dilation	Dependent on findings
Histologist	Liver biopsy	Unexplained liver disease	Learn etiology of liver disease	Dependent on findings

*ERCP = Endoscopic retrograde cholangiopancreatography

symptoms, including AIDS patients. AIDS patients are prone to the common liver diseases, including hepatitis and cirrhosis. The opportunistic infections and cancers of AIDS are infrequent causes of biliary or hepatic disease.[30]

Suspicion of biliary tract obstruction is heightened if the serum alkaline phosphatase concentration is very high. Additional studies to visualize anatomy may include ultrasound and endoscopic retrograde cholangiopancreatography (ERCP).* Surgery may be necessary, first to obtain specimens for diagnosis (confirmation by biopsy and histologic examination), and then for treatment (removal or bypass technique). If data show abnormal liver function in the absence of biliary obstruction, liver biopsy may be necessary to diagnose the cause. Rarely, the cause of liver invasion may be M. *avium-intracellulare,* Kaposi's sarcoma, or CMV. Treatment depends on diagnosis.

Peritonitis.   Often peritoneal fluid can be found by physical examination. Fluid is obtained by paracentesis and its origin determined by cytologists studying the cells and microbiologists culturing the fluid for microbes.

Diarrhea.   Diarrhea reveals an abnormality of the small bowel or colon. Microbiologists and parasitologists determine the cause by examining stool specimens for leukocytes, parasites, and *Clostridium difficile* toxin and culturing for *Salmonella, Shigella,* and *Campylobacter.*[31] If cultures reveal no specific cause, physicians may visualize the colon by endoscopy and obtain biopsy specimens for viral culture and histology. If no microbial cause is documented, the diarrhea is probably a constitutional manifestation of AIDS and not a secondary infectious complication.[32]

Neurologic Infections.   Dementia, depression, and loss of fine motor coordination in patients with HIV infection indicate neuropathy (abnormality of the nervous system). Adequate clinical evaluation for AIDS neuropathy and secondary neurologic infections includes neurologic evaluation by clinical practitioners and psychological testing by clinical psychologists. Anatomic abnormalities are visualized by MRI or CT performed by radiologic technologists. Laboratory technicians study CSF for etiologic clues.

The HIV is associated with many neurologic syndromes. Table 3–6 outlines diagnosis and management for the major syndromes.

Subgroup D: Secondary Cancers: Kaposi's Sarcoma and Lymphoma

Presentation: localized involvement—Kaposi's sarcoma: skin, mouth, gut, and
     lungs; lymphoma: central nervous system
Systemic studies: document HIV infection

---

*ERCP is an endoscopic means of directly visualizing the biliary and pancreatic ducts and injecting them with dye for radiologic visualization.

TABLE 3-6. **Infectious Neurologic Syndromes Associated With AIDS**

Syndrome (Diagnostic Studies) Etiologies	Antimicrobial Treatment
Meningitis (CSF: Gram's stain, latex agglutination, culture, cytology [AFB, crypto, lymphoma])	
Encapsulated bacteria	Individualize
Cryptococcus	Amphotericin B
Mycobacterium tuberculosis	INH + rifampin + pyrazinamide
Lymphoma	Individualize
HIV	No treatment
Encephalitis (CSF studies)	
Toxoplasma	Pyrimethamine + sulfadiazine
Herpes	Acyclovir
Cytomegalovirus	No treatment
Acute HIV	Will clear
Focal Brain Disease (CSF studies, MRI, CT, response to treatment for toxoplasmosis)	
Toxoplasma	Pyrimethamine + sulfadiazine
Primary CNS lymphoma	No treatment
Cryptococcus	Amphotericin B
Mycobacterium tuberculosis	INH + rifampin + pyrazinamide
Myelitis (CSF studies, CT)	
Herpes	Acyclovir
Epidural infection	Individualize
Cytomegalovirus	No treatment

Localizing signs and symptoms: 'skin, mouth, or central nervous system

Abnormal anatomy: skin studied by direct examination; central nervous system studied by MRI or CT

Local specimen needed: specimen for biopsy

How specimen studied: histology

Until the advent of AIDS, Kaposi's sarcoma was an unusual cancer affecting mostly older men of Mediterranean origin and a few younger men in sub-Saharan Africa. Kaposi's sarcoma in AIDS patients involves the head (including the mouth and neck) and the gastrointestinal tract. Radiation may provide palliative (temporary remission) therapy.[33] Lymphoma (cancer of the lymphatics) is relatively common in AIDS patients. Although primary lymphoma of the brain is characteristic, lymphomas also occur in other locations. Lymphomas have a poor prognosis and radiation does not prolong survival.[34]

TABLE 3-7. **Diagnosis of AIDS**

Symptoms	HIV Antibody Test Result	Diagnosis
Primary HIV infection	Seroconversion	Primary HIV infection
Not typical of AIDS	Positive	Asymptomatic with illness
Typical of AIDS	Negative	AIDS if HIV test result previously positive
Typical of AIDS	Negative	HIV-2 or other virus
Typical of AIDS	Negative	Other cause of immune deficiency

Diagnosis of AIDS requires a positive HIV test result* and findings typical of one of the 4 disease courses characteristic of AIDS.[35] Patients with symptoms need immediate testing for HIV. If the symptoms and other findings are typical of AIDS and the test result is positive, then the diagnosis is AIDS. If the symptoms and/or other findings are not consistent with 1 of the 4 courses characteristic of AIDS, then the diagnosis is not AIDS even if the test result is positive. Table 3-7 presents the relationship between symptoms, HIV test result, and diagnosis.

THE NATURAL HISTORY OF HIV INFECTION

Incubation and Communicable Periods

Figure 3-1 illustrates the natural history of HIV infection. Two definitions are important to understanding of this history. The *incubation period* of the disease is the time between organism inoculation and the occurrence of disease.[36] The *communicable period* is the time during which the host is shedding organisms that can infect another susceptible host.[37] For the HIV, the incubation and communicable periods overlap.

Infected people are capable of transmitting the HIV within 3-4 weeks of inoc-

---

*Under certain conditions, the diagnosis of AIDS can be made without an HIV test. See "Revision of the CDC Surveillance Case Definition for Acquired Immunodeficiency Syndrome," MMWR 36:8S, 1987.

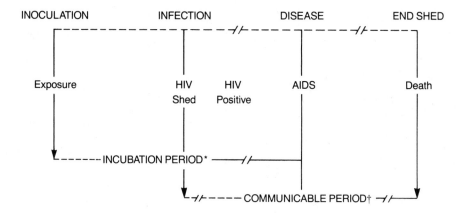

* Incubation Period: Time between organism inoculation and occurrence of disease.
† Communicable Period: Time when host is shedding organisms that can infect another susceptible host.

FIGURE 3-1. The natural history of HIV infection.

ulation and remain infectious for the rest of their lives.[38] They shed the virus in genital fluids and blood.

Very sensitive tests, described later in this chapter, are used when testing for HIV antibody. Usually antibody is detectable within 6–12 weeks of inoculation; occasionally, it takes as long as 26–64 weeks to appear.[39] The antibody titer remains positive for life, although it may become negative in the late stages of AIDS. *A person is infectious before the antibody test result is positive and may be infectious even if the result is negative.*

In adults, the *incubation period* for AIDS varies from 1–10 years or more.[40] In newborns it is usually shorter. During the incubation period, the person may have many minor illnesses, just as do persons without HIV infection. These illnesses do not herald the onset of AIDS.

The time from the onset of symptomatic HIV infection until death varies from 1–4 years.[41] Newborn children die more quickly. Table 3–8 summarizes the course of HIV infection.

Survival of Persons With AIDS

The big question for a person with AIDS is "How long do I have?" The answer is not simple. After the diagnosis of AIDS, about 72% survive the first year and 47% survive the second year. Only 27% live through the third year and less than 17% survive the fourth year. These data apply to survival time from the onset of symptoms typical of AIDS.[42]

TABLE 3–8. **Usual Time Course of HIV Infection**

Event	Time
Inoculation	0
Primary HIV infection	1st–2nd week
Becomes infectious	3rd–6th week
Antibody test result positive	8th–160th week
Typical symptoms appear	2nd–15th year
Incubation period	2–15 years
Symptomatic until death	10–96 months

The most widely used survival statistic is the *case fatality rate*. The case fatality rate is the number of deaths divided by the total number of infected individuals.[43] This is a misleading statistic. The denominator—total number of infected individuals—describes a heterogeneous group that is growing continuously. It includes patients who developed AIDS during the current year (who are unlikely to die within the year), patients who developed AIDS last year (who have a modest chance of dying during the year), and patients who developed AIDS 2 years ago (who have a high chance of dying during the year). "All infected individuals," then, is a category including persons with very different *risks* of dying. The case fatality rate (a composite figure), is, and has been, about 57%[44] (Table 3–9). As long as the number of new patients continues to increase rapidly, the case fatality rate will remain relatively low. Even though most patients die within 4 years, the case fatality rate is only 57%, not 100%, because the number of new patients developing the disease continues to increase.

A better measure of the risk of dying of a given disease is the *survivor rate*, which reflects the proportion of survivors in a population group studied over a

TABLE 3–9. **Case Fatality Rate**

Date	Number of Cases	Number Dead	Case Fatality Rate
Before January 1, 1988	61,753	42,986	0.70
During 1988	23,941	6,775	0.28
Total Cases	85,514	49,761	0.60

From Centers for Disease Control: HIV/AIDS Surveillance Report, March 1989: 1–6.

TABLE 3-10. **Survivor Rate for a Cohort of AIDS Patients**

Year	Survivors/100 patients
1st	60
2nd	30
3rd	7

From Bacchetti, P, et al: Survival patterns of the first 500 patients with AIDS in San Francisco. J Infect Dis 157:1044, 1988.

period of time.[45] Table 3-10 illustrates the survivor rate for a group of AIDS patients.

How long a patient with acute HIV disease, asymptomatic infection, and persistent generalized lymphadenopathy survives depends on the stage of development of AIDS. There are 2 phases of survival: the time from infection until AIDS develops, and the time from the development of AIDS until death. The potential survival period after diagnosis of AIDS is documented in Table 3-10. The time until development of AIDS can be as short as several months or longer than 10 years.

TESTING FOR THE HIV

Antibody Tests

Antibody tests to detect HIV were first licensed by the Food and Drug Administration (FDA) in 1985, primarily as screening tests for donated blood and plasma.[46] These tests were adaptations of a basic serologic method called enzyme-linked immunosorbent assay (ELISA). This test reliably detects the presence of antibody to the HIV and is crucial to ensuring a continued supply of safe blood and blood products. It takes from 6–64 weeks for the body to manufacture detectable amounts of antibody to the HIV.[47] There is a "window" period (3–5 weeks) when the blood contains the virus but the antibody test result is negative.

Figure 3-2 illustrates the principles and steps of the ELISA test. Viral antigen (disrupted HIV) is attached to a solid-phase substrate such as polystyrene beads, microtiter plates, microtiter strips, or ferrous beads. If the specimen to be tested contains antibodies to HIV, they will bind in a classic antigen–antibody binding reaction. Because this reaction cannot be visualized, an indicator system, enzyme-labeled antihuman antibody, is added. If, after washing steps, the second antibody is still bound to the patient's antibody (which was bound to the HIV antigen),

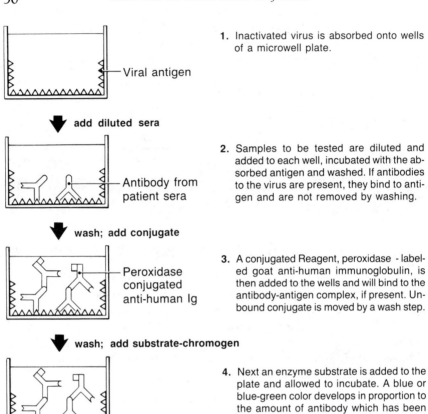

1. Inactivated virus is absorbed onto wells of a microwell plate.

— Viral antigen

add diluted sera

2. Samples to be tested are diluted and added to each well, incubated with the absorbed antigen and washed. If antibodies to the virus are present, they bind to antigen and are not removed by washing.

— Antibody from patient sera

wash; add conjugate

3. A conjugated Reagent, peroxidase - labeled goat anti-human immunoglobulin, is then added to the wells and will bind to the antibody-antigen complex, if present. Unbound conjugate is moved by a wash step.

— Peroxidase conjugated anti-human Ig

wash; add substrate-chromogen

4. Next an enzyme substrate is added to the plate and allowed to incubate. A blue or blue-green color develops in proportion to the amount of antibody which has been bound to the antigen-coated plate.

add H₂SO₄

5. The enzyme reaction is stopped by the addition of acid. This will result in a color change to yellow. The optical absorbance of controls and specimens is determined with a spectrophotometer with wavelength set at 450 nm.

FIGURE 3-2. The microassay ELISA test.

then the substrate will cause a color reaction. If the patient has no antibodies to the HIV, then the enzyme that is linked to the second antibody has no place to bind, and there will be no color reaction. The result will be negative. This technology is sensitive but not specific. It tends to generate false-positive results because it uses nonspecific antibodies.

Confirmatory Testing

All positive results must be substantiated by highly specific confirmatory tests. Often these tests are less sensitive than the ELISA. Two confirmatory tests are the Western Blot (WB) and the direct immunofluorescence assay (IFA). The WB is an expensive, labor-intensive test and is not appropriate for routine screening, but it is the most common confirmatory test currently used. It is the "gold standard" with which all other tests are compared.

The basic principles of the WB test are presented in Figure 3–3. The technique requires that the virus be broken down into its various protein components. The viral proteins are then spread by electrophoresis on a special gel called polyacrylamide. The separated proteins are transferred (blotted) to a nitrocellulose paper by electrophoretic treatment.

A dilution of the serum to be tested is incubated with individual nitrocellulose strips. Antibodies in the serum bind to the different HIV proteins on the strips and precipitate into bands that can be stained and visualized. The presence of antibodies to p24, p31, and gp41 is an unequivocal positive result.[48]

The IFA is also rapidly gaining popularity. HIV-infected and control cells are fixed to glass slides or wells. The slides are flooded with dilutions of the patient's serum. If the patient has produced antibodies, these antibodies will combine with the fixed HIV antigens. Here the indicator system is fluorescein-tagged antihuman antibody. Wherever there is an HIV antibody complex, this second tagged antibody will attach and can be recognized under the fluorescent microscope by its "fluoresce." If the test slides fluoresce and control slides do not, the test result is positive and reported to be HIV positive by IFA.

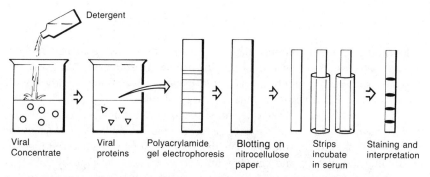

| Viral Concentrate | Viral proteins | Polyacrylamide gel electrophoresis | Blotting on nitrocellulose paper | Strips incubate in serum | Staining and interpretation |

In this technique, the virus is broken down into its parts and then electrophoretically spread on polyacrylamide gel. The antigenic bands are blotted on nitrocellulose paper, which is then cut into strips and incubated in the sample to be tested. Staining reveals the areas where immuno-precipitation has occurred.

FIGURE 3-3. The Western Blot test.

Newer methods include tests to detect not only HIV antigens (proteins) but also HIV genetic components (the genome).

Newer Methods

Listed below are some of the newer HIV detection methods:

Viral culture is a slow, expensive, labor-intensive, and relatively insensitive[49] technique. Viral cultures have been used to detect HIV from many sites including peripheral blood lymphocytes, bone marrow, CSF, semen, and vaginal secretions.

Antigen detection is technically easy to perform, reasonable in cost, and highly sensitive. Antibodies are used in an antigen-capture ELISA system. By this assay it is possible to differentiate various HIV strains.[50]

Nucleic acid hybridization is a slow and difficult method that uses radioactive labels. It is impractical for routine clinical laboratories.

DNA labeling assays is a laboratory method that uses nonradioactive probes.

In Situ Hybridization detects HIV *within* lymphocytes, macrophages, and other cells using polymerase chain reaction (PCR).[51] Computer image analysis permits semi-quantitative assessment of infection within individual cells.

Until the newer tests are generally available, HIV status is determined by initial and repeated ELISA tests and confirmed by WB or IFA. If the ELISA test is not repeated, or if the positive finding is not confirmed by WB or IFA, then the HIV status is indeterminate.

Assays for virus (culture or detection of viral antigen) may not detect the presence of the HIV during some stages of infection. The HIV can establish persistent infection without actively producing viral proteins.[52] Tests are needed that are sensitive enough to detect single HIV genomes within infected cells. When available, such tests could detect HIV during primary HIV disease, possibly before the person becomes infectious.

Sensitivity and Specificity

A desirable test for determining infection will be both highly sensitive and highly specific. Tests results are a way of classifying people. A test that was positive for all HIV-infected people would be a very *sensitive* test. A test that was negative for all people without HIV infection would be a very *specific* test.

Since no test is perfectly sensitive or specific, a test result is not a diagnosis. It *predicts* diagnosis. How good is the predictor? A good test skillfully used results in very few mistakes in classification. Positive results from a very good test identify mostly infected persons and very few uninfected persons (false-positives). (Persons whose test results are false-positive do not have infections; the results are wrong.) Negative results from a very good test identify mostly uninfected persons and very few infected persons (false-negatives). (Persons whose test results are false-negative are not free from infection; the results are wrong.) On the other hand, poor tests and tests used without skill confuse the diagnosis. Many unin-

TABLE 3–11. **Sensitivity and Specificity of HIV Testing**

Test Result	Infection Present	Infection Absent	Total
Positive	True-positive (a)	False-positive (b)	a + b
Negative	False-negative (c)	True-negative (d)	c + d
Total	a + c	b + d	n

Sensitivity = [a/(a + c)]. Sensitivity is the number of true-positive results divided by the total number of infected persons that were tested.

Specificity = [d/(b + d)]. Specificity is the number of true-negative results divided by the total number of uninfected persons that were tested.

fected people are erroneously labeled positive and many infected people are erroneously labeled negative when poor tests are used. Sensitivity and specificity of HIV tests are summarized in Table 3–11.

Positive Predictive Value

Another way of evaluating a test result is to ask how predictive is the test? What percent of persons testing positive have HIV infection, that is, what is the test's positive predictive value?[53]

In the following discussion, HIV testing refers to screening by ELISA and confirmation of positive results with a specific test, either WB or IFA. High sensitivity and specificity are achieved by combining the highly sensitive test with a highly specific test.

The *positive predictive value* of a test is the probability that a patient with a positive test result has an infection. Obviously this depends on the test and on the skill of the technician. Perhaps less obvious is the fact that it depends on the incidence of infection among the people being tested.[54]

To clarify this point, recall that total positives include true-positives plus false-positives. As the incidence of true-positives in a population increases, the ratio of true-positives to total positives increases and the positive predictive value of the test increases. In contrast, as the incidence of true-positives decreases, the ratio of true-positives to total positives decreases and the positive predictive value of the test decreases.

Consider the following examples. In a group of 1 million people with an 0.00013 incidence of HIV infection, there will be 130 infected people. A good test will identify the 130 true-positives. If the specificity of the test is 0.9999 (1 false-positive for every 10,000 of the 999,870 uninfected people tested), the test will produce 100 false-positive results. It will produce a total of 230 positive results (130 true-positives and 100 false-positives). Only 57% of the positives are true-positives (130 out of 230). In this example, a very specific test used on a population with a very low incidence of HIV infection has a positive predictive value of 0.57.

When 1 million people with a 0.20 incidence of HIV infection are tested using the same test, 200,060 results will test positive. Of the 200,000 people actually infected, 199,980 will test positive (sensitivity 0.9999 × 200,000). Eighty of the 800,000 uninfected persons will test false-positive (specificity 0.9999 × 800,000). In this example, a very specific test used on a population with a high incidence of infection has a positive predictive value of 0.9996 (199,980 out of 200,060).

If HIV testing is performed skillfully on a population with a *high* rate of HIV infection, then a positive test result is highly predictive of infection. That is, very few results are false-positive. If the same test is performed skillfully on a population with a *very low* incidence of HIV infection, then the test is less predictive. When testing populations with very low incidence of HIV infection, a positive test result has only a 0.60 positive predictive value. That is, when clinical medicine's best test is performed on this population by the most competent technicians, 6 of every 10 positive results are true-positives and 4 of every 10 are false-positives.

Put in equation format,[55]

$$\text{Positive predictive value} = \frac{(\text{prob dz})_{popul} \times \text{sensitivity}}{[(\text{prob.dz})_{popul} \times \text{sensit.}] + [1 - (\text{prob.dz})_{popul} \times \text{specificity}]}$$

This equation shows that the positive predictive value of a test is proportional to the incidence of disease in the population. If the incidence of disease in the population is high, then the test's positive predictive value is high; if the incidence of disease in the population is low, then the test's positive predictive value is low, all other things remaining constant. Table 3–12 illustrates several of the variables that affect positive predictive value.

Currently, the WB and IFA procedures are not standardized for service laboratories. If personnel perform the tests without adequate experience or quality controls, they may use different end points. State laboratories, reference laboratories, and blood banks provide reference testing for HIV with 0.9999 sensitivity and specificity. Confirmatory tests should be performed at reference laboratories rather than at service laboratories, because the latter often do not adhere to the rigorous quality controls used by reference laboratories to maintain very high sensitivity and specificity. If positive ELISA test results are confirmed by WB at a laboratory without adequate quality controls, the positive test result may have a positive predictive value of only 0.1, that is, only a 10% chance of accurately predicting HIV infection. In other words, 9 out of 10 patients with a positive HIV

TABLE 3–12. **Positive Predictive Value**

Laboratory	Sensitivity	Specificity	Population	Positive Predictive Value*
Service	0.90	0.95	General	10%
Reference	0.9999	0.9999	Very low risk	60%
Reference	0.9999	0.9999	General	90%
Reference	0.9999	0.9999	Moderate risk	99%
Reference	0.9999	0.9999	High risk	99.9%

*Positive predictive value is the likelihood that a positive test result means that the patient is infected.

test result from this laboratory may have false-positive results.

Is the person infected? If infected, what next? HIV testing is the only way a person can determine if he or she became infected after exposure to the HIV. A positive ELISA test result should be confirmed by WB or IFA. If a person who has avoided high-risk practices tests positive by ELISA and WB or IFA, tests should be repeated, that is, ELISA plus confirmation (positive predictive value = 0.6). If both series generate positive results, the positive predictive value rises to 99.99%. That is, if test series (ELISA plus WB or IFA) twice reveal HIV infection and the tests were performed by skilled technicians, even if the person has avoided high-risk practices there is only 1 chance out of 10,000 that the result is a false-positive.

Anonymous testing is a public health tool to determine both incidence and prevalence of HIV infection. It protects infected individuals from potential discrimination and allows for counseling of such individuals.

TREATMENT OF AIDS

Currently, there is no cure for HIV infection.[57] Treatment goals include counseling and support, vaccination against influenza and pneumococcus, medical evaluation, and, when indicated, treatment with zidovudine (azidothymidine, or AZT).

Zidovudine: Treatment and Possible Prophylactic Use

Zidovudine is the first antiviral agent documented to be clinically effective and licensed for use in treatment of serious HIV infections.[58] It is the only medication currently available for the specific treatment of HIV infection. It helps many patients but is toxic to bone marrow and causes neutropenia (severe decrease in the number of white blood cells) and anemia. Despite frequent transfusions, 40% of AIDS patients on AZT must stop because of neutropenia.[59] The cost of AZT treatment is about $7,000/year.

Zidovudine is an effective treatment for AIDS patients for about 1 year, after which time the disease again progresses.[60] During this year, many patients gain weight, feel stronger, and have improved mental function. Zidovudine delays but does not prevent death.[61] The effectiveness of prophylactic treatment with zidovudine is not known. Whether or not zidovudine prevents HIV infection following occupational exposure is currently being studied.[62] Additional studies will evaluate whether or not zidovudine treatment of asymptomatic individuals delays or prevents the symptomatic manifestations of HIV infection.

Supportive care is important to people with AIDS. The prospect of dying is frightening. The prospects of a fragmented body, fractured relationships, and loneliness are frightening. Patients need to know that other people will support them. Allied health professionals can be caring friends for these patients. With courage and hope, many patients with AIDS are able to live remarkable lives, enjoying each day to its fullest.

Although no cure for AIDS currently exists, there are effective treatments for the many opportunistic infections AIDS patients suffer. AIDS patients can live quality lives. Medical science is making rapid progress. Effective treatments that prolong life will eventually become available.

DISCUSSION QUESTIONS

1. Why is it important for allied health professionals to be familiar with the diagnostic schema physicians follow to monitor the various stages of HIV infection?
2. What will be the value of HIV tests that can identify infection within 2 weeks of inoculation?
3. Why does the positive predictive value of a test vary with the frequency of infection among the population being tested?
4. What effect could false-positive test results have on a person's life? What effect could false-negative test results have?
5. What counseling is indicated at each stage of HIV infection? By whom? Why?
6. Why is regular medical monitoring essential during the asymptomatic period?

REFERENCES

1. Brachman, PS: Epidemiology of nosocomial infections. In Bennett, JV and Brachman, PS (eds): Hospital Infections, ed 2. Little, Brown & Co, Boston, 1986, p 1.

2. Brachman, PS: Ibid.
3. Brachman, PS: Ibid.
4. Brachman, PS: Ibid.
5. Revision of the CDC surveillance Case Definition for Acquired Immunodeficiency Syndrome. MMWR 36:1S, 1987.
6. Lifson, AR, et al: The natural history of Human Immunodeficiency Virus Infection. J Infect Dis 158:1360, 1988.
7. Isaksson, B, et al: AIDS two months after primary Human Immunodeficiency Virus infection. J Infect Dis 158:866, 1988.
8. Widy-Wirski, R, et al: Evaluation of the WHO clinical case definition for AIDS in Uganda. JAMA 260:3286, 1988.
9. Classification system for human T-lymphotropic virus type III/lymphadenopathy-associated virus infections. MMWR 35:334, 1986.
10. National Academy of Science: Committee Report. The Nation's Health, July 1988, p 10.
11. National Academy of Sciences: Ibid.
12. Cooper, DA, et al: Acute AIDS retrovirus infection: Definition of a clinical illness associated with seroconversion. Lancet 1:537, 1985.
13. MMWR 35:334 (1986): Ibid.
14. Lifson, AR, et al: Ibid.
15. Kaplan, LD: Pre-AIDS syndrome/ARC. Presentation at symposium: Care of Patients with AIDS. San Francisco, December 8, 1987.
16. Kaplan, LD: Ibid.
17. Greenspan, D, et al: Oral "hairy" leukoplakia in male homosexuals: Evidence of association with both papillomavirus and a Herpes-group virus. Lancet ii:831, 1984.
18. MMWR 35:334 (1986): Ibid.
19. MMWR 36:1S (1987): Ibid.
20. MMWR 35:334 (1986): Ibid.
21. Price, RW and Brew, BJ: The AIDS dementia complex. J Infect Dis 158:1079, 1988.
22. Gabuzda, DH and Hirsch, MS: Neurologic manifestations of infection with Human Immunodeficiency Virus. Ann Intern Med 107:383, 1987.
23. Suffredini, AF, et al: Nonspecific interstitial pneumonitis: A common cause of pulmonary disease in the Acquired Immunodeficiency Syndrome. Ann Intern Med 107:7, 1987.
24. Broaddus, C, et al: Bronchoalveolar lavage and transbronchial biopsy for the diagnosis of pulmonary infection in the Acquired Immunodeficiency Syndrome. Ann Intern Med 102:747, 1985.
25. Fischl, M, et al: Safety and efficacy of sulfamethoxazole and trimethoprim chemoprophylaxis for Pneumocystis carinii pneumonia in AIDS. JAMA 259:1185, 1988.
26. Polsky, B, et al: Bacterial pneumonia in patients with the Acquired Immunodeficiency Syndrome. Ann Intern Med 104:38, 1986.
27. MMWR 36:1S (1987): Ibid.
28. Tavitian, A, et al: Oral candidiasis as a marker for esophageal candidiasis in the Acquired Immunodeficiency Syndrome. Ann Intern Med 104:54, 1986.
29. Rodgers, VD and Kagnoff, MF: Gastrointestinal manifestations of the Acquired Immunodeficiency Syndrome. West J Med 146:57, 1987.
30. Rodgers, VD and Kagnoff, MF: Ibid.
31. Smith, PD, et al: Intestinal infections in patients with the Acquired Immunodeficiency

Syndrome (AIDS). Ann Intern Med 108:328, 1988.

32. Rodgers, VD and Kagnoff, MF: Ibid.
33. Kaplan, LD and Volberding, PA: Treatment of Acquired Immunodeficiency Syndrome and associated manifestations: AIDS from the beginning. American Medical Association, Chicago, 1986, p xxxii.
34. Kaplan, LD and Volberding, PA: Ibid.
35. MMWR 36:S5 (1987): Ibid.
36. Last, JM (ed): A Dictionary of Epidemiology. International Epidemiological Association. Oxford University Press, New York, 1983, p 49.
37. Last, JM: Ibid, p 20.
38. Lifson, AR, et al: Ibid.
39. Ranki, A, et al: Long latency precedes overt seroconversion in sexually transmitted Human Immunodeficiency Virus infection. Lancet 2:589, 1987.
40. Lifson, AR, et al: Ibid.
41. Bacchetti, P, et al: Survival patterns of the first 500 patients with AIDS in San Francisco. J Infect Dis 157:1044, 1988.
42. Centers for Disease Control: United States AIDS programs. AIDS weekly surveillance report, August 22, 1988.
43. Last, JM: Ibid, p 16.
44. AIDS weekly surveillance report: Ibid.
45. Last, JM: Ibid, p 101.
46. Centers for Disease Control: Update: Serologic testing for antibody to Human Immunodeficiency Virus. MMWR 36:833, 1988.
47. Anderson, KC, et al: Transfusion-acquired Human Immunodeficiency Virus infection among immuno-compromised persons. Ann Intern Med 105:519, 1986.
48. Sarngadharam, MG, et al: Antibodies reactive with human T-lymphotropic retroviruses (HTLV-III) in the serum of patients with AIDS. Science 224:506, 1984.
49. Cooper, DA: Ibid.
50. Higgins, JR, Pedersen, NC and Carlson, JR: Detection and differentiation by sandwich enzyme-linked immunosorbent assay of HTLV-III/LAV and ARV-like clinical isolates. J Clin Microbiol 24:424, 1986.
51. Harper, ME, et al: Detection of lymphocytes expressing human T-lymphotropic virus type III in lymph nodes and peripheral blood from infected individuals by in situ hybridization. Proc Natl Acad Sci USA 83:772, 1986.
52. Ho, DD, Pomerantz, RH and Kaplan, JC: Pathogenesis of infection with Human Immunodeficiency Virus. N Engl J Med 317:278, 1987.
53. Last, JM: Ibid, p 81.
54. Ferraro, MJ, et al: Predictive value of microbiologic diagnostic tests. In Lorian, V (ed): Significance of Medical Microbiology, ed 2. Williams & Wilkins, Baltimore, 1982, p 248.
55. Ferraro, J, et al: Ibid.
56. Consortium for Retrovirus Serology Standardization: Serological diagnosis of Human Immunodeficiency Virus infection by Western Blot testing. JAMA 260:674, 1988.
57. Kaplan, LD and Volberding, PA: Ibid.
58. Fischl, MA, et al: The efficacy of azidothymidine (AZT) in the treatment of patients with AIDS and AIDS-related complex. N Engl J Med 317:185, 1987.
59. Bartelett, JA: HIV therapeutics: An emerging science. JAMA 260:3051, 1988.
60. Yarchoan, R, Hiroaki, M and Broder, S: AIDS therapies. Sci Am 259:110, 1988.

61. Creagh-Kirk, T, et al: Survival experience among patients with AIDS receiving zidovu-dine. JAMA 260:3009, 1988.
62. Yarchoan, R, Hiroaki, M and Broder, S: Ibid.

FOUR

TRANSMISSION OF HIV AND PREVENTION OF AIDS

Harvey A. Elder

OUTLINE

61

OBJECTIVES

After reading this chapter, the reader will be able to:
1. Define and describe the role of a reservoir.
2. Distinguish between direct and indirect contact in transmission of the HIV.
3. Rank portals of exit for the HIV according to potential for spread.
4. Rank portals of entry for the HIV according to risk of inoculation.
5. Name host factors that affect resistance to HIV infection.
6. Differentiate among ways in which HIV is spread and ways in which it is not spread, citing supporting evidence.
7. Describe ways in which associated vaginal infections affect transmission of the HIV.
8. Compare and contrast male–male with male–female transmission.
9. List the high-risk sexual behaviors.
10. State reasons why intravenous drug abuse is a potential setting for HIV transmission.
11. Cite reasons why use of blood and blood products has the potential for HIV transmission.
12. Relate pediatric AIDS to the future of the AIDS epidemic.
13. Cite studies and explain the findings related to occupational exposure of HCWs to the HIV.
14. List the primary means of prevention of HIV transmission.
15. List and describe universal precautions for HCWs.
16. Distinguish among infectivity of various body fluids.
17. List and describe appropriate means of decontamination and disinfection.
18. Rate the risk of various kinds of HCWs contracting HIV infections from patients, and vice versa.
19. Outline a model educational program for HCWs.
20. List the components of a model health care facility policy on HIV infection.
21. Explore the current status of vaccine development.

THE EYEGLASS MODEL OF AN INFECTIOUS DISEASE EPIDEMIOLOGY

Figure 4–1 depicts the "eyeglass" model of the epidemiology of an infectious disease. This model includes a reservoir that contains the organism; a host; and a bridge or means of transmission between the two. It also includes a "portal of exit" and a "portal of entry." The eyeglass model helps explain the transmission of the human immunodeficiency virus (HIV).

The HIV cannot multiply outside of living cells (see Chapter 2). When infected blood, semen, or vaginal fluids exit the host and enter the environment, the

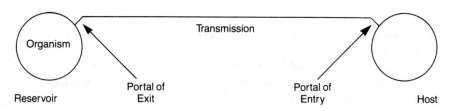

FIGURE 4-1. "Eyeglass" model of infectious disease epidemiology.

virus is unable to survive for more than a few hours under usual environmental conditions.* Most disinfectants readily destroy the HIV.[1]

Humans are the only known reservoir for the HIV—that is, the virus that causes infection comes only from other humans. Any infected human, whether infected with HIV but asymptomatic or suffering full-blown AIDS, can transmit the HIV. People with AIDS are thought to be more infectious than people with asymptomatic infections because their blood contains a higher concentration of the virus.[2] Animals, including insects, are not reservoirs for the HIV and do not have a role in the transmission of AIDS.† Inanimate objects (e.g., dust, water, and food) are not reservoirs.‡

Family members of patients with HIV infection are not at risk for contracting the HIV, with the following 3 exceptions:§ patients' sexual partners; babies born to

---

*Viral cultures survive much longer because they contain higher concentrations of the virus.

†Although HIV can infect chimpanzees, they are not a natural reservoir of this virus.

‡Inanimate objects other than needles and syringes do not ordinarily transmit the HIV. Disinfection of inanimate surfaces is a hygienic practice but not a demonstrated solution to a specific problem of HIV transmission. Disinfection can prevent common-vehicle spread, that is, spread by needles and syringes used by intravenous drug users.

§No other family members developed HIV infection from any other type of exposure, including residence in the same home (sharing the same living, sleeping, bathing, and eating rooms); sharing food, water, eating utensils, laundry facilities, and linen; eating patient-prepared food, and wearing clothes washed in the same machine with the patient's laundry; sharing bathroom facilities, including sink, bath, toilet, razors, and toothbrushes; manifesting human warmth and affection, including touching, hugging, holding, massaging and rubbing tender areas of skin and muscles, and kissing cheek and lips ("dry" kisses).

HIV-infected mothers; and a single case of a mother of an infected baby, in which the mother did not take precautions against exposure to her baby's blood, pus, sputum, and feces.[4]

Transmission is the process by which a microbe spreads from its source to a susceptible person. Infectious disease epidemiologists recognize direct and indirect contact as the 2 mechanisms of transmitting infection.

Spread by Direct and Indirect Contact

Direct contact spread occurs when the victim actively and directly contacts the infection source.[5] The most common example is touching broken skin or mucosal surfaces. In sexually transmitted diseases (STDs), including AIDS, the exit site directly contacts the entry site. Transmissions by blood transfusion and splatter of blood droplets are additional examples of direct contact spread. Droplet splatter is rarely (never yet documented) the mechanism of HIV transmission outside of health care settings. It was the presumed mechanism of transmission for 7 health care professionals who contracted the HIV.[6]

A *vector* is any living carrier, usually a mosquito or other biting insect, that transports an infectious agent from an infected to a susceptible host.[7] Vectors are not mechanisms for HIV transmission. The following data document that mosquitoes do not transmit this virus.[8]

Belle Glade is a town in Florida with a high incidence of AIDS and a major mosquito problem. Careful epidemiologic studies confirmed that the high infection rate was due to a high rate of intravenous drug use. People who were most often exposed to mosquitoes, namely children, were not affected by AIDS or HIV infection.[9] Children exposed to mosquitoes had antibodies to mosquito-borne infections but did not have HIV antibodies. Conversely, persons with HIV antibodies did not have antibodies to mosquito-borne infections. Epidemiologic studies to identify vector spread of HIV infections were conducted in Africa. Most mosquito-borne infections occurred in children 1–10 years of age. HIV infection was limited to sexually active adults and to children under 1 year of age.[10]

The HIV survives a short time and does not multiply in mosquitoes.[11] After mosquitoes eat a blood meal from an HIV-infected person, the ribonucleic acid (RNA) of the HIV can be found in the mosquitoes for only a short time because the RNA quickly disintegrates. The HIV does not even survive, let alone multiply, in mosquitoes. If mosquitoes feeding on HIV-infected blood have their meal interrupted, they do not transmit the HIV to a resumed meal a few seconds later.[12]

For an infectious disease to be transmitted by vector, the infectious agent must survive in the insect (vector) until the host is inoculated. The HIV cannot do this.[13]

Indirect contact spread involves passive transmission from host to victim by intermediate objects.[14] Intermediate objects are often hands or inanimate objects. In this mode, exiting HIV contacts a vehicle that transports it to a portal of entry.

This mechanism of HIV transmission is rare. Airborne transmission by dust and droplet nuclei is undocumented.*

Portals of Exit

The HIV spreads from an infected person to a susceptible person by exiting the infected host through a "portal of exit."[15] Table 4–1 presents virus content, potential for spread, and the chance of inoculation associated with all the possible portals of exit. Whether a person becomes infected with the HIV depends on the chance that body fluid containing the HIV leaves an infected person (by a portal of exit); the concentration of virus particles in the fluid as it exits; the chance that the fluid will come in contact with the susceptible person; the chance that the fluid will reach a portal of entry; and the chance that the HIV will enter the portal of entry and enter host cells. Thus, if a prostitute infected with both the HIV and another STD has intercourse, there is a very high chance (up to 40%, depending on host factors) that her partner will become infected with the HIV.[16]

Most body fluids, such as saliva or tears, have low or very low virus content. "Very low" content means that the virus is rarely, if ever, found in this source. "Very high" content means the fluid is as likely or more likely than blood to contain the HIV. Some fluids transmit the HIV only under specific circumstances; thus their effectiveness is variable.†

Blood, semen, and vaginal secretions are the major portals of exit for the HIV. Blood transmission is usually by direct contact (transfusion or shared needle). The HIV in semen exits during ejaculation, and vaginal HIV exits in vaginal secretions. Sexual transmission of HIV involves direct contact during sexual intercourse. Other body fluids such as sweat, saliva, and tears are only theoretical portals of exit (not shown to transmit the HIV). At the most, they are very inefficient transmitters of the HIV.

Pus contains, among other things, T-helper cells and macrophages.[17] In HIV-

---

*An "undocumented" mechanism of transmission is one that has not been identified in actual conditions; a small number, if any, of unexplained cases have this in common. The home studies referred to by Friedland and Klein[3] are strong evidence against airborne transmission; there are no data supporting airborne spread.

†For example, under ordinary circumstances, tears are an unlikely transmitter of the HIV. Though tears regularly leave the portal of exit, the number of virus particles in tears is relatively low and the probability that the tears will be transmitted to a portal of entry of a susceptible person is very low. Optometrists, however, routinely contact tears. If an optometrist has an open sore on the hand when handling the contact lenses of a patient with HIV infection, then transmission could occur.

TABLE 4–1. **Estimates of Risk of Acquiring HIV
Infection by Portals of Exit***

Portal of Exit[†]	Virus Content[‡]	Potential For Spread[§]	Chance Inoculate[¶]
Respiratory secretions	Very low	Efficient	Very low
Nasal secretions	Very low	Efficient	Very low
Sputum	Very low	Efficient	Very low
Saliva	Very low	Inefficient	Very low
Tears	Low	Variable	Very low
GI			
vomitus	Very low	Variable	Very low
stool	Very low	Variable	Very low
Urine	Very low	Inefficient	Very low
Sweat	Very low	Inefficient	Very low
Skin fomites	Very low	Inefficient	Very low
Wounds			
Intact skin	Very low	Variable	Very low
Broken skin	Low	Variable	Low
Bleeding	High	Efficient	Moderate to high
Fluids exchanged during sexual activity			
Ejaculate	Very high	Efficient	Very high
Vaginal secretions	Moderate	Efficient	Low to moderate
Purulent discharge	Very high	Efficient	Very high
Blood Transfusion	Very high	Efficient	Very high
Shared needles	High	Efficient	Very high
Accidental needle-stick	Low	Inefficient	Low
Body fluids, usually blood-tinged			
Cerebrospinal fluid	Low	Inefficient	Very low
Synovial fluid	Low	Inefficient	Very low
Pleural fluid	Very low	Inefficient	Very low
Peritoneal fluid	Very low	Inefficient	Very low
Pericardial fluid	Very low	Inefficient	Very low
Amniotic fluid	Low	Efficient	Very high
Perinatal	High	Variable	High
Breast milk	Low	Unknown	Low

*Data from: Recommendations for prevention of HIV transmission in health-care settings. MMWR 36:3S, 1987; and from Update: Universal precautions for prevention of transmission of HIV, hepatitis B virus, and other bloodborne pathogens in health-care settings. MMWR 37:377, 1988.

†Route by which HIV leaves infected person

‡Expected virus content for that portal of exit

§Effectiveness with which fluid from that portal of exit spreads

¶Chance that fluid from this portal of exit will transmit to a portal of entry of a susceptible host

infected people, these cells carry large amounts of the HIV. Thus purulent (pus-like) drainage is a portal of exit.

In summary, blood, semen, and vaginal secretions (all with or without pus) are the major portals of exit for the HIV.

Portals of Entry

The site where the HIV enters the host and gains access to the blood is called the "portal of entry." Table 4–2 provides estimates of the risk of acquiring HIV infection by various portals of entry. Intact mucosa and skin block HIV penetration; thus the risk of transmission via these sites is very low.* The major portals of entry are breaks in the mucosa of the genitalia or anus and needle punctures in the skin.

With the exception of maternal–fetal transfer, situations in which the risk of HIV transmission is very high are not random occurrences. Some behaviors epitomize taking risks and other behaviors confine or eliminate risk. Insertive sex with exchange of genital fluids and sharing needles and syringes while using intravenous drugs are very high-risk practices.

During anal-receptive intercourse, the erect penis may tear delicate rectal mucosa, providing vascular access to the ejaculated semen. Anal intercourse thus provides for direct contact transmission. Mucosal tears are the portals of entry, providing the HIV ready access to the recipient's blood stream. The HIV may also gain entry during vaginal intercourse, because vigorous vaginal intercourse can cause mucosal erosions. The mucosa of the mouth has breaks that allow the HIV to enter during oral sex. Thus anal, vaginal, and oral intercourse may all provide the HIV with direct contact to portals of entry (mucosal lesions).

Host

Who is the person with HIV infection? What risks expose a person to infection? More than 95% of AIDS patients are adults who became infected through high-risk behaviors and practices, and 4% are adults who became infected by contact with contaminated blood and blood products. One percent of patients are infants who acquired AIDS from their mothers or from infected blood, and 0.0016% of cases involve work-related AIDS contracted by health care workers.†

---

*Many experts believe that transmission of infectious fluid to broken skin or trauma sites increases risk. This problem is of specific concern to "first responders," including emergency medical technicians, police, and fire fighters.

†If there are about 1,000,000 HIV-infected patients in the United States and 22 had occupationally acquired HIV infections, then 0.0016 of the total infected are occupational infections.

TABLE 4–2. **Estimates of Risk of Acquiring HIV Infection by Portals of Entry***

Entry site[†]	Type Risk[‡]	Risk Gets To Site[§]	Risk Virus Enters[¶]	Risk of Inoculation**
Conjunctiva	Random	Moderate	Moderate	Very low[††]
Oral mucosa	Random	Moderate	Moderate	Low[2]
Nasal mucosa	Random	Low	Low	Very low[2]
Lower respiratory	Random	Very low	Very low	Very low[2]
Anus	Behavior	Very high	Very high	Very high
Skin:intact	Accident	Very low	Very low	Very low
Broken	Accident	Low	High	High
Sexual				
Vagina	Behavior	Low	Low	Medium
Penis	Behavior	High	Low	Low
Ulcers (STD)	Behavior	High	High	Very high
Blood				
Products	Behavior	High	High	High
Shared needles	Behavior	High	High	Very high
Accidental				
needle-stick	Accident	Low	High	Low
Traumatic wound	Accident	Modest	High	High
Perinatal	Accident	High	High	High

*Data from: Recommendations for prevention of HIV transmission in health-care settings. MMWR 36:3S, 1987; and from Update: Universal precautions for prevention of transmission of HIV, hepatitis B virus, and other bloodborne pathogens in health-care settings. MMWR 37:377, 1988.

[†]Potential site where HIV might enter susceptible host

[‡]Type of exposure risk

    random: from victim's perspective risk is not predictable

    accident: risk occurs with events considered to be accidental

    behavior: risk is a recognized high risk behavior

[§]Chance of infected fluid reaching this portal of entry given the type of risk

[¶]Chance that infected fluid reaching the portal of entry gains access to the host's blood stream

**Overall chance that a person will become infected if the person has the usual exposure for this portal of entry

[2]Moderate risk for HCWs with potential exposure to splatter of blood and bloody fluid.

Resistance to HIV infection depends on anatomic integrity, that is, intact skin and mucosa. If the HIV enters the body and gains access to the blood stream, the body is not protected and HIV infection occurs.

All data suggest that every person is susceptible. No one is entirely resistant. Factors that delay or slow the development of AIDS or prolong survival have not yet been identified. Even though infected people make antibodies, they do not develop resistance to the HIV. Rather, as infection progresses, patients become immune-compromised because of loss of T-helper cells (see Chapter 2). No evidence documents the role of nutrition in resistance to the HIV, manifestations of AIDS, or the natural history of HIV infection.

People who practice high-risk behaviors without becoming HIV-positive are not immune or protected. Although they may be lucky for a period of time, unless they cease high-risk behaviors they run a high risk of HIV infection.

REQUIREMENTS FOR AN HIV EPIDEMIC

For an epidemic of HIV infection to occur, there must be a source of the etiologic organism, susceptible hosts, and operative mechanisms of transmission. AIDS could have appeared as a new epidemic only if at least one of the following changed: (1) the organism, (2) host susceptibility, or (3) practices that increase HIV transmission. There is no evidence of a change in host susceptibility, and we may never know if a new or mutant virus developed. In the United States, Western Europe, Australia, and other affluent countries, however, the decades of the 1960s, 1970s, and 1980s were times of liberated sex and intravenous drug experimentation. In sub-Saharan Africa, the same decades were times of independence, increased urbanization, increased population mobility, and increased use of health care facilities without concomitant availability of adequate sterile supplies (needles, syringes, and gloves) or safe blood (screened for hepatitis B and the HIV). These changes in transmission-related *practices* may explain the outbreak of AIDS.

Control of Outbreak

The "eyeglass" model of infectious disease epidemiology suggests 3 methods of outbreak control: remove the source, that is, empty the reservoir; decrease susceptibility of the host; or block transmission.

Food and water-borne epidemics are best controlled by removing the source, but we cannot remove the reservoir for the HIV. It is impossible to find all HIV infected people, let alone isolate or incarcerate them.* If blood samples from every person were tested, the tests would miss HIV-infected people still in the "window" period between infection and becoming antibody positive.[†] Such tests

---

*Not to mention the fundamental cruelty and inhumanity of such an endeavor.

[†]After HIV infection, people become infectious and are capable of spreading the virus within 5 to 10 weeks, and or possibly as long as 14 months, before testing positive. The "window" period is this time when a person is infectious but does not yet test positive. The person with a true-negative test result who is infectious is in the window period (see Chapter 3).

would also miss 1 out of every 10,000 infected persons and patients with advanced infection who have lost their HIV antibodies. If testing were conducted using reference laboratory standards (sensitivity 0.9999 and specificity 0.9999), routine screening of the population would have a positive predictive value of about 70% (see Chapter 3). That is, 30% of the positive results would be false-positives. About 430,000 people in the United States would be falsely identified as infected.* On the other hand, many HIV-infected people who were not identified (false-negatives) would continue to spread the HIV, erroneously believing that they were not infected.

Another means of control would be to decrease peoples' susceptibility to HIV. An effective HIV vaccine would accomplish this. Unfortunately, one is not yet available.

The third option, blocking transmission of the HIV, is a highly effective method of control. Blocking transmission can easily stop the current epidemic. There is no theoretical reason it cannot work; rather, all of the problems are practical.

Only rarely is HIV acquisition random. Pediatric AIDS, occupationally acquired HIV infection among health care workers, and blood- and blood-product associated HIV infection result from accidental transmission. These cases account for 5% of AIDS cases. For the other 95%, transmission occurs because of high-risk behaviors.

It is easy for an individual to avoid HIV infection by practicing lifelong monogamous sex with a noninfected partner and by avoiding using potentially infected needles associated with intravenous drugs. The fact that there are many subcultures in the United States complicates the task of communicating this information.[†] The language and format of messages about blocking the spread of the HIV must be targeted to each subculture in order to inform and motivate members to take individual responsibility for avoiding HIV infection. Many people do not think the message applies to them. Motivating people to take responsibility for preventing HIV transmission must become a national priority.

---

*Assuming that there are 1,000,000 HIV-infected people and that tests have a 0.7 positive predictive rate, if the test were expertly run then the number of true-positive results would be 1,000,000 divided by 0.7, or 1,430,000.

[†]Members of subcultures, even if they use the same language as members of the dominant culture (English), may understand certain words differently, use different symbols, and have different values. Taboos regarding sex and sexual practices may differ. The meaning and practice of drug use may differ. Each subculture must hear about HIV infection and its spread in a manner that is understandable and that communicates the urgency of stopping the spread.

TRANSMISSION OF THE HIV

Epidemiologists discuss risks and probabilities, rather than certainties, about HIV transmission. Labeling a practice "no risk" means that the risk is so close to zero that at this time it cannot be separated from zero. That is, the risk is so low it approximates zero. Means of blocking HIV spread associated with that practice are not known. It is not possible to plan or prevent "zero risk" infections. Likewise, probability may approximate but never reaches 100%. Other (sometimes unknown) factors interfere. We only approximate certainty, but never reach it.

Because humans are the only reservoir for the HIV, only HIV-infected persons can transmit the HIV. Every person with an HIV infection acquired it from another human being, a person who is also infected with the HIV. People do not contract HIV infection from inanimate objects in their homes, restaurants, or in their work places. Tableware, glasses, drinking fountains, and toilet seats[18] are not vehicles for transmission.*

Within a few weeks of exposure an individual who becomes infected with the HIV becomes infectious, that is, capable of transmitting the virus by blood or genital secretions (see Chapter 3). Once infectious, he or she remains infectious until death. No medication will remove the HIV from a person's blood, semen, or vaginal secretions. We need medication that will successfully treat AIDS, medication that will block the spread of the HIV, and medication that will remove the HIV from blood, semen, and vaginal secretions. Treatment that prolongs a patient's life without stopping infectiousness will prolong the communicable period and potentially add to the epidemic.

Role of Associated Vaginal Infections

People who acquire HIV infection from male–female sex often recall having a genital sore (genital herpes, syphilis, or chancroid) when they were exposed.[19] These ulcers provide portals of entry for the HIV to enter and cause infection.

Infected people with Chlamydia urethritis[†] have infected secretions and a

---

*By 1989, there were no cases of HIV infection traced to transmission by inanimate objects other than needles and syringes. Further, the data regarding AIDS patients with "no identified risk" [NIRs] suggest that few, if any, AIDS cases are caused by routes of transmission other than the major ones.

†Chlamydia causes a sexually transmitted disease (STD) most often manifested as non-gonococcal urethritis.

purulent discharge and are more effective transmitters of the HIV,[20] possibly because the cells in the exudate contain large amounts of the virus.[21] Men and women without other STDs, however, may also acquire the HIV during sexual intercourse.

The reasons for the considerable variation in the efficiency of HIV transmission are unknown. Some people are efficient transmitters of the HIV, transmitting it to nearly one half of their sexual contacts, while others are inefficient.

Sexual contact with a person with a heavy virus load (a person who has AIDS or who has HIV infection in addition to urethritis and purulent secretions) increases the risk of HIV exposure. A person with injured genital mucosa (ulcers or erosions) is at higher risk of acquiring the virus, because his or her body has numerous and efficient portals of entry.

Male–Male Sex

Gay men have been the group most afflicted with AIDS. In the past, male–male sex often involved anal-receptive sex and other practices that injure delicate tissues. Injured mucosa provided a portal of entry for the HIV. Each incident of anal-receptive sex with someone infected with the HIV places a person at high risk of contracting the infection. The greater the number of exposures, the greater the likelihood of contracting the infection. Unprotected anal-receptive intercourse is dangerous whether the practice is male–female or male–male. Lesbians who abstain from male–female sex rarely have HIV infection.

Male–Female Sex

Transmission can be in either direction, but in the United States, HIV infection passes more frequently from men to women than from women to men.[22] Male–female sex and male–male sex transmit the HIV by the same mechanisms. Semen and vaginal secretions are the portals of exit and mucosal breaks (sores or ulcers) are the portals of entry. Transmission is by direct contact. The HIV neither knows nor cares about the sexual orientation of the sexual partners.

Skin trauma and other lesions and ulcerative STDs increase the host's susceptibility to HIV infection by creating additional portals of entry. Theoretically, some diseases may increase the host's likelihood of developing AIDS. Some scientists believe that co-infections (other simultaneously occurring infections) such as infections caused by the cytomegalovirus (CMV), or the Epstein-Barr virus (EBV) may trigger the HIV to become productive and lyse the T-helper lymphocytes (see Chapter 2).

A single sexual exposure to the HIV, whether by male–female or male–male intercourse, can lead to HIV infection.[23] Every incident of sexual contact with a potentially infected person increases the risk of exposure to the HIV, and thus the risk of acquiring HIV infection—or another STD. The risk is additive and cumula-

TABLE 4–3. **Risk of Transmission of HIV Infection to Female Partner***

Source Of Male's HIV Infection	Chance That Female Sex Partner With No Other Risk Will Test HIV Positive
Hemophilia	9%
Bisexuality	26%
Transfusion	20%
Intravenous drug abuse	48%

*From: Update: Acquired immunodeficiency syndrome and HIV infection among health-care workers. MMWR 37:229, 1988.

tive. Even though the risk of HIV transmission associated with a single incident of male–female intercourse is small, if the number of incidents is high, then the risk of contracting the infection is high.

Table 4–3 provides an estimate of risks for women associated with different sources of infection in their male sexual partners. Women whose husbands are intravenous drug users have twice the chance of acquiring HIV infection as women whose husbands are not intravenous drug users.[24] Wives of men who have AIDS are more likely to acquire HIV infection than women whose husbands are HIV-infected but do not have AIDS.[25] The risk of acquiring HIV infection is decreased by protection with condoms.

Prostitutes' high rate of HIV infection is usually associated with intravenous drug abuse,[26] but in Africa it is almost exclusively related to sexual transmission.[27] Prostitutes frequently have other STDs and probably are efficient transmitters of the HIV. In Africa, Central America, and most of the Caribbean, prostitutes are major reservoirs of the HIV and are important links in its spread.[28]

In summary, major risk factors for male–female sexual transmission of HIV infection are sex with prostitutes, especially prostitutes who use intravenous drugs, and anal-receptive sex (vaginal and oral sex have less risk).

Intravenous Drug Use and Needles

Intravenous drug use continues to be a major component of the AIDS epidemic. Sharing a needle and syringe for intravenous drug use once is enough to transmit the HIV, because after injecting drugs, intravenous drug users "wash out" with blood the last trace of the drug in the needle. When sharing needles and syringes, subsequent users inject blood and available HIV with the drug. Intravenous drug use is increasing, especially among inner city Hispanic and black youth. As of March 1989, intravenous drug use is the most common mechanism of HIV transmission in the ghettos of large cities, especially, New York City, Newark, and

Miami.

Until the late 1980s, medical practitioners in many Third World countries rarely sterilized needles, syringes, and scalpels between patients. Some tribes and families practice ritual scarification using 1 traditional instrument without sterilizing it between surgeries. These practices are believed to have transmitted HIV.

Transfusion of Blood and Blood Products

Early in the AIDS epidemic, investigators learned that hemophilia[29] and receiving blood transfusion[30] were risk factors for AIDS. Most patients who received a transfusion of HIV-contaminated blood acquired HIV infection.*[31]

Because all blood for transfusion is screened, and because present HIV tests have a sensitivity of 0.9999 (see Chapter 3), the risk of receiving an infected unit of blood is low. However, patients in the "window" period test negative for HIV antibody. The risk from blood transfusion is small, about 1/250,000.[32] Even though the number of new HIV infections spread by blood and blood products is very low and decreasing, many people infected with the HIV by blood transfusions 3–10 years ago have not yet developed AIDS.†

Perinatal Transmission

One percent of AIDS patients are babies and children. Eighty percent acquire HIV infection before, during, or shortly after birth.[33] Usually these babies develop AIDS before their second birthday and die within 2 years. As the number of infected women increases, the frequency of pediatric AIDS will increase. The mother's HIV antibodies enter the baby's cord blood but do not necessarily infect the baby. More than 20% of babies born to HIV-infected mothers are infected.[35,36]

Twenty percent of pediatric AIDS patients received contaminated blood and blood products, usually during late infancy or childhood.[34] The incidence of this method of spreading HIV will decrease with improved blood screening and preparation of blood products free of the HIV.

---

*Retrospective studies showed that two thirds of patients whose cases were followed were HIV positive if they received blood from donors who later donated HIV-contaminated blood. Once donors transmitted the HIV to a recipient, all recipients of subsequent blood, or blood products, developed HIV infection.

†This is because the incubation period is from 2 to over 10 years.

Transmission in Health Care Settings

Reports of HIV infection in health care workers (HCWs) through occupational exposure are summarized in Table 4–4. Just under 7 million people (5.7% of the work force) are employed in health services. The incidence of HIV exposure in this group is not known. The number of "contamination"* exposures probably exceeds the number of "parenteral"[†] exposures. The number of occupationally acquired HIV infections among HCWs is not large. Table 4–5 provides information on transmission categories for HCWs with AIDS. Exposure data are dependent on memory recall of persons reporting exposure. It could be self-serving to over-report occupationally acquired HIV infection. Of the 135 HCWs with no identified risk (NIR),[‡] 20 could not be further evaluated because they died or refused evaluation. Seventy-four cases are still under investigation. Forty-one cases were further investigated but could not be reclassified according to identi-

TABLE 4–4. **Mode of Transmission of Reported HIV Infections in Health Care Workers With No Other Risk Factors***

Country	Number by Parenteral[†]	Number by Contamination[†]	Total
United States	12[‡]	5	17
Other	4[‡]	2	6
Total	16	7	23

*From: Update: Acquired immunodeficiency syndrome and HIV infection among health-care workers. MMWR 37:229, 1988.

[†]Parenteral = needle stick or cut with other sharp object; contamination = splash to mucous membrane, open wound, or broken skin

[‡]Two parenterally exposed workers developed AIDS, 1 from the United States and 1 from another country

---

*"Contamination" is splash to mucous membranes, open wounds, or broken skin.

[†]"Parenteral" exposure is a needle-stick injury or any cut with a sharp object.

[‡]"No identified risk" (NIR) is a technical term used to identify individuals with HIV infection who do not practice high-risk behaviors.

TABLE 4–5. **Transmission Categories for Health Care Workers With Aids***

Category	Health Care Workers	Others	Totals
Identified at risk	2,450	43,678	46,128
Health care workers with occupational exposure	1	0	1
No identified risk (NIR)	135 (5.5%)	1,268 (2.9%)	1,403
NIR after investigation	41		
NIR and reported occupational exposure	17		
NIR and documented occupational exposure with HIV patient	0		

*From: Update: Acquired immunodeficiency syndrome and HIV infection among health-care workers. MMWR 37:229, 1988.

fied risks. Only 1 worker known to be previously uninfected developed AIDS from documented occupational HIV exposure. These data indicate that occupationally acquired AIDS is uncommon among HCWs, but they do not identify occupational risks.

Prospective studies are needed to accurately determine the occupational risk of acquiring HIV infection. The Centers for Disease Control (CDC) began such a prospective study in August 1983. Results through 1987 are reported in Table 4–6. The CDC followed the cases of 1963 workers for more than 180 days. Eight hundred and sixty had parenteral exposure to blood. Four of the 860 contracted HIV infection (indicating the risk was 0.5%). (The upper boundary for the 95% confidence interval is 1.1%). One hundred and three had blood contamination of mucous membranes, open wounds, or broken skin. None of these workers became HIV infected. Therefore, although HIV contamination of mucous membranes may cause infection, the risk appears to be very low.

Table 4–7 summarizes the available literature on the risk of occupationally transmitted HIV infection to HCWs. These numbers are too small to accurately define the occupational risk of acquiring HIV infection by parenteral exposure to HIV-infected blood or other infectious fluids.

Not all needle-sticks inject the same volume of blood; most inject a minimal amount (1.4 microliters[37]). Occasionally a needle-stick accidentally injects a larger volume of blood (1 to several milliliters). An injection of a larger volume is more likely to contain viruses, thus is presumed more likely to successfully transmit HIV infection. Although occupational exposure occurs by contamination

TABLE 4-6. **HIV Infection Among Health Care Workers: CDC Prospective Study, August 15, 1983-July 31, 1988*

Type of Exposure	Number Exposed	Number Infected
Parenteral[†]	860	4
Contamination[†]	103	0
Total	963	4

*From: Marcus, R and the CDC Cooperative Needlestick Surveillance Group: Surveillance of health care workers exposed to blood from patients infected with Human Immunodeficiency Virus. N Engl J Med 319:1118, 1988.

[†]Parenteral = needle-stick injury or cut with other sharp object; contamination = splash to mucous membrane, open wound, or broken skin

(splatter) more frequently than by parenteral (needle-stick) means, the risk associated with the latter is not known.

Other Routes of Transmission

Saliva ineffectively transmits HIV. Studies of dentists and dental hygienists who treat patients with HIV infection show that of those who avoid high-risk practices,

TABLE 4-7. **Risk of Occupationally Transmitted HIV Infection to Health Care Workers According to Available Literature*

Institution or Country Reporting Data	Route of Exposure		Total	Persons Infected
	Parenteral	Contamination		
Centers for Disease Control	963	169	1132	4
National Institutes of Health	103	691	794	0
University of California, San Francisco			235	1
United Kingdom and Canada			220	0
Totals	1066	860	2381	5

*From: Update: Acquired immunodeficiency syndrome and HIV infection among health-care workers. MMWR 37:229, 1988.

only 1 out of more than 2000 became infected.[38] Cuts contaminated by the saliva of HIV-infected persons have not transmitted the HIV.[39]

Transmission by tears is a potential means of infection. The risk associated with tears is probably limited to persons with occupational exposure to tears, such as optometrists. There are no documented episodes of HIV transmission by tears.

PREVENTION OF HIV INFECTION

Compared with other STDs, AIDS is more difficult to contract. The extent of the AIDS epidemic reflects the prevalence of certain human behaviors, not the communicability of the HIV. The risk of contracting AIDS without engaging in high-risk behaviors that transmit the HIV is extremely small. People who avoid high-risk behaviors have little risk of HIV infection unless they work in a health care setting; even there the risk is minimal and can be decreased by taking precautions.

Safe Sexual Practices

Three completely safe sexual practices are lifelong monogamous sex with an uninfected person, practices that do not exchange genital fluids, and abstinence. Persons engaging in these practices do not need condoms to prevent HIV infection.

The risk of acquiring HIV infection by either male–female or male–male sex can be decreased or eliminated by the following practices:

Having sex only with an uninfected, lifetime partner
Ascertaining (by testing) that your partner is not infected with the HIV, and ascertaining (by questioning about high-risk behaviors) that he or she is not in the "window" phase of infection
Using condoms appropriately
Abstaining from all unsafe sexual practices[40-42]

Precautions for Intravenous Drug Use

Prevention of AIDS contracted through intravenous drug use is simple in concept. Public health departments recommend that, if addicts cannot stop intravenous drug use, they should clean needles and syringes between users and disinfect them with bleach. Some health districts are experimenting with making sterile needles and syringes readily available as a way of decreasing HIV infection among drug users. These are desperate measures aimed at solving a desperate problem that is worsening, especially in city ghettos.* As of 1989, education about AIDS, AIDS prevention, and the importance of not sharing needles and syringes has produced only minimal change in behaviors.[43]

Ensuring the Safety of Blood and Blood Products for Transfusions

The number of transfusion-associated AIDS cases should drop because preventive measures are now in place in developed countries. In the United States, Canada, Western Europe, and Australia, transfused blood is usually safe. Blood banks screen by reviewing donor history and by testing for the presence of HIV antibody. Blood testing will miss only 1 infected person out of every 10,000 persons tested.

Factor VIII corrects the clotting deficiency associated with hemophilia A. This product was prepared from the blood of many donors. Since 1985, laboratories have been preparing Factor VIII from HIV-negative donors and processing Factor VIII in a way that kills high titers of the virus, if any are present, and each unit is from one donor. Persons at risk of HIV infection[†] are no longer eligible to donate blood.

Autologous blood transfusion is receiving one's own blood.[‡] Anticipating a need for blood, a person donates his or her own blood, which is stored and made available when needed. Policies and practices vary by blood bank, but it is generally possible to donate blood on multiple occasions; the blood can be frozen and stored for up to several years.

---

*As of 1989, data relevant to the effectiveness of these programs are not available.

†This phrase has a specific meaning in blood banking. Bove lists the following factors related to refusing a donor's blood: if he or she (1) ever injected intravenous narcotics or any drug not so prescribed, (2) ever practiced prostitution, (3) (if a male) had sex with a male since 1977, (4) had sex with a hemophiliac or an intravenous drug user, (5) had intimate (not defined) contact with an individual known to be infected with the HIV or who had a syndrome suggesting HIV infection, (6) had a positive HIV test result or a syndrome suggesting HIV infection, or (7) had an HIV test other than when donating blood. (From Bove, JR: Transfusion-associated hepatitis and AIDS: What is the risk? N Engl J Med 317:242, 1987.)

‡Autologous means "derived from the same individual."

Preventing Spread to Newborns

About half of the babies born to HIV-infected women will contract the infection and develop AIDS. Public health authorities recommend that HIV-infected women not become pregnant.

All women should learn about the HIV and its transmission. Women in their childbearing years should be counseled about the risks to fetuses of maternal HIV infection.*[44] Routine health care for sexually active women should include queries about sexual practices and the sexual practices of their partner(s). Women should be counseled about HIV testing and offered the test as a routine part of pre-pregnancy counseling, particularly if they are at risk of HIV infection. Pregnant women who are at risk of HIV infection need to be counseled about HIV testing. They need to know whether or not they are infected with the HIV and to understand how important it is that they and their health care providers anticipate their babies' health care needs.

Breast-feeding is implicated in a few cases of pediatric AIDS.[45] The risk of transmission is not known but is thought to be small. The magnitude of this problem in the Third World is not known. Breast milk is often the only affordable form of infant nutrition available to a mother. In addition, breast milk provides immune protection and breast-feeding provides the occasion for emotional bonding with the baby.

INCREASING SAFETY IN HEALTH CARE SETTINGS

HIV infection in HCWs is associated with occupational transmission and with high-risk practices. Furthermore, AIDS is only the most current fearful disease that can spread from infected patients to HCWs. Other blood-borne infections, such as hepatitis B, hepatitis non-A, non-B (NANB), syphilis, and CMV infection spread by blood, bloody fluids, purulence, semen, and vaginal secretions. Hepatitis B and hepatitis NANB are more common than AIDS and are at least as important as AIDS. Rational employee health programs seek to prevent the spread of all blood-borne infections to HCWs, by such means as hepatitis B vaccination.

---

*If they have (1) used intravenous drugs, (2) engaged in prostitution, (3) had sexual partners who are infected or are at risk for infection because they are bisexual or are intravenous drug users or hemophiliacs, (4) lived in communities or were born in countries where there is a known or suspected high incidence of infection among women, or (5) received a transfusion between the years of 1978 and 1985, there is risk of maternal infection.

AIDS prevention in health settings depends on 3 major factors:

1. Appropriate precautions
2. Availability of appropriate supplies
3. Personnel knowing and following the precautions

Precautions are aimed at preventing punctures by sharp objects and exposure to splash and splatter of blood and bloody fluids. Policies are institution-specific and should be designed so that it is easier to follow them than not to follow them. Supplies must be available in sufficient quantities, be located so that employees can easily use them, and be of sufficient quality that employees who use them are protected. Health care workers should be taught how to prevent HIV transmission, both in the health setting and in the community. For all hospital personnel to follow the precautions, they must be taught them, receive counseling about them, and see them modeled. They must know that the health care environment is inherently an unsafe place to work and that the employer can establish safeguards but cannot make it completely safe. By following safe practices, however, employees can be relatively safe working in the health care environment. Ultimately, employees are responsible for their own health.

Precautions

Universal precautions[46,47] are based on the assumption that the blood and certain other secretions of any patient may transmit infectious agents. In other words, every patient is potentially infectious. Workers should "treat every patient as if he or she is infected with a blood-borne infection." These precautions represent an attempt to prevent work-associated exposure to blood-borne infectious agents, and reflect the fact that blood and fluids visibly contaminated with blood are the most important sources of these agents. Vaginal secretions and semen are treated as infectious because they are implicated in the spread of many blood-borne infections, although they are not documented occupational risks to HCWs. Breast milk has transmitted the HIV from mother to baby and might be a risk to HCWs in breast-milk banks.

Table 4–8 lists infectious and noninfectious body fluids. Infectious fluids consistently contain the HIV or other blood-borne infectious agents and are believed to be infectious even though their role in transmission has not been documented. These fluids include cerebrospinal, synovial, pleural, peritoneal, pericardial, and amniotic fluids. Epidemiologic studies are not adequate to assess the risk of these fluids to health care workers. Universal precautions do not require treating the following fluids as infectious unless they contain visible blood: sweat, nasal secretions, tears, saliva, sputum, urine, and stool.[49] Employees should use protective barriers to protect themselves from infectious fluids; they do not need protective barriers when working with uninfected fluids.

TABLE 4–8. **Infectious and Noninfectious Body Fluids***

Infectious Fluids	Fluids That Are Usually Noninfectious	Noninfectious Fluids
Blood	Breast milk	Sweat
Bloody fluids		Nasal secretions
Pus and purulent fluids		Tears
Semen		Saliva
Vaginal secretions		Sputum
Cerebrospinal fluid		Urine
Synovial fluid		Stool
Pleural fluid		
Peritoneal fluid		
Pericardial fluid		
Amniotic fluid		

*From: Update: Universal precautions for prevention of transmission of HIV, hepatitis B virus, and other blood borne pathogens in health care settings. MMWR 37:377, 1988.

Practice

Universal precautions supplement but do not replace responsible practice. In addition, universal precautions propose:[48,49]

1. Protective barrier use. Gloves should always be used to protect hands from contamination by blood, bloody fluids, and other infectious fluids. Mask and eyewear (or face shields) should be used to protect mucous membranes from droplets or other splatter. Gowns should be worn to protect from spill and splash.
2. Hands, skin, and mucous membranes should be washed immediately and thoroughly if contaminated with blood, bloody fluids, or other infectious fluids.
3. All HCWs should be careful to prevent injuries with needles and other sharp objects. Needles should not be recapped or manipulated by hand in any way. They should be placed in puncture-resistant containers for disposition.
4. Ventilation devices should be readily available for use during resuscitation. Although there is no evidence suggesting that saliva transmits the HIV, mouth-to-mouth resuscitation should be avoided.
5. Health care workers with open, weeping skin lesions should not give direct patient care or handle patient-care equipment until the lesions heal.
6. Because blood-borne organisms, especially the HIV and CMV, present special

risks to fetuses, pregnant employees should be especially careful to follow universal precautions.

Both latex and vinyl gloves, when intact, are barriers to the HIV and other blood-borne infectious agents. The type of glove to be used depends on the task of be performed. Use sterile gloves when sterility is needed. Examination gloves (non-sterile latex or vinyl gloves) should be used to protect hands from blood or bloody fluids and from major contamination. Use household rubber gloves (utility gloves) when doing housekeeping tasks involving contact with blood, blood spills, or gross contamination, or when exposed to sharp penetrating objects such as those used in autopsies or associated with auto accidents.

Hospitals should interpret universal precautions in view of the prevalence of HIV and other blood-borne infections in their patients. This policy leads to appropriate variations in practice.

Decontamination and disinfection

Decontamination of a large-volume blood spill in an area should follow 3 principles: (1) contain the spill, (2) clean up the spill, and (3) disinfect the area where the spill occurred. The operator should protect his or her hands by wearing rubber utility gloves. Contain the spill by soaking it up with paper towels, removing the paper towels, and placing them in bags for infectious waste. Clean the area with detergent by using paper towels to wash and rinse, and properly dispose of them in bags for infectious waste. To disinfect, wipe the area with paper towels and a tuberculocidal* chemical germicide, and allow to air dry.[50]

Since the HIV is more easily killed than the hepatitis B virus and is present in body fluids in far smaller concentrations than is hepatitis B, guidelines developed to prevent contamination with hepatitis B virus are more than adequate for a worst-case HIV scenario.

Ordinarily, linen used by HIV-infected patients is not a vehicle for transmitting the HIV and is not considered infectious. Thus, laundry needs no special handling. Whether or not patients have HIV infection, moist laundry and laundry contaminated by blood, bloody fluids, or pus should be transported in plastic bags. These bags should be decontaminated before unprotected employees handle the laundry. Heat sterilization of laundry is usually accomplished during the drying cycle, if not during the washing cycle. Chemical decontamination is less dependable and usually more costly.

Dentists and dental personnel should use gloves when touching a patient's

---

*A tuberculocidal agent is lethal to tubercule bacilli. Tubercule bacilli are used as indicator microorganisms for evaluating chemical germicides. Tuberculocidal chemical germicides provide intermediate- and high-level disinfectant, depending on how the germicide is used.

mouth, and dentists should use barriers (mask and goggles or face shields that come to the chin) to protect their own mucosa.[51] All equipment used in patient's mouths should be adequately disinfected between patients. Blood and saliva should be removed from material (such as impressions) that has been in a patients' mouth and that will go to the dental laboratory. Equipment that may be difficult to decontaminate can be protected by covering it with paper backed with an impervious material, and by wiping with an appropriate disinfectant.

Clinical and blood gas laboratory technicians should follow precautions carefully. Specimens should be stored in proper containers that are sealed to prevent spillage. The external surface of the container should be free of specimen and safe for handling. When opening tops and otherwise handling specimens, gloves should be worn and mucous membranes should be protected from splatter (mask and goggles, face shield, or safety cabinet may be indicated). Appropriate safety cabinets should be used whenever procedures can cause splatter or spill. Mouth pipetting should *never* be done. If needles or syringes are used, they should be disposed of in puncture-resistant containers (without recapping needles or otherwise manipulating them by hand). Contaminated laboratory work surfaces, materials, and equipment should be decontaminated in accordance with procedures that will kill the necessary organisms and that are developed for the specific items. All personnel should wear protective clothing when in the laboratory. They should remove protective clothing, wash their hands, and leave the laboratory before eating.

Personnel who are exposed to large volumes of body fluids such as blood without the opportunity of knowing the patient's condition (first respondents—for instance, police, rescue workers, emergency medical technicians, and morticians) should wear utility gloves to protect their hands from injuries that provide portals of entry for the HIV. Sometimes these workers may need face shields to protect mucous membranes. Morticians should wear waterproof aprons and decontaminate their instruments after use. People involved in vehicle accidents have a higher incidence of HIV infection than the rest of the population. Emergency and rescue personnel should protect themselves with adequate utility gloves of a subdued, nonoffensive color. Safety officers such as police and prison guards have a theoretical risk of exposure to the HIV by contact with blood and saliva. Data on bites indicate that they do not transmit the HIV.

Persons with minimal exposure to human blood or infectious fluids (for instance, cosmetologists, beauticians, manicurists, pedicurists, barbers, and electrolysists should avoid contact with clients' blood, infected lesions, and other sores. If the hands will be exposed to blood or bloody fluids, examination gloves should be used.

Ethical Concerns

Precautions in addition to "universal precautions" are in conflict with the patient's right to confidentiality, while serving the wants of HCWs. The ethical issue involved concerns the principle of nonmaleficence (not causing harm to another). Following the principle of nonmaleficence obligates health care institutions to avoid unnecessarily harming patients, and obligates patients to avoid harming HCWs. A breach of confidentiality about a patient's condition could cause emotional, social, and economic harm to the patient. For a patient to withhold critical health information, however, may result in the accidental transmission of a fatal infection to an employee. No employee has the right to breach a patient's confidentiality. No patient has the right to withhold information, if by so doing he or she might endanger an employee in that institution.* Both the employee and the patient must practice nonmaleficence.

Part of the ethical dilemma is resolved by "universal precautions" and the rest by institutional and employee attitude. If prejudice towards any patient or class of patients is not tolerated, if health care institutions teach not only precautions but also humanitarian attitudes, and counsel, warn, and if necessary discipline, then employees will not practice discrimination against HIV-infected patients. See Chapter 9 for further discussion of ethical issues.

In summary, transmission of the HIV in the health care environment is usually either parenteral (by puncture with contaminated needles) or by contamination with blood (or other body fluid) splash or splatter onto mucous membranes. The transmission themes are puncture, spill, splash, and splatter. Care is the only protection against puncture; available gloves do not protect. Whatever the specialty, each employee must apply universal precautions intelligently. Only the employee's own care protects against puncture. Employees should also follow universal precautions and the institution's policies and procedures to protect against spill, splash, and splatter.

Suggestions for Institutional Policies

The risk of HIV transmission from an infected HCW to a patient is very low. Unless the professional involved is a trauma surgeon, the risk is less than 1 in 10 million to 100 million patient contacts. This risk predicts less than 14 excess cases of HIV infection in HCWs occupationally acquired per year nationwide. Risks of this magnitude should be addressed by institutional policies that are friendly and confidential. Various impairment models[†] developed for chemical

---

*Universal precautions do not protect HCWs from puncture injuries. This problem is particularly relevant to surgeons.

[†]Most states have legislation authorizing local committees (hospital-based, county society-based, etc.) that evaluate the problems of impaired practitioners and help them through recovery. Physician impairment committees monitor the progress of chemically impaired and other physicians in therapy. The physician reports regularly to the committee, and is closely supervised by the committee for a period of time, depending on state law. Legislation supports similar impairment committees for other practitioners.

dependency could work. These models would have to be adapted, since HIV-infected HCWs do not recover from HIV infection. Impairment models protect the confidentiality, professional status, and earning ability of cooperative workers while protecting other employees and patients. Noncooperative workers are not protected.

An employee who has a needle-stick injury should be treated according to the routine needle-stick precautions, including evaluation for hepatitis B prophylaxis (per CDC recommendations).[52] The employee should be informed of the potential consequences of the accident, and counseled about the HIV. Informed consent should be obtained if testing is indicated. The patient involved should be counseled about HIV testing. Informed consent should be obtained and the patient tested for HIV. The employee's condition should be monitored clinically during the first 6 weeks for an acute febrile illness consistent with acute HIV infection (see Chapter 3). Depending on the patient's HIV serostatus and the risk that he or she is HIV infected, the employee's condition should be monitored as indicated in Table 4–9. The injured employee has a moral right to know the patient's HIV status.*

If the patient is HIV positive, he or she should be further counseled and treated according to the guidelines presented in Chapter 3. Additionally, the employee should be offered an opportunity to become part of the zidovudine (AZT) prophylaxis protocol.† If the employee is or becomes HIV positive, employee health policies should adequately provide for counseling, continuation of work, and continuation of medical care.

All employees must understand the infection control precautions established by the health care institution. *All* employees includes salaried and nonsalaried personnel and students. Training should be tailored to the needs and expertise of the people being taught. Use different modules when teaching employees in different departments or positions. Do more than overwhelm employees with data. Teach by model and conduct practice sessions to help employees process data and internalize appropriate decisions. Teach so that each employee can make genuinely humane decisions.

The curriculum should include the elements of HIV infection and its natural history, transmission, and prevention. Employees must understand universal precautions. They must realize that any patient could have an HIV infection, how

---

*As a minimum, issues include autonomy and nonmaleficience. How to implement these principles is outside the scope of this text.

†Burroughs-Wellcome Company is studying the effectiveness of zidovudine prophylaxis in preventing HIV infection. HIV-negative employees stuck with a needle carrying HIV may wish to participate in this study. Contact the company at 1-800-HIV-STIK.

TABLE 4–9. **Recommended Follow-up for HCWs Who May Have Been Exposed to HIV**

Serostatus of Source Patient	Intervals for Employee Serological Follow-up
HIV positive	Periodic: 6, 12, 26, 52 weeks
HIV unknown	Periodic: 6, 12, 26, 52 weeks
HIV negative, high risk	Periodic: 6, 12, 26, 52 weeks
HIV negative, not high risk	Not necessary: monitor clinically

infection spreads, and how to prevent the spread. All employees must know how to dispose of sharp objects. Everyone must be trained to avoid punctures, spill, splash, and splatter, and taught how to clean up. Everyone must know how to avoid contamination by blood or other infectious fluid. Employees must understand and internalize the institution's philosophy of patient care. All salaried and nonsalaried personnel and students must make a commitment to providing humane treatment to every patient. Health care institutions must not tolerate discrimination against patients because of disease or lifestyle.

Responsibilities of Health Care Institutions

At their best, health care facilities are not likely arenas for HIV transmission. In hospitals in poorer nations, where blood is not safe, needles and syringes are not sterile, and adequate gloves are not available, the risk of occupationally acquired HIV infection is much higher. Safe blood and needles protect patients, and adequate gloves protect HCWs.

Table 4–10 shows the major determinants of nosocomial HIV infection. Even though severe budgetary restrictions exist in many countries, health care institutions are obligated to stop the spread of HIV infection. They should not transfuse contaminated blood even if testing for HIV is not fiscally possible;* they should avoid administering blood products except when absolutely essential. The risk posed by unscreened blood varies geographically. In some countries, the chance that unscreened blood is infected with HIV is as high as 8%. That is, a person receiving a transfusion of 1 unit of blood has a chance of 1 in 12 of getting HIV infection from that transfusion. Multiple transfusions almost guarantee HIV infec-

---

*In many areas of the world, HIV testing is supported by WHO funds.

TABLE 4–10. **Major Determinants of Nosocomial HIV Infection***

Factor	Proper Procedure	Proper Procedure Minimum Risk[†]	Improper Procedure: Maximum Risk[†]
Blood for transfusion	Determine by testing that specimen is HIV negative	1/40,000	1/12
Needles and syringes	Sterilize	1/1,000,000	1/100
Gloves	Choose type adequate for function	1/1,000,000	1/100

*From: Elder, HA: Health care workers infected with HIV. Paper presented to Presidential Commission on Human Immunodeficiency Virus epidemic on May 12, 1988.

[†]Risk is expressed as number of exposures necessary to have one chance of acquiring HIV infection.

tion. Properly screened blood is more than 10,000 times safer than unscreened blood.

In health care facilities in some Third World countries, needles and syringes are reused without sterilization. All needles and syringes that become contaminated can transmit HIV infection.* Using sterile needles and syringes decreases the risk of transmitting HIV infection by at least 10,000-fold. Facilities that cannot provide sterile needles and syringes should not allow personnel to administer injections. They should restrict themselves to oral therapy.

Unless they wear adequate gloves, practitioners who deliver babies, clean and dress wounds, drain abscesses, and perform pelvic examinations have a modest risk of acquiring HIV infection. The risk is at least 1 in every 100 such exposures.[†]

---

*Rural clinics often see several hundred patients per day and almost everyone gets an injection from the same needle and syringe, unless the needle becomes dull. In an area with 5% HIV infection incidence, the needles and syringes will probably become contaminated with HIV by the 20th patient. From then until the end of the day, all subsequent patients are injected with a contaminated needle and syringe. The risk of HIV spread associated with parenteral medication is not known, but may be as high as 1 out of every 100 injections.

[†]The risk is proportional to the incidence of HIV infection in the population, the risk of defective gloves, and the chance of skin breaks. In many poor countries, the incidence of HIV infection in obstetric practitioners is more than 10%. If the risk of a glove defective at the site of a skin break is 10%, then the predicted number of exposure is 1%.

Using adequate gloves decreases the risk of transmission of the HIV to HCWs by more than 10,000-fold. Health care facilities that cannot provide adequate gloves must limit their activities (deliveries, cleaning and debriding wounds, and so forth) to protect their workers from a high risk of HIV infection.

VACCINATION

Vaccination is the hope. Many experts believe that vaccination is the ultimate protection against HIV infection. Scientists have tested many different vaccines. As of March 1989, they have not reported a vaccine that effectively stimulates antibody against the HIV.[53] Antigenic variations in HIV strains make developing candidate vaccines difficult. When a vaccine is finally ready, it is likely it will be effective only against HIV-1 and not against HIV-2. Research efforts are intense, and large amounts of money are being invested in vaccine research. Once a vaccine is developed, investigators must test its effectiveness and demonstrate its safety and efficacy. How long will that take? Since it takes 5 to 15 years to develop AIDS, complete documentation of vaccine efficacy may take a long time. Because controlling the HIV epidemic and preventing AIDS is urgent, a vaccine would probably be released when it had been adequately tested but before documentation was completed.

SUMMARY

HIV-infected patients can be safely cared for by health care workers. Nonetheless, they do present a small risk to workers. Each worker must adhere to the proper techniques when working with needles and other sharp objects and use barriers when dealing with blood and other infectious fluids. Family members and friends who care for AIDS patients do not acquire HIV infection by caring for, helping, or assisting patients.

DISCUSSION QUESTIONS

1. Compare the risk of HIV infection for health care workers associated with practicing their profession with the risks associated with personal lifestyle.
2. What precautions would you recommend to travelers to Third World countries that have high incidences of HIV infection?
3. If you were going as a health care worker to a Third World country with a high incidence of HIV infection, what precautions would you follow?
4. If you were an infection control practitioner in a health care institution, how

would you balance the rights of patients with the rights of health care workers? How would the need for this balance affect the policies you would develop?
5. Who is ultimately responsible for protecting health care workers?

REFERENCES

1. Resnick, L, et al: Stability and inactivation of HTLV-III/LAV under clinical and laboratory environments. JAMA 255:1887, 1986.
2. Goedert, JJ, et al: Heterosexual transmission of Human Immunodeficiency Virus (HIV): Association with severe T₄-cell depletion in male hemophiliacs (abstr). Third International Conference on AIDS, Washington DC, 1987, p 106.
3. Friedland, GH and Klein, RS: Transmission of the Human Immunodeficiency Virus. N Engl J Med 317:1125, 1987.
4. Apparent transmission of HTLV-III/LAV from a child to a mother providing health care. MMWR 35:76, 1986.
5. Brachman, PS: Epidemiology of nosocomial infections. In Bennett, JB and Brachman, PS (eds): Hospital Infections, ed 2. Little, Brown & Co, Boston, 1986, p 12.
6. Update: Acquired Immunodeficiency Syndrome and HIV infection among health care workers. MMWR 37:229, 1988.
7. Last, JM: A Dictionary of Epidemiology. International Epidemiological Association. Oxford University Press, New York, p 108.
8. Miike, L: Do insects transmit AIDS? Staff paper, Office of Technology Assessment, United States Congress. US Government Printing Office, Washington, DC, September 1987.
9. Castro, KG, et al: The Belle Glade field-study group: Transmission of HIV in Belle Glade, Florida: Lessons for other communities in the United States. Science 239:193, 1988.
10. Castro, KG, et al: Ibid.
11. Jupp, PG and Lyons, SF: Experimental assessment of bedbugs (Cimex lectularius and Cimex hemipterus) and mosquitoes (Aedes aegypti formosus) as vectors of Human Immunodeficiency Virus. AIDS 1:171, 1987.
12. Brachman, PS: Ibid.
13. Brachman, PS: Ibid.
14. Brachman, PS: Ibid.
15. Brachman, PS: Ibid.
16. Simonsen, JN, et al: Human Immunodeficiency Virus infection among men with sexually transmitted diseases: Experience from a center in Africa. N Engl J Med 319:274, 1988.
17. Levy, JA: The transmission of AIDS: The case of the infected cell. JAMA 259:3037, 1988.
18. Lifson, AR: Do alternate modes for transmission of Human Immunodeficiency Virus exist? JAMA 259:1353, 1988.
19. Haverkos, HW and Edelman, R: The epidemiology of Acquired Immunodeficiency Syndrome among heterosexuals. JAMA 260:1922, 1988.
20. Simonsen, JN, et al: Ibid.
21. Levy, JA: Ibid.
22. Levy, JR: Ibid.

23. Peterman, TA, et al: Risk of Human Immunodeficiency Virus transmission from heterosexual adults with transfusion-associated infections. JAMA 259:55, 1988.
24. Human Immunodeficiency Virus infection in the United States: A review of current knowledge. MMWR S-6 36:1, 1987.
25. Geodert, JL et al: Ibid.
26. Antibody to Human Immunodeficiency Virus in female prostitutes. MMWR 36:157, 1987.
27. Mann, JM, et al: The international epidemiology of AIDS. Sci Am 259:82, 1988.
28. Haverkos, HW and Edelman, R: Ibid.
29. Pneumocystis carinii pneumonia among persons with hemophilia A. MMWR 31:365, 1982.
30. Possible transfusion-associated Acquired Immune Deficiency Syndrome (AIDS): California. MMWR 31:652, 1982.
31. Ward, JW, et al: Risk of Human Immunodeficiency Virus infection from blood donors who later developed the Acquired Immunodeficiency Syndrome. Ann Intern Med 106:61, 1987.
32. Ward, JW, et al: Ibid.
33. Heyward, WL and Curran, JW: Ibid.
34. Quarterly report to the Domestic Policy Council on the prevalence and rate of spread of HIV and AIDS in the United States. MMWR 37:223, 1988.
35. Heyward, WL and Curran, JW: Ibid.
36. Editorial. Vertical transmission of HIV. Lancet 2:1057, 1988.
37. Friedland, GH and Klein, RS: Ibid.
38. Update: Universal precautions for prevention of transmission of Human Immunodeficiency Virus, Hepatitis B virus, and other blood borne pathogens in health-care settings. MMWR 37:377, June 24, 1988.
39. Lifson, AR: Ibid.
40. Haverkos, MW and Edelman, R: Ibid.
41. Lundberg, GD: The age of AIDS: A great time for defensive living. JAMA 253:3440, 1985.
42. Kus, RJ: Sex, AIDS, and gay American men. Holistic Nursing Practice 1:42, August, 1987.
43. Fineberg, HV: Education to prevent AIDS: Prospects and obstacles. Science 239:592, 1988.
44. Public health service guidelines for counseling and antibody testing to prevent HIV infection and AIDS. MMWR 36:509, 1987.
45. Friedland, GH and Klein, RS: Ibid.
46. Recommendations for prevention of HIV transmission in health-care settings. MMWR 36:3S, 1988.
47. Update: Universal precautions for prevention of transmission of HIV, hepatitis B virus, and other bloodborne pathogens in health-care settings. MMWR 36:377, 1987.
48. Recommendations for prevention of HIV transmission in health-care settings. MMWR 36:3S, 1987.
49. Update: Universal precautions for prevention of transmission of HIV, hepatitis B virus, and other bloodborne pathogens in health-care settings. MMWR 37:377, 1988.
50. Garner, JS and Favero, MS: Guideline for handwashing and hospital environmental control. Centers for Disease Control, Public Health Service, US Department of Health and Human Services, publication no. 99-1117. Springfield, VA, National Technical

Information Service.

51. Recommendations for preventing transmission of infection with Human T-Lymphotropic Virus Type III/Lymphadenopathy-Associated Virus in the workplace. MMWR 34:681, 1985.

52. Recommendations for prevention of HIV transmission in health-care settings. MMWR 36(2S):1S, 1987.

53. Koff, WC and Hoth, DF: Development and testing of AIDS vaccines. Science 241:426, 1988.

FIVE

PSYCHOSOCIAL ASPECTS OF AIDS

Eunice Diaz, Marianne Hart,
Juliette Monique So'Brien van Putten

OUTLINE

*Suggested Approaches to AIDS
in the Hispanic Community*
Asians, Pacific Islanders, and Native
Americans

A FRAMEWORK FOR INTERVENTION
Systems Theory

OBJECTIVES

By the close of this chapter, the reader will be able to:

1. Describe the emotional climate in which a person with HIV infection or AIDS must often function.
2. Cite and describe 2 psychosocial problems particular to health care workers who must treat AIDS patients.
3. Describe the relationship of persons with AIDS to the ecosystem in which they function.
4. Cite 6 major categories of psychosocial problems persons with AIDS must face and give examples of appropriate interventions for each.
5. List 6 universal needs of persons with AIDS.
6. Identify the special needs of gay men with AIDS.
7. Describe the special needs of bisexual men with AIDS.
8. Identify the special needs of intravenous drug users with AIDS.
9. Explore the special needs of hemophiliacs with AIDS and the needs of their families.
10. Identify the special needs of women and children with AIDS.
11. Discuss issues relevant to patient care for black persons with AIDS.
12. List and describe factors that affect Hispanic persons with AIDS.
13. Using general systems theory, plan an intervention a member of your profession could use in treating an AIDS patient.

AIDS is a disease that involves every aspect of life, with implications for the fields of medicine, microbiology, neurology, psychology, sociology, psychiatry, pharmacology, nursing, social work, politics, religion, ethics, morality, and thanatology. This chapter addresses the psychological and sociological aspects of AIDS. The term *psychosocial* expresses the complex and intricate relationship between individuals and their environment.

HEALTH CARE WORKERS AND QUALITY OF LIFE FOR PERSONS WITH AIDS

The most crucial psychosocial factor that has negatively affected HIV-infected persons and persons with AIDS (PWAs) has been society's reaction—namely fear.

Society's fear has caused unnecessary anxiety, fear, and stress among infected persons. Health care workers' (HCWs) fear has caused many workers to abandon professional ethics and their ability to act as caring, compassionate, and civilized human beings. Some HCWs have refused to treat persons dying of AIDS; others have emotionally or spiritually abused PWAs. Some have accused PWAs of a crime (acquiring AIDS), or judged them and sentenced them to die as ostracized people. That ostracism has come at the time when PWAs most need the support and understanding of HCWs.

Surgeon General Everett Koop[1] of the United States Public Health Service admonishes citizens and HCWs thus:

> At the beginning of the AIDS epidemic, many Americans had little sympathy for people with AIDS. The feeling was that somehow people from certain groups "deserved" their illness. Let us put those feelings behind us. We are fighting a disease, not people. Those who are already afflicted are sick people and need our care as do all sick patients.

HCWs need to be part of the solution to the epidemic, not part of the problem. There are 2 essential ways in which HCWs can make a positive impact on the AIDS epidemic: by educating, and by providing compassionate care. HCWs should spread accurate information about AIDS, not fear. They can counteract the hysterical reactions many people display, including their colleagues in the health care professions. HCWs can positively affect the quality of life for HIV-infected persons and PWAs by addressing the following areas.

AIDSophobia

According to Freed,[2] AIDSophobia is the fear of catching AIDS. This fear can be alleviated through education and through contact with PWAs. After caring for PWAs, workers find that AIDSophobia diminishes. They find they begin to care for and about the person, rather than dread the disease. HCWs should protect themselves against contracting the virus,[3] but using precautions need not prevent them from rendering competent and compassionate care.

Homophobia

Homophobia, the fear, dislike, and hatred of gays and lesbians, and of homosexuality,[4] is another attitude that prevents some HCWs from competently caring for PWAs. It is insufficient merely to identify the problem; HCWs need to develop ways of eliminating homophobia.

Moses and Hawkins[5] suggest that "personal homophobia is best combated in 2 ways. First, gather information through reading, talking to people, and listening to music created by lesbians and gays; secondly, get to know some lesbian women and gay men personally. Research has shown that the best way to combat stereotypes is to have contact with people about whom one holds such stereotypes."

Denial of Death and Dying

Denial of death and dying is a third issue HCWs must confront when working with PWAs. At this time, there is no cure for HIV infection or for AIDS. HCWs are oriented toward healing persons, rather than helping them to die. Workers must first explore their thoughts and feelings about their own mortality. This process is difficult in a culture that often denies dying, death, and bereavement. Attending a hospice training program or a class on death and dying is a good way to explore personal feelings on the topic. Reading and sharing thoughts and feelings with colleagues is another way. Thoughts and feelings about death and dying are not stagnant; the death of a relative, close friend, or associate may affect how a worker feels about death.

Countertransference

Countertransference is a problem HCWs may not recognize. Macks[6] describes this phenomenon as "the health care worker's conscious or unconscious behavioral, cognitive, or emotional reaction to the circumstances, emotions, or behaviors presented by the client." Mental health workers have long recognized the occurrence of this phenomenon. For example, if a 55-year-old female physical therapist is caring for a 25-year-old man with AIDS, the physical therapist may react or feel toward the patient the same way she reacts to her 25-year-old son.

Countertransference can have negative or positive consequences for the HCW's professional conduct. It is important for a HCW to identify any signs of countertransference when working with a PWA. Evaluate whether the countertransference has a positive or negative influence on providing care to the patient. If it enhances care, it is a positive development. If it exerts a negative influence on care, seek help from a mental health worker or attend a support group for persons who care for PWAs.

Demanding Nature of Caring for Persons with AIDS

Caring for PWAs is time- and energy-consuming. PWAs suffer many different opportunistic infections; the severity of these infections may vary from hour to hour. A patient may enter the hospital with a primary diagnosis of *Pneumocystis carinii* pneumonia (PCP), but may also have the wasting syndrome and candidiasis as well as a mild case of AIDS dementia. The patient may not be able to eat because of the candidal infection. Twenty to 25 episodes of diarrhea a day are not uncommon for patients with the wasting syndrome. An unstable pulmonary condition will necessitate cardiopulmonary supervision and treatment. The patient may need to be placed on a respirator. Multiple tests—blood gases, CBC, chest x-ray, CT scan, urinalysis, bronchoscopy—may be required. The HCW needs to inform the patient about each test—what it is, and why it is being done. Convincing the patient to authorize the various tests may sometimes be difficult.

During all of this treatment, the patient is likely to be extremely afraid of dying, afraid of the pain, afraid of not knowing what test or procedure to expect next, and afraid of having a HCW refuse to care for him or her. Such patients need the compassion and care of HCWs. Little wonder, though, that HCWs experience burnout when rendering care to PWAs. A team approach is important in caring for PWAs, because team members may help support each other. Leukefeld and Fimbres[7] suggest using a voluntary system of staff rotation.

HCWs themselves need support as they support persons affected by this epidemic. Involvement in a support group can prove very helpful; if such a group does not exist in your institution or agency, contact the nearest community AIDS project for assistance.

Persons With AIDS and Their Ecosystems

After diagnosis, PWAs usually have more difficult psychosocial needs to meet than at any other time in their lives. These needs also affect the lives of people around them. Patients may experience feelings of hopelessness, helplessness, fear, anxiety, depression, grief, anger, loss, and despair. Yet some also are able to express feelings of completeness, acceptance, harmony, meaningfulness, peace, and hope. PWAs can and do experience a full range of emotions. A person's emotional reactions may vary as his or her illness progresses.

Each person's method of dealing with a personal crisis such as AIDS is different, and depends on age, sex, ethnicity, family, friends, religious beliefs, educational background, employment experiences, socioeconomic status, and life experiences. PWAs progress or regress in their ability to cope with the crisis according to the reactions of persons with whom they associate. A patient's financial situation, living arrangements, level of independence, and role changes all affect coping, as do the complications of the disease and the course it takes in the body. These situations are all fluid.

Figure 5–1 shows the PWA at the center of his or her ecosystem surrounded by a number of spheres representing the patient's family, support system, society, work or school, HCWs and mental health care workers, and social and community services. As changes occur in these aspects of the person's life, they force the PWA to shift focus. Shifting focus or adjusting takes time and a great deal of energy. Needless to say, the less often change occurs, the better able the patient will be to adjust and cope with his or her environment.

Providing quality care to PWAs includes taking a thorough and indepth history. Such histories should include the person's lifestyle before becoming ill, including work history, significant relationships, sexual history, use of alcohol and drugs, especially intravenous drugs, psychiatric history, defense mechanisms, and responses to other crises in their lives.

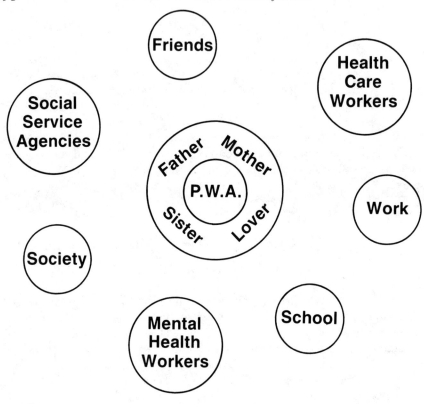

Fill in connections where they exist.

Indicate nature of connections with a descriptive word or by drawing different kinds of lines:
——————— for strong, ---------- for tenuous, + + + + + + + + for stressful.

Draw arrows along lines to signify flow of energy, resources, etc. → → → . Identify significant people and add empty circles as needed.

FIGURE 5-1. Eco-map. (Adapted from Social Work Processes, revised edition, by Beulah Roberts Compton and Burt Galaway © 1979, 1975 by The Dorsey Press. Reprinted by permission of Wadsworth, Inc.)

Major Problems of Persons With AIDS

Patients have 6 major problems:

1. Managing distressing feelings
2. Managing crises
3. Loss of status
4. Loss of social support

5. Managing the grieving process
6. Managing care and treatment

HCWs can effectively intervene in each of these areas as detailed below.

Managing Distressing Feelings

Patients need help managing anxiety, depression, anger, guilt, and fear. These feelings are normal responses to a life-threatening disease. The person may be anxious about the meaning of the diagnosis, how family and friends will react, how he or she will cope, what treatments will be needed, and what will happen next.

Symptoms of anxiety may be somatic, cognitive, or behavioral, and include a feeling of tightness in the chest, headaches, diarrhea, poor appetite, sweating, poor concentration, feelings of unreality, avoidance, and apprehensiveness. Interventions for managing anxiety include encouraging the patient to talk about his or her anxieties; providing factual information; explaining the various symptoms of anxiety; encouraging relaxation and stress-reducing activities; and helping the patient plan enjoyable activities.[8] If the patient is unable to control anxiety, anti-anxiety medication may be necessary.

Issues about sex and sexuality can cause a great deal of distress. By nature, humans are sexual beings; the AIDS crisis does not change that fact. For AIDS patients, however, sexual attitudes and behavior can and must change. Sex can represent many things: an expression of emotions or intimacy; a desire for procreation; a need to feel loved or desirable; physical release; a way to pass time; a habit; or a way to escape from uncomfortable feelings.[9] Many people have a narrow belief that the only sexual options are shaking hands and having intercourse.[10] Between the extremes of shaking hands and having intercourse are an incredible number of intimate sexual options that the body and imagination are capable of producing.[11] Many of these activities, such as cuddling, holding, "dry" or "social" kissing, masturbation, and mutual masturbation involve little or no risk of transmitting the HIV.

Persons facing death, loss of independence, and the progressive nature of AIDS are frequently depressed. Symptoms of depression may also be somatic, cognitive, or behavioral and include poor appetite, significant weight loss or gain, loss of interest in usual activities, decreased sex drive, fatigue, insomnia or sleep disturbance, feelings of worthlessness, poor concentration, indecisiveness, reduced activity, and social withdrawal. It is important to distinguish between *secondary* depression and anxiety, and depression and anxiety caused by the disease process of AIDS, particularly its neuropsychiatric effects (see Chapter 6).

Intervention to combat depression include increasing the patient's activity level; encouraging a hopeful attitude; encouraging a positive perspective (e.g., "the glass is half full rather than half empty"); and encouraging the patient to control the illness rather than letting the illness control him or her. For example, ask the patient to imagine the immune system as "Pac-man" eating up all the virus particles and to focus on what he or she can do to strengthen the body's defenses. Another intervention involves planning rewards for accomplishing a task, such as getting an ice cream cone after a short walk or other form of exercise.

Encourage the patient to plan an evening with friends or to attend an AIDS support group. Help the patient to re-establish as normal a lifestyle as possible.[12] Constantly evaluate for suicidal ideation. Antidepressant medicine may be needed. Be aware that it takes time for such medication to be effective, however, and that the medication can be used as an overdose to commit suicide. Also, make the patient's caregivers aware of any suicide ideation.

Anger is another feeling AIDS patients may experience. The patient may be angry about the injustice of contracting the virus, about not being able to fulfill life plans and dreams, or about loss of control. Anger may be directed at the spouse or lover for transmitting the virus, or at himself or herself for engaging in high-risk activities. Anger may be expressed passively or aggressively or both ways. Indications include social withdrawal, continuing to engage in high-risk activities, becoming emotionally and physically abusive, and blaming or being extremely critical of others or of self.

There are many interventions to combat anger. HCWs should help patients express their feelings, identify destructive behaviors, and develop a plan to re-place these behaviors. Workers will often find that the anger is directed at them. Do not take it personally or be defensive. Listen and be empathetic and caring. Usually this response will improve the situation.

Guilt feelings must also be addressed. The patient may feel guilty about being gay or bisexual, about using intravenous drugs, or about transmitting the virus to a spouse, lover, or child. Symptoms of guilt include social withdrawal, obsessive thoughts or behaviors, feelings of powerlessness, and a negative and defeatist outlook. Effective interventions include encouraging catharsis, or expression of feelings, and encouraging the client to accept himself as gay or bisexual (if appli-cable). Counseling by a spiritual or religious representative is occasionally useful. Be sure to refer the patient to a nonjudgmental counselor. Encourage the patient to live in the present and let the past go, since the past cannot be changed and no one is assured of a tomorrow.

Fear is omnipresent with PWAs. Their fears are many. Methods of dealing with fear are discussed later in this chapter.

Managing Crises

The patient will experience a number of crises during the course of HIV infection and illness. Crises most commonly occur when the person learns the test result is positive; when AIDS is diagnosed; at the onset of opportunistic infections; with loss of independence; with rejection by family and friends, if this occurs; and at the realization of impending death. In general, interventions such as enhancing the patient's adaptive skills and helping the patient integrate his or her coping skills are essential to help the patient learn to manage crises.[13]

Loss of Status

Loss of status is a major problem that occurs in the areas of occupation, role in the family, power, control, and independence. At some point during the course of the illness, a patient will no longer be able to continue to work. Loss of employment means loss of finances and a loss of the esteem that comes from identifying with his or her occupation or profession.

Medical social workers are indispensable members of the interdisciplinary health care team, because they can educate and assist the patient in applying for financial assistance. They can redirect patients from focusing on loss of identity to focusing on being an AIDS survivor rather than an AIDS victim. They can assist in overcoming the loss of social support PWAs often experience. Family and friends may fear the contagion of the virus; they may feel overwhelmed with the issues the patient has to face. Social workers can help other team members work with family members to meet the extra emotional and financial demands placed on them. Occupational therapists can help patients find alternative, meaningful occupational roles.

Loss of Social Support

Another problem patients face is loss of social support. Family and friends may already have withdrawn support from the patient when they learned the patient is gay or bisexual. They may withdraw support for the reasons discussed above. Also, many patients are not able to go out socially because of fatigue and diarrhea, and may back away from a support system. Family and friends may feel there is nothing they can do to support the patient. HCWs need to educate the patient's family and friends about the fears they may have about contagion. Encourage the patient to communicate why he or she may not feel like going out with family and friends, rather than just withdrawing. Listen to family members where they express feelings of being overwhelmed and inadequate to provide assistance to the patient. Encourage the family and friends to understand that the most significant thing they can do for the patient is show their willingness to go through this experience with the patient.

Managing the Grieving Process

Every PWA must face the grieving process. Resolving issues about death and dying is difficult in a society that denies death. One of the foremost experts in leading this society to recognize the need for understanding and accepting death is Dr. Elisabeth Kübler-Ross.[14] She identified 5 stages of dying, namely denial, anger, bargaining, depression, and finally acceptance. Ways to intervene to help a dying person in each of these stages are discussed later in this chapter.

Managing Care and Treatment

Managing care and treatments after discharge from inpatient facilities is the province of HCWs. Many PWAs recently discharged from the hospital need follow-up appointments for chemotherapy, laboratory work, CT scans, counseling, or physical, occupational, and speech therapy. Some need assistance in locating services from community AIDS projects, home health care agencies and hospice agencies.

Everyday needs—adequate nutritional intake, transportation, medications, home nursing care—can be overwhelming for a PWA without assistance or support to manage. Workers can help patients organize their needs according to priority and plan for ongoing care. Chapter 7 provides further information for planning home care.

Major Needs of Persons with AIDS

PWAs have many needs and problems. Not all patients have the same needs, but 6 needs appear to be universal for PWA: alleviation of fear and uncertainties; working through the grieving process; reduction of stress; receiving emotional support; having someone to listen; and needing to be touched.

Alleviation of Fears and Uncertainties

Persons with HIV infection fear or wonder about the following:

Which opportunistic infection will strike next
How family and friends will react to the HIV+ or AIDS diagnosis
Which high-risk activity or activities resulted in infection
Whom they may have infected with the HIV
Whether they will die alone
Whether they will die in pain
How long they will survive
Whether there will be a cure before they die
How they will cope financially
How the disease(s) will affect their bodies
Whether they will go crazy
How long will they be able to continue to work or go to school
Who will care for them
How HCWs will treat them

These fears and uncertainties cause a great deal of stress, which HCWs can help alleviate. For example, HCWs may provide information on medicines that can ease pain, new and promising treatment drugs, or cofactors that can increase or decrease life expectancy.

Working Through the Grieving Process

For each of the stages of death and dying,[15] the HCW can use specific interventions. Examples of interventions for each stage follow.

A patient in the stage of *denial* may tell you, "I don't have AIDS; someone has made a mistake in my diagnosis." Denial is a way of coping with the devastating diagnosis. Do not directly confront the patient, but help him or her to resolve other questions about the illness.

The patient may report, "The doctor said nothing about my having AIDS. He said he would start me on chemotherapy, and this will help me." In an instance like this, it may be necessary to recommunicate the diagnosis of AIDS.

The *angry* PWA may ask, "Why me? What kind of a God would allow this disease to exist?" Gently assist the patient to explore his or her beliefs and past experiences. You may share your beliefs, but do not force them on the patient. Having pat answers is not necessary to help a person through this stage, but listening is necessary. Even though anger may be directed toward you as a HCW, do not react. Allow the person time to adjust his or her thinking.

Bargaining usually involves bargaining with God. "I know I am dying, but if God will only let me live until my next birthday," or "until my family arrives." Again, listen emphathetically.

Depression is a feeling many people experience at different points in their lives. It is understandable for a PWA to feel depressed. During this stage, the patient acknowledges, "Yes, I am dying of AIDS. There is no cure, and I am dying." In this stage, the patient begins to face the crucial reality of what is happening.

Acceptance is the stage in which the person comes to terms with what is happening. Not all patients reach this stage, but those who do will exhibit a sense of harmony and peacefulness.

Patients may move between these various stages. You may even find a person moving between stages during a brief encounter. This rapid movement requires you to listen and be alert to what the patient is expressing, which requires considerable energy. Consider the following example from one of the author's experiences.

> In one of the first situations I encountered, I went to the hospital to visit R.M., who had just been diagnosed with AIDS and was having great difficulty accepting the diagnosis. When I introduced myself as coming from the AIDS Project, he exclaimed, "Great! Someone who can understand what I am going through."
>
> As we moved out to the lawn, where he had asked for the visit to take place, he became very upset. "I don't know why the staff requested that you see me because I don't have AIDS. These doctors are stupid and just misdiagnosed me!"
>
> I listened and asked if there was anything I could do for him. To this, he replied, "Yes, I have certain things I want done at my funeral. Will you help me with these plans? I don't know how long I can live with this diagnosis of AIDS."
>
> I agreed to help him with the funeral arrangements. Within the hour's visit, R.M. fluctuated between denial, bargaining, and acceptance. This took me by surprise. I had worked with many terminal patients, but never had I experienced such fluctuation in a short period of time. Since that time, I have

*worked with countless PWAs and find this movement to occur frequently. I
expect it now.*[16]

During the grief process the patient will experience both positive and negative
emotions. Such emotions can be healthy. If the negative emotions are intense,
however, they can render the patient emotionally immobile or self-destructive.
You can help the patient in this stage by listening, allowing expression of feelings,
and permitting silences, if necessary. Often the patient wants to discuss such
feelings with a HCW, because family and friends may be too uncomfortable. The
family may say to the patient, "What's all this talk about dying? You're going to be
OK." Patients fear that family members may not be able to handle thinking or
talking about death.

Stress Reduction and Management

Stress reduction and management are important. There is evidence that stress can
reduce the effectiveness of the immune system.[17] Since modern medicine has few
ways of healing or strengthening the immune system, HIV-infected persons
should keep their immune systems as healthy and strong as possible.

The use of alcohol and drugs also has a negative effect on the immune system.
Convincing patients to reduce or discontinue the use of these substances is a
major task, because AIDS is probably the most stressful thing they have ever
faced—and some may be accustomed to handling stress by using drugs or alcohol.
Discontinuing smoking is also a powerful health promotion measure. Other
health promotion measures include good nutrition, exercise, and a regular sleeping pattern. Chapter 7 further discusses health promotion measures.

Pacing activities and managing time help to reduce stress. While the patient is
in the acute care setting, the HCW can schedule tests, x-rays, and various procedures so that the patient has time to eat and rest between procedures. When
outside an institution, PWAs should plan ahead to avoid being "on the run" all the
time. They should schedule activities to allow adequate time for exercise, sleep,
and rest.

Other stress-reducing techniques that PWAs can learn include progressive
relaxation, self-hypnosis, meditation, imaging, "thought stopping," refuting irrational ideas, breathing exercises, biofeedback training, and assertiveness training.

Emotional Support

The traditional support systems (family, friends, home) may be partially or completely lacking for PWAs. You can assist patients by helping them locate support
for the problems they face. Support can be found through anonymous groups for
substance abusers; AIDS support groups for both the patient and his or her caregivers, and home health care agencies or hospices, if appropriate.

Active Listening

Active listening may be the strongest support a HCW can offer. A laboratory
technician can listen to a patient express fear of having blood drawn. A nurse,

while dressing a wound, can listen to a patient express concern over how he will tell his father he is bisexual. A physical therapist can listen to a patient's concerns while ambulating the patient.

Touching

One of the most important needs of PWAs is the need to be touched. The importance of this need cannot be overemphasized. Because of the widespread fear of the virus, infected persons have often been treated as lepers—no handshakes, no hugs, no physical contact. Touching by a HCW helps patients know we are treating them as people, not as a disease. We can still touch patients, even though we must follow the guidelines for adequate protection. Gloves should be worn when you will come in contact with body fluids, not when you are shaking hands, placing a hand on the arm, or giving a hug.

The following experience of a social worker[18] demonstrates the value of touching:

> This man had been a licensed clinical social worker in inpatient psychiatric facilities for 17 years. He prided himself on the fact that he never touched a patient—never shook a patient's hand, placed his hand on a back, or gave a hug. He believed that touching contaminated the therapeutic process. This belief reflects the Freudian theoretical approach.
>
> Then he learned he had AIDS. The lesions on his body proved to be Kaposi's sarcoma. He was devastated. He called me a day after learning his diagnosis, wanting my help in figuring out how to tell his 3 sons. He met me at the door of his home, and I saw the tears, fear, and hopelessness in his eyes. I reached up and gave him a big hug while he cried.
>
> At the end of my visit, he said, "I've professionally prided myself on not touching my clients . . . and now I realize I have denied them the most therapeutic skill I could have used."

Most HCWs touch patients while providing care. We touch them when we draw blood, position a person for an x-ray, provide respiratory therapy, provide passive range of motion, or provide wound care. Touching the patient becomes therapeutic, however, when we touch *caringly* and *compassionately*. Touching does not cost money or take extra time, and it is not a difficult skill. So provide your patients with therapeutic touching.

NEEDS AND PROBLEMS OF SPECIAL GROUPS

Gay Men

Gay men and AIDS are synonymous in the minds of many people, but not all gay men have AIDS or are HIV positive, and not all PWAs are gay. However, because over half of the PWAs in the United States at this time are gay or bisexual men, it is important to understand the psychosocial issues that affect them.

Issues gay men must face include homophobia, "coming out," and discrimination. What we call gay men is an important issue to gay patients. Woodman and Lenna[19] point out that *homosexual* is frequently viewed as a clinical term with negative connotations, and many gay people do not identify with the term easily or comfortably. Many gay people feel that the term *homosexual* emphasizes certain aspects of their lives (namely, sexual practices) at the expense of others. Apparently because the term *gay* evolved among members of the gay culture, clients generally find the term more acceptable.

The term *gay* usually applies to gay men but not to lesbians. Discussion about AIDS issues (as in this book) usually focuses on gay men because female–female sexual behaviors do not place women at high risk for HIV infection. According to a brochure published by the San Francisco AIDS Foundation,[20] "a woman who only has sex with other women is at low risk. There are no proven cases of female-to-female sexual transmission of AIDS."

Homophobia is a term developed by behavioral scientists to describe fear, dislike, and hatred of gays, lesbians, or homosexuality. Homphobia has been at the root of blaming gay men for AIDS. Gay men themselves may verbalize internalized homophobia, if they have not resolved their own feelings. Gay men who have not resolved their feelings may appear repressed, withdrawn, and depressed.[21] These feelings can lead to self-destructive means of coping.

"Coming out" or "coming out of the closet" is a gay argot for acknowledging one's gayness to oneself, or being open about or asserting one's gay identity.[22] Conor-Ryan[23] states:

> *Ordinarily, coming out represents a lifelong process of self-actualization, discovery and growth. Being forced to acknowledge one's gay identity when a disease like AIDS is diagnosed can present an additional burden and shock for the patient and family.*

This process is easier for patients if they do not encounter homophobia on the part of HCWs. Patients may need to role-play telling family and friends about their gay identity if it is not already known. HCWs should be aware of the immense emotional, psychological, and physical energy it takes to "come out" about gayness, and at the same time "come out" about a diagnosis of AIDS.

Some gay men have experienced much trauma and pain because of their gayness. They may have been disowned by family and friends. They may have been victims of various forms of discrimination, in housing, employment, education, and medical care. Gays have been beaten, abused, and even killed solely because they were thought to be gay. Such "queer/gay bashing" provides a realistic basis for their fears.

Bisexual Men

Bisexuality is "sexual attraction, emotion and/or physical attraction and behavior that are directed to persons of both genders."[24] People who are bisexual have some of the same problems gay men and lesbians have. But they also have some unique distresses. They are not openly accepted and supported by gays or lesbians any more than they are accepted by non-gays. The gay community often thinks that a bisexual person is using this label to hide his or her gayness, and sometimes this is true. On the other hand, non-gays feel that a bisexual person is really gay and is trying to "pass" as part of the non-gay/straight community, and sometimes this is true. Bisexual men face the possibility of transmitting the virus to their female partners or to their infants, as well as to male partners. Often the bisexual man does not tell his wife or female partners that he is bisexual, so they may have no idea they are having sex with someone who has engaged in high-risk behaviors for AIDS. "Coming out" in this instance can be very stressful.

HCWs should encourage bisexual PWAs to be honest with any person with whom they are or have been intimate. Education is essential to ensure that the PWA does not transmit the virus in the future. A bisexual man may suffer extreme guilt or become suicidal if he fears or discovers he has infected his wife and child, especially if he is asymptomatic.

Wives or female partners of bisexual men also have many issues to face when they learn of their partner's illness. Auerbach and Moser[25] state that common responses are anger, homophobia, feeling betrayed, and feeling hurt. Depression often precedes anger toward the man for altering the marital relationship and for his infidelity. Women may feel betrayed when they learn about their partner's bisexual identity. They may also feel the whole relationship has been based on a lie.

Intravenous Drug Abusers

Intravenous drug abusers are the second largest group of PWAs. Half of the women with AIDS are in this category. The majority of children with AIDS have parents who were or are intravenous drug users or partners of such users. Many intravenous drug users with AIDS continue with their drug habit. It is important to encourage HIV-positive drug abusers to enroll in a substance abuse treatment program. Substance abuse treatment has many purposes. Drugs suppress the immune system. Brown[26] states that drugs such as heroin increase a person's susceptibility to infection.

Furthermore, current or previous drug addiction can cause complex medical treatment problems because pain medications, psychotropic drugs, and some anti-emetic drugs may not be tolerated by a person addicted to certain substances. It is difficult to maintain addicts on methadone while administering medication to treat them for AIDS.[27] Continuous drug use impairs a person's thought processes and increases the possibility that he or she will make potentially life-threatening decisions, such as not to use sterilized needles when shooting up.

Drugs are costly, and a sizable proportion of intravenous drug users, particularly women but sometimes men, earn the money to buy drugs by prostitution.[28] Also, because of their drug use, many addicts have distressed or alienated the people who had previously constituted their support systems.

Many substance abuse treatment centers have long waiting lists, making access to treatment difficult, particularly for persons with low incomes who cannot pay for private care. Many public programs are outpatient oriented; even inpatient programs allow only a few days for detoxification and therapy before discharging patients. Many intravenous drug users need several weeks of inpatient care for effective rehabilitation.

Another problem characterizing available programs is that they are often oriented to white men and insensitive to the needs of ethnic minorities and women. Sometimes the workers in such centers have AIDSophobia, and deny HIV-positive persons access to care when they learn the diagnosis.

Another concern of HIV-infected persons undergoing treatment is the drug withdrawal process. This process can negatively affect the disease process of AIDS. Also, recovery from substance abuse is a lifelong process; once an addict, always an addict. A person who has an addiction needs to work on recovery continually, 1 day at a time. A diagnosis of AIDS can be stressful enough to cause a recovering addict to return to previous ways of handling stress, that is, by using drugs.

Addiction is part of life for substance abusers, but with AIDS it is a deadly part of life that demands immediate attention. As health care workers, we can educate other professionals about substance abuse and AIDS through our professional organizations and institutions. According to Cancellieri,[29] drug abusers are at the worst end of the spectrum of intactness of ego functioning. Abusers tend to have poor psychological coping mechanisms.

Denial is the chief defense used by substance abusers with AIDS in regard to their drug use and the fact that they have AIDS. Faltz and Madover[30] indicate that interventions that should be used to address denial are different for substance-abusing and non-substance-abusing patients. They state that the most effective time to address the substance abuse issue is when the patient has accepted the AIDS diagnosis.

Substance abusers often manipulate the people around them, including HCWs. Manipulation may be passive or aggressive; if one method does not work, they will try another. Pregnant drug abusers may demonstrate more severe regression and more overt psychopathology than nonpregnant women who abuse drugs, according to Cancellieri.[31]

Hemophiliacs

Hemophiliacs with AIDS have a dual medical diagnosis and need treatment for both conditions. Kernoff and Miller[32] have this to say about hemophiliacs:

Before AIDS, the prospects of a normal life had to many never seemed so bright, a mood of optimism which was fueled not only by the expectations and hopes of the patients themselves, but also by health care professionals and commercial interest.

But since the appearance of AIDS, life seems bleaker, and pessimism again replaces optimism. For the hemophiliac, pain, bleeding, restricted activities, stigmatization, and isolation had been common before blood transfusions became readily available. With the AIDS crisis, transfusions themselves became life-threatening. Hemophiliacs have very high anxiety about developing AIDS. Presently the methods used to treat blood products, such as heat treatment and monoclonal absorption, have been found to eliminate the HIV and the hepatitis virus. Anger about exposure to the virus and about the unfairness of having been exposed may be additional issues. The fear of having transmitted the virus to a spouse or to offspring is an additional stress. Dietrich,[33] a physician who treats hemophiliacs, advises that the wives of hemophiliacs (who are mostly men) postpone pregnancy until more is known about perinatal transmission.

Some hemophiliacs are children. Their parents need support facing issues related to AIDS. Whether these children attend school is a significant issue that school officials and communities must address (see Chapter 7 for further discussion of AIDS in schools).

Most persons with hemophilia use the services of a particular clinic that specializes in treating hemophilia. Workers in such clinics may have followed their patients' cases for years and become a special support to the patients. These workers can continue to be a significant support to hemophiliacs who develop AIDS.

Women and Children

Women and children with AIDS are a growing population with special concerns. The growing number of cases of women with AIDS includes mostly women whose sexual partners are intravenous drug users or who are drug users themselves. Shaw and Paleo[34] indicate there are 3 areas of concern for women with AIDS:

1. Women respond differently to illness than men do.
2. Women may get pregnant.
3. Women have the primary social role of mothering.

Women are more likely to contract an opportunistic infection such as PCP. The opportunistic infections that affect women are often those that are severely incapacitating and that have a serious short-term prognosis in terms of fatality rates.[35] Part of the reason women with AIDS do not survive as long as men with AIDS is that the diagnosis is often not made as early as it is for men. Because the number of women affected has been smaller than the number of men, there have been fewer resources for women.[36] For example, there is a limited number of inpatient drug rehabilitation facilities that treat only women.

Another problem for women is pregnancy. Should a woman with AIDS postpone pregnancy, or run the risk of transmitting the virus to an infant? Most of the new cases of pediatric AIDS result from *in vivo* transmission. If pregnant and HIV positive, should a woman abort or continue with the pregnancy? According to the CDC,[37] women infected with the HIV have a 65% chance of having an infected child at birth.

Macks[38] points out:

> *A woman who chooses to terminate her pregnancy or to postpone pregnancy indefinitely may experience profound grief and loss; a woman who chooses to continue a pregnancy or become pregnant may not only experience opposition from providers, family members, and community, but must endure the long wait to know whether her child is healthy.*

Religious beliefs, ethnic background, whether the women already has other children, her relationship to the baby's father, and her socioeconomic status all influence the decision the woman makes. The decision-making process itself can be extremely stressful. HCWs should be careful not to impose their own beliefs on women in this situation but instead should try to assist in a nonjudgmental way.

Another major concern is how pregnancy affects the course the virus takes. Stroller-Shaw[39] states that "pregnancy can accelerate the course of illnesses associated with AIDS and perhaps also the underlying disease syndrome itself." Research continues in this area, and it is important that HCWs remain informed of the latest findings and share them with such women.

A diagnosis of AIDS may affect a woman's role as a mother. When a woman who is the primary caregiver to a child, children or other adults in the household develops AIDS-related illnesses, her role is immediately affected. AIDS may make the woman too ill to care for her children and household. If someone else in the family also has AIDS, this problem further complicates her ability to offer care. Care of children becomes even more difficult if the mother has the dual diagnosis of AIDS and substance abuse. She may be hospitalized numerous times. Alternative child care is needed in this situation, either on an intermittent or permanent basis.

Foster home placement of *children with AIDS* is often difficult. Children who develop AIDS in the first year of life frequently suffer developmental delays and failure to thrive.[40] Children and adolescents with AIDS need treatment for opportunistic infections as well as other therapies. A multidisciplinary team approach is essential when working with children with AIDS, because it assists caregivers in providing maximum care for the children.

Be honest and open when treating children with AIDS. Answer their questions clearly and in age-specific language. They will have questions about death from AIDS, perhaps their mother's or a sibling's death. They will have questions about their own death. Fielding such questions from children is emotionally stressful for HCWs; the possibility of burnout is high for workers who must do this. Pediatric oncology workers can assist by providing insight and support.

Children need to be emotionally prepared for problems they will face if they attend school. Sending the child with AIDS to school without properly preparing him or her can result in an emotional and physical crisis for the child.

An issue for health care workers is the possibility of becoming emotionally attached to children with AIDS. In many parts of the country, infants and young children with AIDS are spending much or all of their lives in hospitals. The HCW becomes the child's mother, father, brother, or sister. Such attachments are normal, but they take a toll on the HCW.

Blacks

The AIDS epidemic poses a unique set of biomedical, educational, public health, and social challenges to black communities already under siege from a variety of social and medical problems. The disease has changed American society and culture by influencing public policy and by reinforcing stigmas and tolerating discrimination against people affected by the disease. It has provoked new tensions about sexual mores, about individual versus public rights, and about medical treatment for persons with HIV infection or symptomatic AIDS.

Although statistics and epidemiological data predict an epidemic with far-reaching consequences for all segments of society, AIDS is exacting a much higher toll on the black community than on other segments. The black community has been historically underserved medically, economically, and educationally. AIDS is devastating a community whose members have experienced chronic unemployment, inadequate income, and inferior educational experiences. It further complicates and jeopardizes the quality of life for people who have always been poorly served by health and social programs.

Although AIDS is often discussed in terms of its effect on the black community as a whole, it is imperative to recognize that blacks come from a variety of cultural backgrounds, including American, Carribean, and Africa. Each nationality within the broader ethnic group displays differences in community structure, language, religion, and cultural values. There are also many socioeconomic classes within the black community. These differences explain the differences HCWs observe among blacks in behavior, attitude, and thinking related to AIDS.

"The Haitian community, for example, illustrates the effect of AIDS on a specific group within the black population," states Honey.[41] "Because at one time they were labeled a risk group, Haitians have experienced a great deal of ostracism by the general public. Individuals have reported losing their jobs solely because they were Haitian."

The AIDS epidemic poses significant challenges to medical, public, and allied health professionals who work within black communities. These challenges include:

1. Identifying specific factors critical to fostering understanding and changing behavior
2. Developing effective and appropriate culturally sensitive prevention strategies
3. Using the community organization approach to build local coalitions and forums to set priorities and address health problems associated with AIDS

The AIDS epidemic challenges the black community's ability to address the broader issues raised by this disease in society and to develop strategies for community mobilization. The community must organize to encourage lifestyle modification and behavioral risk reduction for persons at risk for AIDS.

Population at Risk

Although the public continues to perceive AIDS as a white, gay male disease, it is disproportionately affecting blacks.[42] Blacks compose approximately 12% of the United States population; however, 36% of all persons diagnosed with AIDS are black.[43] Blacks and Hispanics accounted for 70% of the cases in heterosexual men, 70% of those in women, and 75% of those in children[44] (Fig. 5–2).

The CDC[45] estimates that the proportion of AIDS cases involving racial and ethnic minorities has remained relatively constant since 1981. The rate or number of reported cases of AIDS among all racial and ethnic backgrounds, however, continues to rise. It is estimated that between 1% and 1.4% of the black population may be infected with the virus, a rate approximately 3 times that of whites. The epidemiologic pattern of viral infection in the black population differs significantly from the pattern in the white population; among blacks, AIDS has made a greater incursion into the heterosexual population.[46]

Bakeman and colleagues[47] describe factors influencing differences in the epidemiology of AIDS among whites and minorities. They compared the cumulative incidence (CI) of AIDS cases (the number of cases per million relevant population reported to the CDC since 1981) between minority and white populations as of April 6, 1987.[48] These data show that AIDS has affected black and Hispanic men disproportionately to white men and to women of all ethnic backgrounds. There were 764 and 730 cases per million adult black and Hispanic men, respectively, but only 291 cases per million adult white men. The CIs among black and Hispanic women, 105 and 73 cases per million, respectively, were substantially lower than the corresponding incidences among men. However, the CI for white women, 8.6 per million, was even lower.[49] The overall CI among black men is thus 2.6 times the CI among white men, and the CI among black women is 12.2 times the CI among white women. The CI among black children under age 12 is 14.1 times the CI among white children in the same age group. Higher CIs among blacks than among whites were found in urban as well as other areas.

Behavioral Risk Factors

Factors that probably put blacks at higher risk for HIV transmission include intravenous drug use involving sharing of needles and drug paraphernalia (leads to

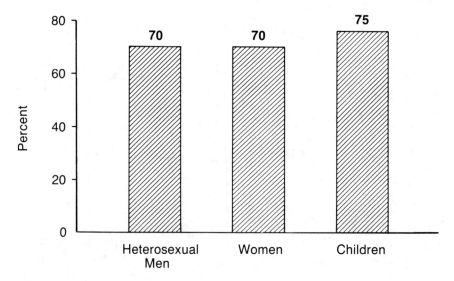

FIGURE 5-2. Proportion of reported AIDS cases contributed by blacks and Hispanics to cases among heterosexual men, women, and children in the United States as of July 1988. (From Centers for Disease Control, *MMWR* 37 (SS-3) July 1988, p 1.)

parenterally acquired infections, as well as to secondary sexual and perinatal transmission);[50] greater likelihood of engaging in high-risk practices, especially among adolescents, because of different perceptions of risk;[51] differing patterns of sexual behavior and social affiliations among black gay and bisexual men compared with white gay men; and engaging in same-sex sexual behaviors and/or drug use while incarcerated and resuming heterosexual involvement upon release.[52]

While gay and bisexual men account for 46.3% of all AIDS cases among blacks (compared with 88.9% among whites), heterosexual IV drug users account for 35.4% (compared with 5.2% among whites).[53] Most researchers acknowledge that intravenous needle sharing and drug use account, either directly or indirectly, for the magnitude of the difference between the incidences of AIDS in minority and white communities. Drug use is a major factor in male–female transmission of the virus; 54% of AIDS cases among blacks are associated with drug abuse. Also, the sexual partner of a non-drug-using black woman with AIDS is often an intravenous drug user[54] (Fig. 5–3). Unfortunately, drug treatment has not been readily available or affordable for black persons who need assistance. In most major cities, waiting lists for treatment programs are long, and no solutions to this problem appear likely in the near future.

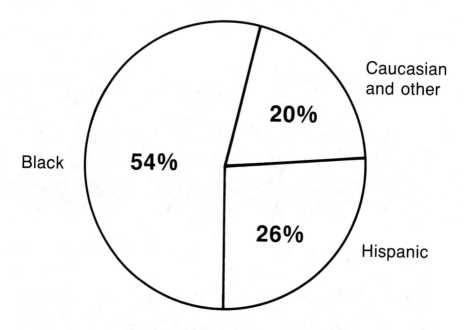

FIGURE 5-3. Proportion of reported AIDS cases among heterosexuals. Contributed by Hispanics and blacks to cases associated with intravenous drug abusers as of July 1988. (From Centers for Disease Control, *MMWR* 37 (SS-3) July 1988, p 2.)

Peterson and Bakeman[55] reviewed several articles about minorities and AIDS and concluded that "the disproportionately high number of AIDS cases within black and Latin communities apparently results from the greater prevalence of IV needle sharing and unsafe sexual practices than it does from some genetic predisposition to become infected with the HIV."

Social Influences

The problem is made more complex by the many social and economic problems within black communities, especially among adolescents and young adults. Gibbs[56] analyzed 6 major social indicators (education, unemployment, delinquency, substance abuse, teenage pregnancy, and suicide) and found that black youths had more problems than white youths in all but 1 of the indicators. Black youths are relatively worse off at the end of the 1980s than they were in 1960.

In 1980, approximately 50% of the total black population was under 24 years of age. The median age for blacks was 25 years, compared to 41 years for whites. As a result, the black population, composed of relatively young persons, is deeply affected by the interrelated factors that reduce the quality of life for black youth, and increase their risk of HIV exposure. Gibbs[57] comments:

> Although there are currently more middle-income black families and more black college students than during any previous period in U.S. history, there are also more blacks on welfare and more severe problems among the majority of black youth who are neither middle class nor college bound.

In 1983, the overall national rate of unemployment was 8.8%, but unemployment among black youth had risen to 48.3%, more than twice the rate among all teenagers (21.6%).

Educational statistics suggest some improvement in test scores in the past decade among black youth. An alarmingly large number of black high school graduates, however, are functionally illiterate or do not possess basic skills necessary for entry-level jobs. Studies by the Urban League and the Population Council[58] show that "black male teenagers leave high school primarily for family economic problems, academic difficulty, or disciplinary problems, while females often dropout due to pregnancy."

Although the number per year of out-of-wedlock births to black teenage mothers has decreased since 1960, black girls and women continue to become pregnant at rates almost twice as high as those of white girls and women. Approximately 59% of black women ages 15–19 have had premarital intercourse, and 45% of those women have had at least 1 premarital pregnancy, with a mean age of 16.6 years at conception.[59] Untimely parenting usually has negative consequences for their educational and career opportunities; they are likely to experience chronic unemployment and inadequate income throughout their lives.

Increasing drug use has created an infrastructure and an underground economy within the black community based on crime and victimization. Drug use and addiction inevitably lead individuals into other activities, such as gang affiliation, prostitution, or dealing drugs, all of which increase their risk of HIV exposure.

In 1980, 27% of the clients admitted to federally funded drug-abuse treatment centers were black, and approximately 12% of these addicts were under age 18. Three out of five persons in this group were addicted to heroin and nearly 50% had been arrested at least once. These statistics graphically illustrate the relationship between drug abuse and delinquency.[60] Black juveniles account for 21% of all juvenile arrests and a higher proportion of the prison population than is warranted, given their numbers in the general population. The statistics clearly show that blacks become involved in the justice system at earlier ages and with greater frequency than do whites.

While in prison, a person may either initiate or continue drug use. Because drug use in prison is an illegal activity conducted in a closed environment, the likelihood of sharing drug paraphernalia and the subsequent risk of HIV transmission are quite high. In addition, prisoners may engage in same-sex sexual activities but upon release not view themselves as either bisexual or gay. It is uncommon for them to recount the experiences that were a part of prison life to their families, intimates, or sexual partners. As a result, the sexual partner of a person who has been incarcerated may be at extremely high risk for HIV exposure.

The sociocultural milieu in many black communities has created an environment in which rapidly increasing numbers of unemployed and unemployable urban youth are socialized to a nonproductive life on the streets.[61] These adolescents and young adults are at high risk for HIV exposure. This problem threatens further to cripple members of a group that is already disadvantaged in several significant social dimensions.

Issues in Patient Care

Mays and Cochran[62] provide an excellent overview of the special psychosocial needs of blacks from 3 perspectives: psychosocial resources (personality, coping resources, support); sociocultural factors (social stigma, external resources); and aspects of medical care (symptoms, patient–physician relationships, treatment decisions).

While the diagnosis of AIDS is a disruptive emotional experience for members of all racial and ethnic groups, Mays and Cochran document that black Americans appear to differ with respect to available coping resources and cultural norms that influence access to health care. Many blacks, especially those from lower socioeconomic groups, have a history of negative experiences with health care systems. Due to financial constraints, access to health care services may be limited to public clinics and hospitals. Treatment at these facilities is often characterized by long waiting periods, impersonal care, and/or staffing patterns involving mostly health care workers from majority cultures.

The dominant influences on health behavior for many blacks are family and friendship networks.[63] The strength and importance of a black person's informal kinship group may heighten the sense of rejection that the diagnosis of AIDS creates. The diagnosis may result in the disclosure of previously hidden, stigmatized behaviors. The sense that tangible emotional and social support has been withdrawn may be more severe for black than for white patients.

Until recently, most support groups and programs for PWAs were sponsored by predominantly white gay organizations, located in white neighborhoods, and staffed primarily by whites. As a result, referrals for blacks from traditional health care systems to AIDS support organizations were generally not heeded. The presence of comprehensive minority AIDS projects has been a significant factor in reducing barriers to support and care. Nonetheless, trends indicate that time of survival after diagnosis is shorter for blacks because treatment is often initiated in advanced stages of the disease. Thus black PWAs frequently need more intensive medical and psychosocial support than white PWAs.

Therapeutic alliances may be difficult to build, however, for the following reasons: perceived or actual cultural barriers in communication; feelings of embarrassment about lack of knowledge or familiarity with medical terminology; or a sense that the HCW is too busy to talk or is not personally interested in the patient. Including family and friends (if the patient approves) is important when dispensing information. Also, creating an atmosphere that encourages open-ended questioning by the patient may assist in the development of a therapeutic relationship.

Intervention Strategies

The design of AIDS intervention strategies to assist blacks has been slow due to a lack of descriptive data on health beliefs, attitudes, and prevention practices on minorities in general, and specifically on blacks. Only recently have federal and state funds been targeted for intervention programs specific to black communities. Given the interrelated nature of drugs, crime, and AIDS within black communities, it is unfortunate that these approaches are still segmented and noncomprehensive.

Recent polls show that blacks are more likely than whites to have misconceptions about the modes of transmission of AIDS.[64,65] These misconceptions cause a high amount of anxiety, which makes effective and constructive community action difficult.

Interventions among black persons at high risk are difficult. Black gay and bisexual men, for instance, are not as visible or well organized a community as the white gay and bisexual community. In addition, many of the persons at risk within poor inner city neighborhoods participate in a "street culture" devoid of strong community ties or organizations. AIDS compaigns that use traditional organized channels of communication, and rely heavily on print media, are generally ineffective with these populations.

The black church, traditionally a focal point for community interventions, has recently turned its attention to AIDS. The church has focused on support of persons with AIDS rather than on prevention or promoting behavior change. Church leaders have chosen this focus because educational and preventive interventions involve openly discussing behaviors that often contradict fundamental religious standards and beliefs.

The magnitude of the AIDS problem within the black community underscores the fact that no easy techniques, quick fixes, or short-term strategies will adequately address the complex social, economic, and health factors that put this population at risk for HIV transmission. Fundamental components of a long-term solution to AIDS within the black community include: culturally relevant education that emphasizes recognizing personal vulnerability and avoiding risk-taking behaviors; coalition building to strengthen cooperation and communication among community and health care workers across disciplinary lines; advocacy and policy development to integrate approaches to health problems and facilitate access to health services; and community development to create a cadre of individuals who are professionally trained and committed to restructuring public policy priorities for AIDS research, health care, and education within a culturally diverse society.

In order to effectively address the AIDS issues within black communities, allied health professionals must be sensitive to the complex web of factors that place blacks at increased risk of contracting AIDS. Workers must seek formal and informal leaders, both professional and nonprofessional, in order to form effective alliances for culturally appropriate interventions. In doing so, they must explore their own values and constrain tendencies to judge their patients' behavior.

Hispanics

There are 18 million Hispanics in the United States. This minority represents 7% of the population, but accounts for 16% of the AIDS cases[66] (Fig. 5–4). By 1992, the National Science Foundation[67] projects that there will be over 365,000 AIDS cases in the United States, 100,000 of which will involve ethnic minorities. As discussed in the previous section, blacks and Hispanics are affected by AIDS disproportionately to their numbers in the population. AIDS may affect minority communities much more in the future. In a study of HIV infection among civilian applicants for the United States military services (1985–1986),[68] prevalence rates among applicants in 5 counties were over 1%. Of the 306,061 applicants tested, the highest antibody incidence (3.89%) was found among non-Hispanic blacks, and the lowest incidence (0.88%) among whites. The incidence among Hispanics was 1.07%, and the incidence among other racial and ethnic groups was 2.42%. These findings suggest that minority communities contain disproportionate numbers of individuals who are infected with the HIV or have AIDS.

Hispanics are concentrated in the largest metropolitan areas, such as New York City, Miami, and Los Angeles, where the highest incidences of AIDS are found.

Yanklovich and Skelly,[69] in a nationwide study of Hispanics in 1984, describe the following characteristics of this population:

a. Hispanics are generally a younger age group than the United States population as a whole.
b. Hispanics place a high value on the family, on children, and on maintaining the high reputation of the family name.
c. Hispanics hold on to the traditional values of their various subcultures and countries of origin. Sixty percent of the Hispanics in the United States are of Mexican or Mexican–American descent; the remaining 40% are Cuban, Puerto Rican, or Central or South American.
d. Approximately three fourths of Hispanics regularly use or prefer to use the Spanish language. Over half would like their children to develop fluency in the "mother tongue."
e. As a people, they depend heavily on the church and the home to transmit cultural, ethical, and moral values.
f. Parents and elders are held in high esteem and respected throughout their lives.

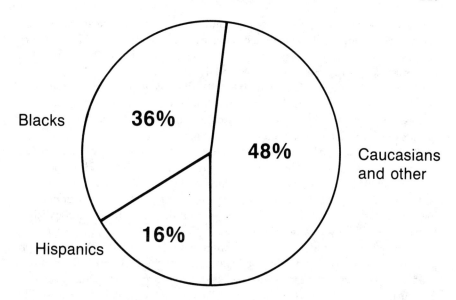

FIGURE 5-4. Proportion of reported AIDS cases among blacks and Hispanics in the United States as of September 1988. *Note:* In September 1987, the AIDS case definition was revised to include a broader spectrum of HIV-associated diseases; this led to an increase in the proportion of reported AIDS cases among blacks and Hispanics. (From Centers for Disease Control.[66])

g. Hispanics depend heavily on certain communication media to obtain information; television and radio are prime sources, print media less useful sources.

h. Hispanics are generally a proud people who work hard to provide a better life in this country for future generations.

i. Hispanics are usually resourceful and take pride in "taking care of their own" within the context of the family and community. In times of crisis, they seem to show their best attributes—compassion, caring, and unequaled devotion to anyone in "la familia," which includes members of the extended family.

These factors affect how the Hispanic community reacts to the AIDS epidemic.

Factors that Affect AIDS Among Hispanics

AIDS ("SIDA" in Spanish) is perceived differently by Hispanics. Many Hispanics still feel it is a white gay male disease that will not affect them.[70] Their communities are 3–5 years behind the white community in terms of information. Most do not realize the inroads the epidemic has made in their community. Few Hispanics who habitually engage in high-risk practices have made the behavioral changes necessary to halt the transmission of the HIV.

Hispanics have difficulty identifying AIDS as a potential risk to themselves or their families. There is considerable denial, apathy, and embarrassment about addressing AIDS in the Hispanic community, apparently reflecting the belief, "This cannot touch me, since I am neither Anglo nor gay."

Cultural factors such as religion, education, socioeconomic conditions, social customs, norms, beliefs, and values all play significant roles in the Hispanic community's reluctance to practice risk reduction and preventive behaviors. It is difficult to discuss AIDS openly with most Hispanics because of taboos about discussing sexual subjects, and because of their societal disapproval of homosexuality. Denial of bisexuality is widespread.

Many Hispanics find it difficult to comprehend diseases with long incubation periods. The concept that a behavior engaged in tonight might place them at risk 5–15 years later, as is the case with AIDS, is difficult to grasp. Hispanics also tend to wait until the disease is far progressed before seeking medical services. The average life span for a white man after AIDS is diagnosed is 2 years, but for Hispanic men it is 6 months.

Often language, fear, and economics present barriers to obtaining health care. Hispanics often do not trust health care providers or feel they can be frank and open with them about their sexual orientation or behaviors. They do not expect workers to provide them with risk-reduction information without being judgmental.

Within the Hispanic community, there is considerable reluctance on the part of community leaders to be associated with the AIDS issue. Hispanic physicians have essentially been quiet thus far; only a few have become spokespersons or advocates for Hispanics with AIDS.

Suggested Approaches to AIDS in the Hispanic Community

Professionals and others working with the AIDS issue among Hispanics must be motivated solely by a desire to save lives and reduce the number of potentially infected individuals. HCWs should review their own motives and values before embarking on an educational or treatment program.

AIDS prevention information must be provided in simple terms within culturally relevant parameters. The message must be clear and concise and communicated by credible health professionals in order to raise the level of perceived susceptibility among persons who engage in high-risk behaviors.

Hispanics are most effectively reached in community settings, such as churches, schools, and work sites, rather than at special forums or community conferences on AIDS. They may refrain from attending such conferences because of the inferences others may draw from their being seen in attendance.

There should be no further alienation or stigmatization of Hispanics because of AIDS. Speak of high-risk *behaviors,* not high-risk *groups.* Engaging in specific behaviors can put anyone at risk. Counsel persons who are sexual partners or clients with AIDS about their risks. Families of PWAs can become powerful educators within the Hispanic community.

Generally, Hispanics prefer that families provide home care for AIDS patients, reflecting their "care for our own" philosophy. Increased support is needed within the Hispanic community for families who are caring for AIDS patients at home. Encourage community action to provide hospice care, respite care, and home are assistance; these services are often difficult for Hispanics to obtain in white communities.

Information provided to the Hispanic community should be culturally relevant and in the Spanish language. Bilingual "hot lines" should be established. Whenever possible, Hispanics should be employed to provide education, information, and services.

It is very important that service providers and health educators acquire as much knowledge about and acquaintance with the Hispanic community as possible. Any group or individuals seeking to serve the Hispanic community should request consultation with experienced professionals. Organizations that offer information and technical assistance are listed in the Appendices.

Asians, Pacific Islanders, and Native Americans

The incidence of AIDS among Asians and Pacific Islanders, according to a 1988 study in San Francisco, is significantly lower than the incidences among whites (Relative Risk [RR] = 0.05), blacks (RR = 0.16), Latinos (RR = 0.14), and Native Americans (RR = 0.42).[71] In San Francisco, the number of AIDS cases among Asians and Pacific Islanders has increased 176% since 1985 (compared with 41% among whites, 114% among blacks, and 70% among Latinos). Asians and Pacific Islanders with AIDS are more likely to be transfusion recipients (RR = 10.1) than are AIDS patients from other racial and ethnic groups. Each of these ethnic communities is seeking culturally sensitive ways of educating and treating PWAs.

A FRAMEWORK FOR INTERVENTION

Pincus and Minahan[72] define intervention skills as "those techniques used by the worker to influence and effect change in action and target systems on behalf of client system."

Systems Theory

General systems theory provides a good model for intervention because it considers all aspects of a person's situation. For example, when working with a PWA who expresses fear of dying, according to this theory you should consider not just the patient's fear, but also his or her environmental deficiencies, disabilities, living arrangements, and ethnicity. A practitioner of general systems theory considers the total patient and works toward satisfying the patient's total needs.

According to McPheeters and Ryan,[73] general systems theory is practiced by

> *the person who plays whatever roles and does whatever activities are necessary for the person or family when the person or family needs them. His concern is the person in need, not specific tasks or techniques or professional prerogatives. He is an aide to individual or family, not an aide to an agency or to a profession.*

Figure 5–5 presents the basic framework of social welfare and human service problem areas, and explains the significance of viewing the patient in the context of his or her environment. The framework includes 3 important elements: domains of living, status of functioning, and obstacles to functioning. By understanding these elements and how they impact on each other, HCWs will be better able to care for the wide range of problems experienced by the PWAs they encounter.

In this framework, no one type of HCW has more power or responsibility than any other in caring for the patient. The system allows each team member to use his or her skills and abilities to the greatest extent possible, and provides for maximum utilization of the team's energy. It also provides the highest quality of care to PWAs and their families.

Klenk and Ryan[74] state 12 objectives and goals that can be used by HCWs: detection, linkage, advocacy, mobilization, evaluation, instruction, behavior change, consultation, community planning, information processing, administration, and providing continuing care.

Detection involves identifying the patient experiencing difficulty or crisis and identifying issues contributing to the problem. The goal is to reduce or alleviate the problem or crisis. For example, if it appears that the patient does not understand the information you have provided and if you have determined that the patient understands Spanish better than English, numerous problems will be alleviated by speaking in Spanish.

Linkage involves steering the person toward existing services from which he or she can benefit. The goal is to provide him or her with any support service that can improve the quality of life. Reaching this objective can also reduce the stress on the HCW. Linkage might involve contacting an AIDS project that provides support and concrete services to patients, such as arranging transportation to outpatient treatments.

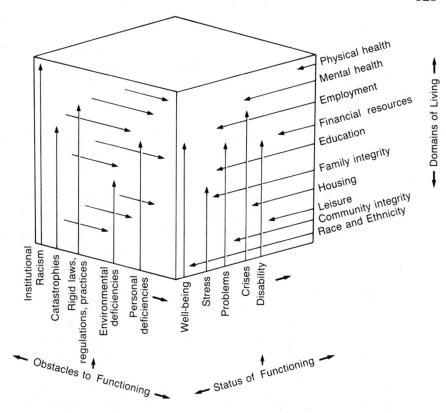

FIGURE 5-5. Basic framework of social welfare human services problem areas. (From Klenk, RW and Ryan, RM,[74] with permission.)

Advocacy involves attempting to gain rights and services for PWAs, with the goal of removing barriers and developing services. For instance, a physical therapist who confronted a durable equipment provider who refused to provide specially needed supplies for a PWA was practicing advocacy. (The patient subsequently received the supplies.)

Evaluation involves gathering information on patients' needs and on the availability and effectiveness of present services. It also includes determining priorities for needs and services. The goal is to ensure both quantity and quality of services for PWAs. For instance, the California Nurses Association evaluated the knowledge of nurses practicing in California and discovered gaps. As a result of this evaluation, the association now provides a 2-day conference teaching nurses about AIDS, so that nurses can promote AIDS awareness among their coworkers.

Mobilization brings together existing groups, institutions, and resources to collectively fight the battle against AIDS. The purpose of mobilization is to maximize the effectiveness of existing services. A group of women in San Francisco effectively mobilized to serve women with AIDS. They convinced a group of agencies traditionally serving women that women with AIDS needed the specialized care they could—and subsequently did—provide.

Instruction involves conveying information and knowledge about the prevention and treatment of HIV infection. The goals are to relieve fears, provide support, and to stop the spread of this devastating virus. The dean of a southern California school for allied health professionals mandated AIDS education for all students was acting with these goals in mind.

Promoting *behavior change* includes attempting to change patterns, habits, and perceptions. The purpose is to alleviate or moderate behaviors that negatively affect patients' health. When mental health counselors work with a PWA to help him or her develop coping skills to replace intravenous drug use, they are promoting behavior change.

Consultation involves assisting patients, other HCWs, and agencies to increase their skills. A neuropsychiatrist may consult with a patient care team to help identify symptoms and signs that signal HIV infection of the brain.

Community planning helps to ensure that human service needs of the community and patients are met. The goal is to assist the community with service development. A social worker may initiate an AIDS project in the community before the needs and numbers of PWAs become overwhelming.

Information processing is particularly important in the AIDS epidemic. Its purpose is to keep HCWs updated on the latest developments in the field of AIDS. Another purpose is to keep the lines of communication open. There are a number of systems available for processing AIDS information; one of the more common is the Computerized AIDS Information Network (CAIN).

The purpose of *administration* is to provide leadership and direction to agencies, institutions, or programs servicing PWAs. Directors of AIDS projects or AIDS clinics are examples of persons pursuing this objective.

The final objective is providing *continuing care*. Caring for patients in the hospital is not sufficient; HCWs must also provide for care when the patient is discharged or released to another agency. The purpose of continuing care is to provide continuity and an ongoing support system for the patient.

Caring for PWAs is like fighting a war, and it is by no means an easy endeavor. But it is a war that can be won by people working together in scientific research, in health care institutions and agencies, and in the community.

An AIDS pamphlet published by the National Association of Social Workers[75] said it well:

> *The foundation of civilization rests in part upon our ability to care for others, who are part of our collective self. Failing to understand the needs of others and to provide what is required to meet those needs diminishes our claim to be a civilized people.*

DISCUSSION QUESTIONS

1. Why is an interdisciplinary health care team the best approach to providing care to PWAs?
2. How can a community best respond to the needs of special groups such as blacks? Hispanics? Women with AIDS? Children with AIDS?
3. Why does the general systems approach offer a good framework for dealing with the AIDS epidemic?
4. Should the development of community services for PWAs be the sole responsibility of tax-supported agencies?
5. What advocacy steps can allied health professionals take to assist PWAs?
6. What recommendations would you make to your professional organization about its responsibility to PWAs?

REFERENCES

1. Koop, CE: The surgeon general's report on acquired immune deficiency syndrome. The Los Angeles Times, December 7, 1987.
2. Freed E: AIDSophobia. Medical Journal of Australia 2:479, 1983.
3. Update: Universal precautions for prevention of transmission of human immunodeficiency virus, hepatitis B virus, and other blood-borne pathogens in health care settings. MMWR 37:377, June 24, 1988.
4. Hidalgo, H, Peterson, TL, and Woodman NJ (eds): Lesbian and Gay Issues: A Resource Manual for Social Workers. National Association of Social Workers, Silver Spring, MD, 1985, p 2.
5. Moses, AE and Hawkins, RO: Inservice training session on homophobia. In Hidalgo, H, Peterson, TL, and Woodman NJ (eds): Lesbian and gay Issues: A Resource Manual for Social Workers. National Association of Social Workers, Silver Spring, MD, 1985, p 156.
6. Macks, J: Women and AIDS: Counter-transference issues. Social Casework: The Journal of Contemporary Social Work, June 1988: 340, 1988.
7. Leukefeld, CG and Fimbres M (eds): Responding to AIDS: Psychosocial Initiatives. National Association of Social Workers, Silver Spring, MD, 1987, p xii.
8. Miller, D: Psychology, AIDS, ARC and PGL. In Miller, D, Weber, J, and Green J (eds): The Management of AIDS Patients. Macmillan, New York, 1986.
9. Reece, R: Expression of sexuality. In Moffat, BC, et al: AIDS: A Self-Care Manual. AIDS Project Los Angeles. IBS Press, Santa Monica, CA, 1987.
10. Gochros, HL: Risk of abstinence: Sexual decision making in the AIDS era. Social Work 33:254, 1988.
11. Gochros, HL: Ibid.
12. Miller, D: Ibid.
13. Macks, J: Ibid.
14. Kubler-Ross, E: On Death and Dying. Macmillan, New York, 1969.

15. Kubler-Ross, E: Ibid.

16. MR: Personal communication, 1985.

17. Moffatt, BC, et al: AIDS: A Self-Care Manual. AIDS Project Los Angeles. IBS Press, Santa Monica, CA, 1987.

18. CA: Personal communication, March, 1986.

19. Woodman, NJ and Lenna, HR: Counseling with Gay Men and Women. Jossey-Bass, San Francisco, 1980, p 11.

20. San Francisco AIDS Foundation: Women and AIDS, ed 2. Autumn Press, 1986.

21. Kaplan, S and Saperstein, S: Lesbian and Gay Adolescents. In Hidalgo, H, Peterson TL, and Woodman, NJ (eds): Lesbian and Gay Issues: A Resource Manual for Social Workers. National Association of Social Workers, Silver Spring, MD, 1985.

22. Woodman, NJ and Lenna, HR: Ibid.

23. Conor-Ryan, C: Gay issues: Oppression is a health hazard. In Hidalgo, H, Peterson, TL, and Woodman, NJ (eds): Lesbian and Gay Issues: A Resource Manual for Social Workers. National Association of Social Workers, Silver Spring, MD, 1985, p 64.

24. Hidalgo, H, Peterson, TL, and Woodman, NJ (eds): Ibid.

25. Auerback, S and Moser, C: Groups for the wives of gay and bisexual men. Social Work 32:312, 1987.

26. Brown, RK: AIDS, Cancer and the Medical Establishment. Robert Speller, New York, 1986.

27. Moynihan, RT and Christ, GH: Social, psychological and research barriers to the treatment of AIDS. In Leukefeld, CG and Fimbres, M (eds). Responding to AIDS: Psychosocial Initiatives. National Association of Social Workers, Silver Spring, MD, 1987, p 90.

28. Green, J: Reduction of risk in high-risk groups. In Miller, D, Weber, J, and Green, J (eds): The Management of AIDS Patients. Macmillan, New York, 1986.

29. Cancellieri, FR et al: Psychological reactions to human immunodeficiency virus infection in drug using pregnant women. In Schinazi, RF, and Nahmias, AJ (eds): AIDS in Children, Adolescents and Heterosexual Adults: An Interdisciplinary Approach to Prevention. Elsevier, New York, 1988.

30. Faltz, BG and Madover, S: Substance abuse as a cofactor for AIDS. In McKusick, L (ed): What to Do About AIDS: Physicians and Mental Health Professionals Discuss the Issues. University of California Press, Berkeley, CA, 1986.

31. Cancellieri, FR: Ibid.

32. Kernoff, PBA and Miller, RR: AIDS-related problems in the management of hemophilia. In Miller, D, Weber, J, and Green J (eds): The Management of AIDS Patients. Macmillan, New York, 1986, p 81.

33. Dietrich, SL: Medical impact of AIDS on hemophilia. In Moffat, BC, et al: AIDS: A Self-Care Manual. AIDS Project Los Angeles. IBS Press, Santa Monica, CA, 1987.

34. Shaw, N and Paleo, L: Women and AIDS: Risks and Concerns. In McKusick, L (ed): What to Do About AIDS: Physicians and Mental Health Professionals Discuss the Issues. University of California Press, Berkeley, CA, 1986.

35. Stroller-Shaw, N: Women and AIDS: Risks and Concerns. In Moffat, BC et al (eds): AIDS: A Self-Care Manual. AIDS Project Los Angeles. IBS Press, Santa Monica, CA, 1987.

36. Shaw, N and Paleo, L: Ibid.

37. Centers for Disease Control: Recommendations for assisting in the prevention of perinatal transmission of human T-lymphotropic virus type III/lymphadenopathy-associated virus and acquired immunodeficiency syndrome. MMWR 34:721, 1985.

38. Macks, J: Ibid.
39. Stroller-Shaw, N: Ibid.
40. Scott, GB: Management of HIV infection in children. In Schinaz, RF and Nahmias, AJ (eds): AIDS in Children, Adolescents and Heterosexual Adults: An Interdisciplinary Approach to Prevention. Elsevier, New York, 1988.
41. Honey, E: AIDS and the inner city: Critical issues. Social Casework: The Journal of Contemporary Social Work 365, June 1988.
42. Houston-Hamilton, A: A constant increase: AIDS in ethnic communities. Focus: A Review of AIDS Research 1:1, 1986.
43. Center for Disease Control: Trends in reported cases of AIDS. MMWR 37(36):552, 1988.
44. Selik, RM and Pappaioanou, M: Distribution of AIDS cases by racial/ethnic group and exposure category. MMWR 37(SS-3):1–10, July 1988.
45. Centers for Disease Control: Acquired immunodeficiency syndrome (AIDS) among Blacks and Hispanics: United States. MMWR 35:655, 1986.
46. Mays, VM and Cochran, SD: Acquired immunodeficiency syndrome and Black Americans: Special psychosocial issues. Public Health Rep 102:224, 1987.
47. Bakeman, R., et al: Ibid.
48. Mays, VM and Cochran, SD: Ibid.
49. Bakeman, R, et al: Ibid, pp 922, 923.
50. Hopkins, DR: AIDS in minority populations in the United States. Public Health Rep 102:677, 1987.
51. DiClemente, RJ, Boyer, CB, and Morales, ES: Minorities and AIDS: Knowledge, attitudes, and misconceptions among Black and Latino adolescents. Am J Public Health 78:55, 1988.
52. Mays, VM and Cochran, SD: Ibid.
53. Mays, VM and Cochran, SD: Ibid.
54. Bakeman, R, et al: Ibid.
55. Peterson, J and Bakeman, R: The epidemiology of adult minority AIDS. Multicultural Inquiry and Research on AIDS 2:1, 1988.
56. Gibbs, JT: Black adolescents and youth: An endangered species. Am J Orthopsychiatry 54:6, 1984.
57. Gibbs, JT: Ibid, p 7.
58. Gibbs, JT: Ibid, p 7.
59. Dawson, DA: The effects of sex education on adolescent behavior. Fam Plan Perspect 18:162, 1986.
60. Gibbs, JT: Ibid.
61. Gibbs, JT: Ibid.
62. Mays, VM and Cochran, SD: Ibid.
63. Neighbors, HW and Jackson JS: The use of informal and formal help: Four patterns of illness behavior in the Black community. Am J Community Psychol 12:629, 1984.
64. Hopkins, DR: Ibid.
65. DiClemente, RJ: Ibid.
66. Centers for Disease Control: Trends in reported cases of AIDS. MMWR 37(36):552, 1988.
67. Institute of Medicine, National Academy of Science: Confronting AIDS: Directions for Public Health, Health Care and Research. National Academy Press, Washington, DC, 1986, p 8.

68. Centers for Disease Control: HTLV-III/LAV antibody prevalence in U.S. military recruit applicants. MMWR, July 4, 1986, p 421.
69. Yankelovich, Skelly, White: A Study of the USA Hispanic Market: Spanish USA. New York Life—AIDS Communications Study, November 17, 1987. Yankelovich, Skelly & White, Washington, DC, 1987.
71. Woo, JM, et al: AIDS Among Asian and Pacific Islander Populations in San Francisco. Paper presented at American Public Health Association, Boston, November, 1988.
72. Pincus, A and Minahan, A: Toward a model for teaching a basic first-year course in methods of social work practice. In Gilbert, N and Specht, H (eds): The Emergence of Social Welfare and Social Work. FE Peacock Publishers, Itasca, IL, 1978, p 448.
73. McPheeters, HL and Ryan, RM: A Core of Competence of Baccalaureate Social Welfare and Curricula Implications. Southern Regional Education Board, Atlanta, 1971, p 22.
74. Klenk, RW and Ryan, RM (eds): The practice of social work, ed 2. Wadsworth Publishing Co, Belmont, MA, 1974.
75. National Association of Social Workers: AIDS: We Need to Know, We Need to Care. National Association of Social Workers, Silver Spring, MD, 1988, p 1.

SIX

NEUROPSYCHIATRIC ASPECTS OF AIDS AND HIV INFECTION

Marianne Hart

OUTLINE

OBJECTIVES

By the close of this chapter, the reader will be able to:
  1. Recognize the neuropsychiatric aspects of HIV infection.

2. Cite examples of central nervous system and peripheral nervous system disorders associated with HIV infection.
3. Cite common neuropsychiatric side-effects of drugs used in treatment of AIDS and opportunistic infections.
4. List the symptoms of AIDS dementia complex.
5. Describe interventions for AIDS dementia complex that your profession might use.
6. Name ways you might intervene to prevent the suicide of an HIV-infected patient.
7. Cite categories of psychiatric diagnosis associated with HIV infection.
8. List and describe potential effects of HIV infection on the peripheral nervous system.
9. Differentiate between types of central nervous system involvement in children with AIDS.
10. Summarize interventions health care workers can employ with HIV-infected persons to improve their psychosocial environment.

The neuropsychiatric aspects of AIDS represent one of the more complex issues developing around infection by the human immunodeficiency virus (HIV). Weber and Pinching[1] point out that "the central nervous system is the third major organ system to be infected by opportunistic pathogens or tumours in AIDS." For health care workers (HCWs) to provide optimum and comprehensive care for the HIV-infected patients, they must be well informed about the neuropsychiatric aspects of HIV infection. HCWs should be able to differentiate between persons having reactionary depression when told they have AIDS and persons experiencing depression resulting from AIDS dementia complex (ADC), because the treatments and interventions for these conditions differ.

For example, after Mary learned she had AIDS, she became depressed. She experienced reactionary depression in response to an external situation, the diagnosis of AIDS. The depression was *psychological,* not physiological. Mary was effectively treated with counseling and the assistance of a support group for persons with AIDS (PWAs). In contrast, Raymond had a mild case of ADC, and suffered depression as a result. His depression was *physiological.* The primary intervention in Raymond's case was to treat the AIDS virus and the resulting dementia. He was placed on a regimen of zidovudine (azidothymidine, or AZT, an antiviral agent) and amitriptyline (Elavil, an antidepressant) and received counseling to assist him in problem solving. With this treatment, his symptoms were alleviated. Counseling alone would not have affected Raymond's depression because its etiology was physiological.

Reported clinical experiences and neuropathologic data indicate that neurologic complications occur in most HIV-infected persons.[2-6] Clinical studies show that approximately 40% of AIDS patients develop clinical neurologic syndrome.[7,8]

Autopsy studies show that at least 70% of AIDS patients have central nervous system (CNS) disease at the time of death.[9,10] Approximately 10% of persons in the studies developed a neurologic syndrome as the first manifestation of HIV infection before developing symptomatic AIDS.[11] Research indicates that manifestation of CNS involvement can occur up to 12 months before symptomatic AIDS develops.

It has been documented that the HIV may reach the brain. The receptors on brain cells are identical to those found on the lymphocytes infected by the HIV[12-15] (see Chapter 2). As result, the HIV must be considered as much an infection of the nervous sytem as of the immune system.[16]

Within the Centers for Disease Control (CDC) modified classification for HIV infection, subgroup IV-B is neurologic disease caused by direct HIV infection of the CNS. In subgroup IV-B there are 2 categories:

Central Nervous System Disorders:
  Dementia
  Acute atypical meningitis (occurring after initial infections)
  Myelopathy
Peripheral Nervous System Disorders:
  Painful sensory neuropathy
  Inflammatory demyelinating polyneuropathy

Subgroups IV-C and IV-D include secondary infections and cancers that cause CNS complications.[17] The CDC has not been more precise in defining HIV-related CNS disease; the nomenclature is still evolving in this area.

CENTRAL NERVOUS SYSTEM COMPLICATIONS IN ADULTS

The most common HIV complication affecting the brain is ADC. ADC is followed by a number of other HIV complications. These are listed in Table 6–1, ranging from the most common to the most rare. Some of the less common viral, bacterial, fungal, protozoal, and helminthic infections of the CNS associated with HIV infection are listed in Table 6–2.

HIV-infected persons may suffer a wide variety of CNS complications. HCWs encounter many of these conditions in non-HIV-infected persons. The picture is not the same, however, for a HIV-infected patient with one of these diagnoses. In the past, rehabilitation professionals have not always treated AIDS patients because referrals were not always made and therapists were not always on the care team for a HIV-infected patient. As the number of cases of HIV-related CNS disease grows, however, multiple therapies, treatment modalities, and creative interventions by therapists will be needed.

TABLE 6–1. **HIV Complications of the Central Nervous System**

Brain
  Most common
    AIDS dementia complex (ADC)
  Common
    Cerebral toxoplasmosis
    Cytomegalovirus (CMV) encephalitis
    Primary CNS lymphoma
  Uncommon
    Progressive multifocal leukoencephalopathy (PML)
    Varicella-zoster virus (VZV) encephalitis and vasculitis
    Fungal abscesses: candidal and cryptococcal
  Rare
    Herpes simplex virus (HSV) encephalitis
    Tuberculosis *(Mycobacterium tuberculosis)*
    Kaposi's sarcoma (KS)
Leptomeninges
  Common
    Aseptic meningitis
    Cryptococcal meningitis
  Uncommon
    Lymphomatous meningitis
    Tuberculous meningitis
Spinal Cord
  Common
    Vacuolar myelopathy
  Uncommon
    Viral myelitis: VZV, HSV, and CMV
Peripheral Nerve and Root
  Common
    Distal, predominantly sensory polyneuropathy
  Uncommon
    Mononeuritis multiplex
    Demyelinating motor polyneuropathy (Guillain-Barré Syndrome [GBS])
    CMV polyradiculopathy
    Segmental herpes zoster

From Navia, BA, Jordan, BD, and Price, RW: Central nervous system complications of immunosuppression. In Parrillo, JE and Masur, H (eds): The critically ill immunosuppressed patient. Aspen, Rockville, MD, 1987. Used by permission.

Treatment

Many of the neuropsychiatric and secondary CNS diseases in HIV-infected patients are treatable (Table 6–3). In evaluating drug-related neurotoxicities, it is important to know the neuropsychiatric side-effects of drugs used to treat the

TABLE 6–2. Less Common HIV Infections of the Central Nervous System

Viral
    Measles virus
    Enteroviruses
Bacterial
    Monocytogenes
    Nocardia asteroides
    Gram-negative bacilli
    Mycobacterium tuberculosis
Fungal
    Cryptococcosis
    Aspergillosis
    Candidiasis
    Mucomycosis
Protozoal and Helminthic
    Toxoplasma gondii
    Strongyloides stercoralis

From Navia, BA, Jordan, BD, and Price, RW: Central nervous system complications of immunosuppression. In Parrillo, JE, and Masur, H (eds): The critically ill immunosuppressed patient. Aspen, Rockville, MD, 1987, p 122, with permission.

TABLE 6–3. Treatable Infections of the Central Nervous System

Infection
    Toxoplasmosis
    Cryptococcosis
    Herpes encephalitis
    Progressive multifocal leukoencephalopathy (Papillomavirus)
    Mycobacterium tuberculosis (disseminated tuberculosis)
    Atypical mycobacterial infection
Cancer
    Primary brain lymphoma
    Burkitt's lymphoma
    Disseminated Kaposi's sarcoma
    Other sarcomas
Other Causes
    Drug-related neurotoxicities
    Nutritional deficiencies
    Depression
    Psychosis

From Ostrow, D, Grant, I, Atkinson, H: Assessment and management of AIDS patients with neuropsychiatric disturbances. J of Clin Psych 5:14, 1988, with permission.

various HIV-related opportunistic diseases. The side-effects of AZT are headache, restlessness, severe agitation, and insomnia. Vincristine may produce hallucinations, headache, ataxia, and sensory loss. Acyclovir can cause visual hallucinations, depersonalization, tearfulness, confusion, hyperesthesia, hyperacusia, thought insertion, and insomnia. Isoniazid may produce depression, agitation, hallucinations, paranoia, and impaired memory. Procarbazine can cause mania, loss of appetite, insomnia, nightmares, confusion, and malaise. The side-effects of amphotericin include delirium, peripheral neuropathy, diplopia, weight loss, and loss of appetite.

AIDS DEMENTIA COMPLEX

The term *AIDS dementia complex* was adopted by Navia and colleagues[18] in 1986. The term evolved as their research indicated dementia was a frequent complication of AIDS. Encephalitis and subacute encephalitis did not include the full range of AIDS-related neurologic complications they observed, namely progressive cognitive impairment with accompanying motor and behavioral disturbances.

Pathophysiology

ADC appears to be a subcortical dementia. Navia and colleagues[19] autopsy studies revealed abnormalities primarily in the subcortical structures. Certain manifestations are unique to ADC. The areas of disturbance are attention, intelligence, language, memory, visuospatial skills, reasoning, motor abilities, and personality.[20]

In a study of 70 patients, Navia and colleagues[21] report that 66% of the patients' clinical records indicated some unexplained cognitive or behavior change before their deaths. Autopsies revealed subcortical dementia in two thirds of the patients. Of the 46 patients in the sample with ADC, AIDS was diagnosed before dementia in 29 cases; for 6 patients, AIDS and dementia diagnoses were established concurrently. In 11 patients, the dementia manifested before AIDS was diagnosed; in 4 of the 11, dementia was the only clinical sign of AIDS. The temporal profile shows an insidious onset and progression, from a few weeks to months, in 30 of the patients. In 19 of the 30 patients there was an abrupt acceleration of the dementia. In 16 of the patients, onset was acute or subacute, occurring in a matter of days.

Signs and Symptoms

Navia and colleagues[22] recorded early as well as late signs and symptoms of ADC. Early symptoms of ADC involved impairment of cognitive, motor, and behavioral function (Table 6–4). Twenty-nine patients had cognitive symptoms in the

TABLE 6–4. **Early Signs of AIDS Dementia Complex in 44 Patients***

Symptoms	Number of Patients Affected
Cognitive	29
Forgetfulness	17
Loss of concentration	11
Confusion	10
Slowness of thought	8
Motor	20
Loss of balance	15
Leg weakness	9
Deterioration in handwriting	6
Behavioral	17
Apathy, social withdrawal	16
Dysphoric mood	5
Organic psychosis	2
Regressed behavior	1
Other	
Headache	6
Seizures	3

*It was possible to accurately characterize the early features of the illness in 44 of the 46 patients; the other 2 patients were seen late in the course of their illness.

From Navia, BA, et al: The AIDS dementia complex: I. Clinical Features. An Neurol 19:520, 1986, with permission.

early stages of ADC. Characteristic complaints included difficulty remembering recent events, difficulty maintaining attention to conversations, and difficulty with writing and language. These patients also reported losing their train of thought in midstream. It took them a longer time and increased effort to organize their thoughts, complete tasks, and respond to questions.

Motor symptoms were a problem for 20 of the 44 patients in Navia's study. In 12 patients, motor symptoms were the predominant complaint; 6 suffered progressive loss of balance or leg weakness 1–6 months before developing cognitive difficulty. Behavioral symptoms were found in 17 of the 44 patients. In 10 of the patients, behavioral changes were the sole initial complaint. Patients with organic psychosis first developed agitated psychosis and visual hallucination. Six patients had bilateral chronic headaches and 3 had generalized seizures. Four patients had transient episodes of speech disturbance, which was the initial presenting symptom for 3 patients; the fourth patient had a recurrence after the first episode. Figure 6–1 presents the results reported by Navia and colleagues[23] of routine bedside mental status testing of the 44 patients with ADC. Major findings during

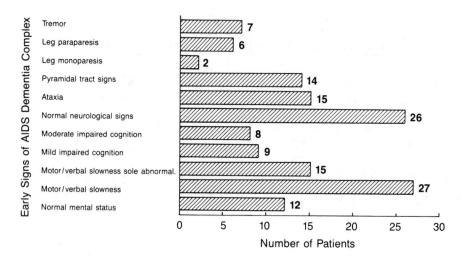

FIGURE 6-1. Early signs of AIDS dementia complex in 44 patients. It was possible to accurately characterize the early features of the illness in 44 of the 46 patients; the other 2 were only seen late in their course. (Adapted from Navia et al.[18])

the late stage of ADC as reported by Navia and colleagues[24] are shown in Figure 6–2.

Navia and colleagues also noted significant associated neurologic findings. Of the original 70 patients, none of the 24 nondemented patients had signs of peripheral neuropathy; 22 of the 46 demented patients did. Burning, painful paresthesias, and/or numbness were the most typical symptoms. Lower and upper motor neuron dysfunction signs coexisted. Of the 46 demented patients, 14 had retinopathy involving cotton-wool spots as first described by Newman and colleagues[25] as their only symptom.

Interventions

HCWs should provide environmental aids, assist the patent in structuring his or her activities of daily living, educate caregivers, secure assistance in estate planning, and refer the patient for psychotherapy assessment and treatment if the patient is depressed. Table 6–5 presents the practical considerations and recommendations for persons with ADC.

Caregiving

Patients with ADC need structure to limit their level of confusion and to ensure maximum independence in activities of daily living. An occupational therapist

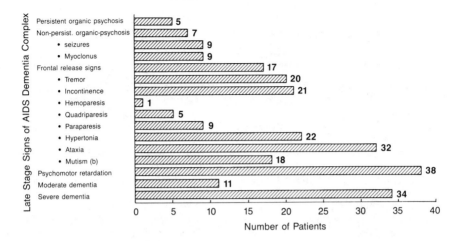

FIGURE 6-2. Late stage signs of AIDS dementia complex in 45 patients. One patient in this series succumbed to systemic illness shortly after early dementia was recognized. (b) = Mutism consisted of either no verbal output or only occasional 1- or 2-word expression. (Adapted from Navia et al.[18])

can be a significant resource in this area. It may be helpful to map out daily activities and place a written record in the patient's bedroom. Patients' days are often difficult to schedule because of the number of medical, therapeutic, and diagnostic appointments and services they need. Many patients are motivated to perform certain activities but lack the mental ability. In such cases, the HCW should direct the patient or help him or her begin a task, such as tooth brushing.

HCWs should educate caregivers about what to expect and how to handle various patient care issues that arise. They should explain early symptoms such as forgetfulness, and help caregivers plan ways of coping, such as reminding the patient of important appointments. Workers should constantly monitor depression, because it can signal other symptoms to come, such as suicide ideation.

Monitoring for Suicide Risk

Marzuk and colleagues[26] have provided the first epidemiologic documentation of a connection between AIDS and increased risk of suicide. This report from Cornell University Medical College and the Office of the Chief Medical Examiner of New York City states that the rate of suicide in 1985 among New York City residents with AIDS was 66 times higher than that of the general population of New York residents in the same age group. Men 20–59 years of age with AIDS were 36 times more likely to commit suicide than their counterparts in the general population of New York City.

TABLE 6–5. **Practical Considerations and Recommendations for Persons with AIDS-Related Dementia Complex**

Forgetfulness

1. Use calendars and appointment books.
2. Place Post-It notes in conspicuous places.
3. Make lists (questions for your physician, groceries, etc.).
4. Develop list for important things to check when leaving the house (gas, stove, lights, etc.).
5. Use alarm clock as a reminder for medication.
6. Keep a log or journal for complex projects.
7. Maintain a telephone log and keep important telephone numbers near the telephone.
8. Maintain a medication log.
9. Use a cassette tape recorder to dictate thoughts and questions.
10. Purchase a noise-activated key chain.

Slowed Speech

1. Allow more time for conversation.
2. Don't hurry; give yourself permission to take your time.

Visuospatial Problems

1. Don't drive if unable to do so.
2. If able to drive, plan routes in advance, allow plenty of time, and take a friend along when you can.

Depression and Social Withdrawal

1. Plan recreational activities.
2. Be an active participant.
3. Rekindle interest in hobbies and activities.

Concentration Problems, Inattentiveness Distractability

1. Limit distractions (*e.g.*, turn off television when talking).
2. Meet with people one at a time.
3. Break large tasks into smaller, more manageable tasks.
4. Don't drive in heavy traffic.

Problems with Sequential Reasoning or Multistep Tasks

1. Don't take on new or unfamiliar job responsibilities.
2. Avoid tasks for which speed of performance is important.
3. Don't drive in heavy traffic.
4. Simplify activities (*e.g.*, don't plan a 7-course meal; use prepared foods.)
5. Plan activities at the time of day when you are at your best.

From Buckingham, SL and Van Gorp, WG: AIDS-Dementia complex: Implications for practice. Social Casework: The Journal of Contemporary Social Work 19:373, 1986, with permission.

According to Glass,[27] the documentation of increased suicide risk among PWAs raises 2 important issues: the question of "rational suicide," including assisted suicide and active euthanasia, and the suicide risk for healthy persons when informed of positive HIV test results. There have been a number of anecdotal reports[28] indicating that suicides have occurred as part of the devastation that can result from the news of a positive test result. For this reason, it is essential that testing be accompanied by information and counseling.

PWAs with a psychiatric diagnosis may have symptoms of depression and delirium. Suicidal ideation is more apt to be present when these symptoms exist. Patients who have CNS complications may also be more suicidal. According to Buckingham and van Gorp,[29] psychosocial trauma combined with a biologic cause of depression creates a fertile ground for suicidal intent and planning.

It is important to take preventive measures to reduce the risk of suicide in persons who are HIV positive and in AIDS patients. Measures should include the same measures used for patients who have other serious diseases or illnesses.[30] Risk reduction includes encouraging and allowing patients to verbalize their feelings and thoughts, including those about suicide. Encourage patients, and their families and important others to attend an AIDS support group. Refer patients to mental health workers for counseling. At times, referral for psychiatric evaluation and treatment may be needed.

Suicide ideation is not a problem for all HIV-positive or AIDS patients. Most of these patients want to live, and to live life to its fullest.

Psychotherapy

Psychotherapy can be helpful to patients and caregivers. A psychotherapist can assist in developing interventions for a wide range of symptoms the patient may have. Psychotherapy assists in problem solving, designing adequate structure and limits, decreasing level of hypochrondriacal preoccupation, and reducing family conflict.[31]

Other specialists who can provide indepth intervention for ADC patients include speech pathologists, psychiatrists, physical therapists, occupational therapists, dietitians, social workers, nurses, and mental health workers (see Chapter 10 for specific interventions).

Evaluation Tools

Tools used for diagnosis and treatment include serology tests, hematology tests, electroencephalograms (EEGs), computed tomographic (CT) scans, neuropsychological tests, neurologic tests, routine bedside mental status tests, magnetic resonance imaging (MRI) scans, cultures of blood and spinal fluid, electron microscopic studies, brain biopsies, and clinical assessments. Currie and colleagues,[32] report that recording eye movements may be a valuable technique for early detection of neurologic dysfunction in asymptomatic patients who are HIV positive or in patients with AIDS before other clinical evidence of ADC is apparent.

Neuropsychological tests that have been helpful in diagnosis are the Wechsler Memory Scale Semantic Recall, the Trail Making A and B test, the Wechsler Adult Intelligence Scale, the Shipley Vocabulary Test, the Controlled Oral Word Association Test, the Finger Tapping and Thumb-Finger Sequential Touch Test, the Zung Depression Scale, Speilberger's State Anxiety Scale, and the Minnesota Multiphasic Personality Inventory.[33] In some situations 1 of a number of tools could be used. The team should decide in advance which tools and tests will provide the best data with the least amount of effort by the patient.

PSYCHIATRIC DIAGNOSIS ACCOMPANYING HIV INFECTION

Psychiatric diagnoses have been reported in HIV-infected persons.[34-37] These diagnoses have ranged from adjustment disorder with depressed mood (the most frequent), to major depression, dementia, delirium, and panic disorders. Differential diagnosis can be acute existential crisis, chronic depression with acute exacerbation, grief (acute or chronic), chronic stress syndrome, organic mental disorder, major depression, physical exhaustion and disability, and acute interpersonal conflict.[38] The *Diagnostic and Statistical Manual of Mental Disorders,* Third Edition-Revised (DSM-III-R), provides information on each of these diagnoses.[39] The DSM-III-R provides a comprehensive and detailed explanation of what differentiates one diagnosis from another. For example, an adjustment disorder with depressed mood is predominantly manifested by symptoms of depression, tearfulness, and hopelessness. In an adjustment disorder with anxious mood, the symptoms are nervousness, worry, and jitteriness.

Adjustment Disorder

An adjustment disorder involves a maladaptive reaction to an identifiable stressor—the diagnosis of HIV infection or AIDS—that occurs within 3 months of the diagnosis. The maladaptive reaction can be impairment in social or occupational functioning or symptoms that exceed a normal and predictable reaction to the stressor. This disturbance persists beyond one instance, but it is expected that the person will eventually achieve a new level of adaptation.

Major Depression

Major depression may develop over several days or weeks, or it may develop suddenly. Depressed patients may exhibit any number or combination of the following symptoms: dysphoric mood, loss of interest or pleasure in usual activities, sadness, hopelessness, irritation, poor appetite, significant weight loss or weight gain, insomnia, hypersomnia, psychomotor agitation, retardation, decrease in sexual drive, loss of energy, and fatigue. Other symptoms include feelings of worthlessness, self-reproach, excessive or inappropriate guilt, diminished ability to think or concentrate, slowed thinking, indecisiveness, incoherence, recurrent thoughts of death or suicide, and suicide attempts.

Dementia

The dominant feature of dementia is a loss of intellectual abilities so severe as to interfere with social or occupational functioning. It also involves memory impairment and at least 1 of the following deficits: impairment of abstract thinking, impaired judgment, personality change, or other disturbances of higher cortical function, such as aphasia or apraxia. The patient's state of consciousness is not clouded.

Delirium

Clinical features of delirium include a clouded state of consciousness, difficulty shifting focus or sustaining attention, and difficulty engaging in conversation. Perceptual disturbances include misinterpretations, illusions, and hallucinations. Disturbance in the sleep-wakefulness cycle is almost always a symptom. Psychomotor activity, such as restlessness, hyperactivity, groping, stroking nonexistent objects, increased or decreased motor activity, sluggishness, or even catatonic stupor are symptoms HCWs may observe. The AIDS patient frequently experiences delirium, often caused by metabolic or toxic medical abnormalities. The major difference between dementia and delirium is that dementia is a persistent disturbance, and delirium is not.[40]

Panic Disorders

Panic disorders do not often affect PWAs, but occasionally do. Panic attacks are manifested by any 4 of the following symptoms: dyspnea, palpitations, chest pain or discomfort, choking or smothering sensations, dizziness, vertigo or unsteady feelings, feelings of unreality, paresthesias, hot and cold flashes, sweating, faintness, trembling or shaking, fear of dying, fear of going crazy, or fear of doing something uncontrolled during an attack.

Substance Use Disorders

At least 17% of AIDS patients also have a substance use disorder, which includes abuse and dependence, as well as a substance-induced organic mental disorder, because one of the major high-risk behaviors for HIV infection is sharing blood-contaminated needles and syringes in intravenous drug abuse. "Also, because at present most PWAs in the United States are gay men, and because alcoholism and related chemical dependencies are believed to afflict between 20%–33% of gay men, it is likely that the incidence of substance abuse disorder is actually much greater than 17%."[41] The DSM-III-R definition of this disorder includes abuse of alcohol.[42] Psychoactive substance use disorders are abuse and dependence on alcohol; amphetamine; cannabis; cocaine; hallucinogen; inhalant; opioid; phencyclidine (PCP); a sedative, hypnotic, or anxiolytic; and nicotine. Substance-induced organic mental disorders are the direct effects on the nervous system the above list of substances causes. This differs from Psychoactive Substance Use Disorders, which refers to the behavior associated with drug use.[43]

NEUROMUSCULAR DISEASE

Neuromuscular aspects of HIV infection occur less frequently than CNS manifestations. The peripheral nervous system (PNS) is involved in at least 15% of AIDS cases, and neuromuscular disease can complicate all stages of HIV infection.[44-48] Dalakas and Pezehkpour[49] emphasize that neuromuscular manifestations of HIV infection are important because some of these diseases may: coincide with HIV seroconversion; be the only indication of a chronic silent HIV infection, or the presenting sign of symptomatic AIDS; be treatable if diagnosed early; occur concurrently with another neurologic illness such as ADC, worsening the patient's disability and complicating the overall neurologic picture.

Three classifications of neuromuscular disease are peripheral neuropathies, inflammatory myopathies, and less common neuromuscular manifestations such as type II muscle fiber atrophy and nemaline myopathy.

Peripheral Neuropathies

The 6 subtypes of peripheral neuropathies are:

1. Acute Guillain-Barré syndrome (GBS)
2. Chronic inflammatory demyelinating polyneuropathy (CIDP)
3. Mononeuritis multiplex
4. Distal axonopathy
5. Ganglioneuronitis
6. Progressive inflammatory polyradiculoneuropathy

GBS in a HIV-seronegative person is clinically indistinguishable from acute demyelinating inflammatory sensorimotor polyradiculoneuropathy.[50] In HIV-seropositive persons with GBS, the cerebrospinal fluid is often pleocytotic.[51,52] Therefore, a finding of acute GBS should prompt a search for HIV infection. CIDP usually follows a progressive course, and is often found in HIV-infected patients who are otherwise asymptomatic.[53] It is appropriate to test every CIDP patient for the presence of HIV.

Mononeuritis multiplex in HIV-infected patients involves sensory or motor deficiency.[54] A differential diagnosis of mononeuropathy or mononeuritis multiplex should include ruling out varicella zoster virus in spinal or cranial nerves, viral meningitis of cranial nerves, and brachial or lumbar plexopathies caused by viral infection. Distal axonopathy, a disease of the impulse-conducting neurons (found furthest from the cell body), is very painful and is the most common neuropathy occurring with full-blown AIDS.[55] The etiology is suspected to be toxic, metabolic, or nutritional.

Sensory ataxic neuropathy due to ganglioneuronitis has been reported in only 1 patient with HIV infection; therefore, we are not able to define the development of this disease yet. Progressive inflammatory polyradiculoneuropathy predominantly affects the lower extremities and often involves asymmetrical, flaccid paraparesis, accompanied by sphincteric dysfunction, areflexia, flexor plantar responses, and diffuse hypoesthesias in the legs.[56] This neuropathy invariably leads to death.

Inflammatory Myopathies

Polymyositis is the most common myopathy occurring with HIV infection.[57] It may be the presenting sign of HIV infection, preceding AIDS by several months.[58] Persons with AIDS who have polymyositis develop proximal muscle weakness and elevated creatine kinase.[59-61] HIV-associated polymyositis shows inflammatory infiltrates when a muscle biopsy is performed.[62] The etiology of polymyositis in HIV-positive patients is speculative, but it could be the result of the virus directly invading the muscle but not causing a cytopathic effect on the muscle fibers. Or it could be caused by immune-mediated mechanisms initiated by presences of HIV infection, which invades the muscle, according to Dalakas and Pezehkpour.[63]

Less Common Neuromuscular Manifestations

Less common neuromuscular manifestations are type II muscle fiber atrophy, amyotrophic lateral sclerosis, and nemaline myopathy.[64] In patients with proximal muscle weakness with normal creatine kinase, biopsies showed severe type II fiber atrophy.[65,66] Causes of this weakness could be poor nutrition, rapid weight loss, prolonged bed rest, or remote effects of lymphomas or sarcomas.[67]

In amyotrophic lateral sclerosis, muscles in the upper and lower extremities and bulbar muscles are progressively involved with significant wasting of muscles.[68] Nemaline (rod) myopathy presents with subacute onset of progressive muscle weakness and elevated creatine kinase.[69]

An increasing variety of neuromuscular manifestations will probably emerge as more HIV-infected persons are identified.

Treatment Modalities

Treatment modalities for neuromuscular disease vary. Chronic demyelinating polyneuropathy responses to plasmapheresis, and inflammatory myopathy responds to corticosteroids. Hyperalimentation and mobilization are effective treatments for type II fiber atrophy. The literature thus far reveals little research on the effects of physical, occupational, speech, or diet therapy on any of these diseases.

CENTRAL NERVOUS SYSTEM COMPLICATIONS IN CHILDREN

The pattern of CNS involvement associated with HIV infection in children is similar to the pattern in adults. There are differences, however, in children's HIV symptoms. Researchers report a progressive encephalopathy in 30%–50% of infected infants and children.[70,71] This symptom is believed to be a direct result of HIV infection of the brain.[72] Neurologic classification of HIV infection in children is divided into 3 categories: normal neurologic findings; progressive encephalopathy; and static encephalopathy. Children with HIV infection have fewer occurrences of brain infections than do adults with HIV infection.

Progressive Encephalopathy

There appears to be a direct correlation between the neurologic symptoms of HIV infection in children and children's mortality levels, as indicated by Epstein and colleagues[73] (Table 6–6). Children with progressive encephalopathy have a poor prognosis and almost invariably die.

TABLE 6–6. **Mortality of Children With Human Immunodeficiency Virus Infection Compared to Neurological Status***

Classification	Number of Patients	Number Alive	Number Dead
Progressive encephalopathy	34	11	23
Static encephalopathy	23	21	2
Neurologically normal	22	22	0
Total	79	54	25

*Fisher's exact test comparing numbers alive and dead among children with progressive encephalopathy and static encephalopathy or normal neurologic findings demonstrated a significant association ($p < 0.001$).

From Epstein LG, Sharer LR, Goudsmith J: Neurological and neuropathological features of Human Immunodeficiency Virus infection in children. Annals of Neurology 23:S20, 1988. Used by permission.

Static Encephalopathy

Children with static encephalopathy present with normal brain growth but with developmental delays or nonprogressive motor deficits. In Epstein and colleagues' study, all of the 34 children with progressive encephalopathy failed to achieve normal developmental milestones or suffered subcortical dementia and impaired brain growth. Epstein and colleagues' findings are presented in Table 6–7.

Implications of early and persistent brain infection in HIV-infected children, according to Epstein, Sharer, and Goudsmit,[74] include the following:

1. Brain infection will be difficult, if not impossible, to eradicate, particularly while the virus is in the latent stage.
2. Treatment of CNS involvement will probably depend on control of viral latency and expression.
3. Because of the increased morbidity and high mortality associated with HIV brain infection, and the therapeutic problems posed by such infection, the most useful approach is prevention.

The limited number of children with AIDS and CNS disease studied thus far makes it difficult to offer specific diagnostic and therapeutic modalities to HCWs.

TABLE 6–7. **Neurological Findings of Progressive Encephalopathy in 34 Children With Human Immunodeficiency Virus Infection**

Neurological Finding	Percent of Patients
Loss of developmental milestones, or subcortical dementia	100
Impaired brain growth	94
Secondary microcephaly	68
Cerebral atrophy on computed tomographic scan	88
Generalized weakness with pyramidal signs	94
Pseudobulbar palsy	35
Ataxia	18
Seizures	18
Myoclonus	9
Extrapyramidal rigidity	9

From Epstein LG, Sharer LR, and Goudsmith J: Neurological and neuropathological features of Human Immunodeficiency Virus Infection in children. Ann Neurol 23:S20, 1988. Used by permission.

Increased experience and research should prove productive as the epidemic increasingly involves infants born with HIV infection.

INTERVENTIONS: SUMMARY

Interventions HCWs can employ with HIV-infected persons and persons with symptomatic AIDS include the following:

1. Inform patients which tests and evaluations will be performed and explain the rationale for performing them. This helps to ensure patient and family cooperation. Even if the patient's mental capacity for understanding is questionable, explaining and educating may prevent a crisis from occurring during the evaluation or in the future.
2. Discuss results of the tests and evaluation with the patient and family. They will feel less like guinea pigs. Help them to recognize that they are contributing to knowledge of the disease. At the same time, assure the patient that the knowledge and the clinical skills HCWs gain by conducting specific tests can result in interventions to help them.
3. A multidisciplinary team of health professionals should provide care. Use the services of consultants and specialists in assessment, diagnosis, and therapeutic planning.

Because knowledge about the emerging nature of AIDS and associated neuropsychiatric disorders continues to evolve, HCWs are urged to keep abreast of new approaches to the diagnosis, treatment, and care for HIV-infected persons. Allied health professionals should collaborate with physicians, nurses, psychiatrists, psychologists, social workers, and mental health workers specializing in HIV infection, both in clinical practice and in research, for the ultimate benefit of their patients.

DISCUSSION QUESTIONS

1. What kinds of research can you and other members of your profession conduct that would prove helpful to HIV-infected persons with CNS disease, ADC, or neuromuscular disease?
2. What health professionals can you identify in your community with whom you could work to assist HIV-infected persons with the various neuropsychiatric problems requiring inpatient care? Requiring outpatient or home care?
3. In what ways can allied health professionals become more involved in diagnosis and therapeutic interventions for HIV-infected persons with neuropsychiatric involvement?

4. Which community agencies are most likely to respond to the needs of an HIV-infected person who also has a neuropsychiatric problem?
5. What effect will the increasing number of HIV-infected persons with neuropsychiatric involvement have on the health care system?

REFERENCES

1. Weber, J and Pinching, A: The clinical management of AIDs and HTLV-III infection. In Miller, D, Weber, J, and Green, J (eds): The Management of AIDS Patients. Macmillan, New York, 1986.
2. Tross, S, et al: Psychological and neuropsychological function in AIDS spectrum disorder patients (abstr). The International Conference on the Acquired Immunodeficiency Syndrome. American College of Physicians, Philadelphia, 1983.
3. Snider, WD, et al: Neurological complications of acquired immune deficiency syndrome: Analysis of 50 patients. Ann Neurol 14:403, 1983.
4. Petito, CK, et al: Vascular myelopathy pathologically resembling subacute combined degeneration in patients with the acquired immune deficiency syndrome. N Engl J Med 312:874, 1985.
5. Shaw, GM, et al: HTLV-III infection in brains of children and adults with AIDS encephalopathy. Science 227:177, 1985.
6. Jordan, BD, et al: Neurological complications of AIDS: An overview based on 110 autopsied patients (abstr). The International Conference on the Acquired Immunodeficiency Syndrome. American College of Physicians, Philadelphia, 1985.
7. Levy, RM, Bredesen, DE, and Rosenblum, ML: Neurological manifestations of the acquired immunodeficiency syndrome (AIDS): Experience at UCSF and review of the literature. J. Neurosurg 62:475, 1985.
8. Weber, J, and Pinching, A: Ibid.
9. Levy, RM, Bredesen, DE, and Rosenblum, ML: Ibid.
10. Weber, J and Pinching, A: Ibid.
11. Levy, RM, Bredesen, DE, and Rosenblum, ML: Ibid.
12. Pert, CB, et al: Octapeptides deduced from the neuropeptide receptor-like pattern of antigen T_4 in brain potently inhibit human immunodeficiency virus receptor binding and T-cell infectivity (abstr). Proc Nat Acad Sci USA 83:254, 1986.
13. Levy, J, et al: Isolation of AIDS-associated retroviruses from cerebrospinal fluid and brain of patients with neurological symptoms. Lancet 2:586, 1985.
14. Gartner, S, et al: Virus isolation from and identification of HTLV-III/LAV-producing cells in brain tissue from a patient with AIDS. JAMA 256:2365, 1986.
15. De la Monte, SM, et al: Subacute encephalomyelitis of AIDS and its relation to HTLV-III infection. Neurology 37:562, 1987.
16. Ostrow, D, Grant, I, and Atkinson, H: Assessment and management of AIDS patients with neuropsychiatric disturbances. J Clin Psychiatry 5:14, 1988.
17. The Centers for Disease Control: Revision of the case definition of acquired immunodeficiency syndrome for national reporting: United States. MMWR 36:15, 1987.
18. Navia, BA, et al: The AIDS dementia complex: I. Clinical features. Ann Neurol 19:517, 1986.

19. Navia, BA et al: Ibid.
20. Buckingham, SL and Van Gorp, WG: Essential knowledge about AIDS dementia. Social Work 33:517, 1988.
21. Navia, BA, et al: Ibid.
22. Navia, BA, et al: Ibid.
23. Navia, BA, et al: Ibid.
24. Navia, BA, et al: Ibid.
25. Newman, NM, et al: Clinical and histologic findings in opportunistic ocular infections—part of a new syndrome of acquired immunodeficiency. Arch Ophthalmal 101:396, 1983.
26. Marzuk, PM, et al: Increased risk of suicide in persons with AIDS. JAMA 259:1333, 1988.
27. Glass, RM: AIDS and suicide. JAMA 259:1369, 1988.
28. Underscore urgency of HIV counseling: Several suicides follow positive tests. Clinical Psychiatry News, October 1987:1.
29. Buckingham, SL and Van Gorp, WG: AIDS dementia complex: Implications for practice. Social Casework: The Journal of Contemporary Social Work 39:371, 1988.
30. Glass, RM: Ibid.
31. Buckingham, SL and Van Gorp, WG: Ibid, p 112.
32. Currie, J, et al: Eye movement abnormalities as a predictor of acquired immunodeficiency syndrome dementia complex. Arch Neurol 45:949, 1988.
33. Janssen, RS, et al: Neurological complication of human immunodeficiency virus infection in patients with lymphadenopathy syndrome. Ann Neurol 23:49, 1988.
34. Barbuto, J: Psychiatric care of seriously ill patients with acquired immune deficiency syndrome. In Nichols, SE and Ostrow, DG (eds): Psychiatric Implications of Acquired Immune Deficiency Syndrome. American Psychiatric Press, Washington, DC, 1984.
35. Hoffman, RS, Prudic, J, Fiori, M, and Freedman, EP: Psychopathology complicating acquired immune deficiency syndrome. Am J Psychiatry 142:95, 1984.
36. Hoffman, RS: Neuropsychiatric complications of AIDS. Psychosomatics 25:393, 1984.
37. Dilley, JW, Ochitill, HN, Perl, M, and Volberding, PA: Findings in psychiatric consultation with patients with acquired immune deficiency syndrome. Am J Psychiatry 142:82, 1985.
38. Wolcott, D (workshop leader): Neurological and psychological manifestations of AIDS. AIDS: Practical Applications for Nurses and Social Workers Conference, San Diego, CA, September 3, 1987.
39. Diagnostic and Statistical Manual of Mental Disorders, Third Edition-Revised (DSM-III-R). American Psychiatric Association, Washington, DC, 1987.
40. Buckingham, SL and Van Gorp, WG: Ibid.
41. Kus, RJ: Personal communication, December 5, 1988.
42. DSM-III-R: Ibid.
43. DSM-III-R: Ibid.
44. Dalakas, MC: Neuromuscular aspects of AIDS. American Academy of Neurology Lecture Series 173, 1987.
45. Dalakas, MC: Neuromuscular complications of AIDS. Muscle Nerve 9:92, 1986.
46. Lipkin, WI, Parry, G, Kiprov, D, and Abrams, D: Inflammatory neuropathy in homosexual men with lymphadenopathy. Neurology 35:1479, 1985.
47. Eidelberg, D, et al: Progressive polyradiculopathy in acquired immune deficiency syndrome. Neurology 36:912, 1986.

48. Cornblath, DR, McArthur, JC, and Griffin, JW: The spectrum of peripheral neuropathies in HTLV-III infection. Muscle Nerve 9:76, 1986.
49. Dalakas, MC, and Pezehkpour, GH: Neuromuscular diseases associated with human immunodeficiency virus infection. Ann Neurol (Suppl) 23(7):S38–S48, 1988.
50. Arnason, BGW: Acute inflammatory demyelinating polyradiculoneuropathies. In Dyck, PJ, Thomas, PK, Lambert, EH, and Bunge, R (eds): Peripheral Neuropathy. WB Saunders, Philadelphia, 1984.
51. Cornblath, DR, McArthur, JC, and Griffin, JW: Ibid, p 76.
52. Cornblath, DR, et al: Inflammatory demyelinating peripheral neuropathies associated with human T-cell lymphotropic virus type III infection. Ann Neurol 21:32, 1987.
53. Dalakas, MC (1987): Ibid.
54. Dalakas, MC (1987): Ibid.
55. Dalakas, MC and Pezehkpour, GH (1988): Ibid.
56. Eidelberg, D, et al: Ibid.
57. Dalakas, MC and Pezehkpour, GH (1988): Ibid.
58. Dalakas, MC (1988): Ibid.
59. Dalakas, MC (1987): Ibid.
60. Dalakas, MC (1986): Ibid.
61. Dalakas, MC, Pezehkpour, GH, Gravell, M, and Sever, JL: Polymyositis associated with AIDS retrovirus. JAMA 256:2381, 1986.
62. Dalakas, MC (1988): Ibid.
63. Dalakas, MC (1988): Ibid.
64. Dalakas, MC (1988): Ibid.
65. Dalakas, MC (1987): Ibid.
66. Dalakas, MC (1986): Ibid.
67. Dalakas, MC (1988): Ibid.
68. Dalakas, MC (1988): Ibid.
69. Dalakas, MC (1988): Ibid.
70. Belman, AL, et al: Calcification of the basal ganglia in infants and children. Neurology 36:1192, 1986.
71. Epstein, LG, et al: Neurologic manifestations of HIV infection in children. Pediatrics 78:678, 1986.
72. Epstein, LG, Sharer, LR, and Goudsmit, J: Neurological and neuropathological features of human immunodeficiency virus infection in children. Ann Neurol (Suppl) 23:S19, 1988.
73. Epstein, LG, Sharer, LR, and Goudsmit, J (1988): Ibid.
74. Epstein, LG, Sharer, LR, and Goudsmit, J (1988): Ibid.

SEVEN

*SUPPORTIVE MEASURES: LIVING WITH AIDS**

*Kathleen R. Guindon, Joyce W. Hopp,
Elizabeth A. Rogers, Edwinna May Marshall*

OUTLINE

FOCUS ON QUALITY LIVING
PATIENTS' RESPONSES TO LIVING WITH
 AIDS
NEEDS OF FAMILIES, FRIENDS, AND
 SIGNIFICANT OTHERS
SUPPORTIVE MEASURES
Support Groups
Health Promotion Measures
 Sexual Counseling
 Nutrition

Exercise
Stress Management
Alternative Therapies
HOME CARE
 Daily Care
 Respite Care
REHABILITATION TEAM MEMBER
 CONTRIBUTIONS
THE CHILD WITH AIDS
Schools and Day Care Centers

OBJECTIVES

By the close of this chapter, the reader will be able to:
 1. State the focus health care workers should seek to foster in HIV-infected
  individuals.

*Home Care Plans contributed by Cindy L. Kosch, Robert L. Wilkins, Edwinna May Marshall, Delia Gutierrez.

151

2. List the stages of HIV infection during which responsive interventions are most appropriate.
3. Describe the special needs of families and friends of persons with AIDS.
4. Outline the benefits of support groups.
5. List and describe appropriate health promotion measures for persons with AIDS.
6. Describe general measures for home care of persons with AIDS.
7. Cite and describe components of a home care plan that a specialist in your profession could implement for an AIDS patient, if appropriate.
8. Define respite and describe ways of providing it.
9. Cite the specific contributions of various members of the rehabilitation team.
10. Cite and describe special problems of children with AIDS.

FOCUS ON QUALITY LIVING

Today, persons with AIDS (PWAs) learn to live with the disease rather than give up to death. Although the fatality rate remains high for this infectious disease, an AIDS diagnosis is not an immediate death sentence. When working with PWAs, it is important not to destroy hope. The key is to focus on the person's life today, not on the distant future.

The outlook for the patient may seem bleak. Each bout of illness may appear to be terminal. But many AIDS patients do "bounce back"; they do go home from the hospital. Health care workers (HCWs) should plan for discharge, not for death. In the early days of the epidemic, workers did not do this. Thus many patients failed to receive the physical, occupational, and emotional therapy essential for living with AIDS.

The physical and psychological benefits of focusing on quality living are many. The attitude and outlook of the HCWs are quickly communicated to the patient. If workers imply by look or action that they are caring for a person with no hope of recovery, their belief can be a self-fulfilling prophecy; their patient may give up hope of living.

On the other hand, a bubbly overcheerfulness may depress the patient. "Who does she think I am? Can't she tell I'm dying?" or "Doesn't he know I am really sick? This is no time for jokes!" The HCW walks a narrow line between unrealistic optimism and unwarranted pessimism.

PATIENTS' RESPONSES TO LIVING WITH AIDS

AIDS is a continuum extending from initial infection with the HIV to death from diseases resulting from the depression of the immune system. The time from inoculation with the HIV to the development symptomatic AIDS may be as long as 15 years. The HIV-infected person's response to learning his or her diagnosis will vary according to how far the disease has progressed.

Learning of a positive HIV test result can be one of the most traumatic things to happen to a person. A person may be angry about being infected or afraid of developing full-blown AIDS and dying. Some people deny the test results. The most important interventions during this crisis state are providing information and emotional support. The person needs information about health care practitioners and clinics that specialize in treating persons with HIV infection. He or she needs to learn about HIV infection, how the virus is transmitted, and precautions to take to avoid further exposure or transmission. (Chapter 4 provides the informational base for such teaching.) Emotional support from family, significant other, and HCWs is essential. Participation in an AIDS support group can show the patient how others have coped with this kind of crisis.

HIV-infected persons should be encouraged to establish a relationship with a personal physician, one who understands their cares and concerns. When an illness develops, the person can be reassured that the illness does not signal the beginning of AIDS, if that is the case; receive prompt treatment of opportunistic infections; or receive drugs such as zidovudine (AZT) in the early stages to help control the progress of the disease.

HIV-infected persons who have symptoms but have not yet been diagnosed with AIDS may be caught in a difficult "in limbo" time. "Do I have it? Is this the 'Big A'? What if I can't work? What about my insurance? What about my job?" Social workers or AIDS project volunteers can bring information about available means of financial support and about emergency short- or long-term care. Most states have some form of disability assistance, although eligibility criteria vary. Assistance from some insurance, state, or federal aid programs is not available until the person is declared disabled.

When a diagnosis of AIDS has been made, patients usually experience another crisis. At this point they no longer have the hope of avoiding full-blown AIDS, but must focus on ways of living with AIDS. Some patients become suicidal, feeling they would rather die immediately than let the disease run its course. HCWs should monitor for suicide attempts and teach family and significant others to do the same.

Some patients initially deny the diagnosis of AIDS. During this period, they may refuse to follow any advice from HCWs. Referral to a mental health counselor can be beneficial in such an instance. Other patients actually experience feelings of relief when they learn of an AIDS diagnosis, because under many current health care plans they can then receive financial assistance and health care services not available without an AIDS diagnosis.

With the onset of the various opportunistic infections, patients find themselves once again in crisis. Suffering these infections and the many complications that accompany them makes patients wonder how severe the infection will become. Patients realize that such infections can be life-threatening. This fear causes some to overutilize health care services, and others to avoid such services altogether. Intervention at this stage includes educating the patient about the signs and symptoms of the various opportunistic infections they may suffer (see Chapter 4).

When people are faced with their mortality, they must re-evaluate how they are going to live. They need to know they have options. They can focus on living for the present, or become obsessed with horror of the future. People can take control of their own situations—be in charge. They need not rely on health professionals to take the initiative, but instead should use professionals as resources. Death is not a failure, but failing to take on the challenge of living is.

Persons with symptomatic HIV infection may experience a loss of independence. They may lose their jobs and financial resources. They may lose control over various body functions, such as the ability to walk or to control their bladders. HCWs should encourage patients to concentrate on the control or function they have remaining, rather than on what they have lost. They should be encouraged to be as independent as possible. Occupational therapists, physical therapists, nurses and social workers on the health care team can be especially helpful during this time.

Some persons experience rejection when they reveal to family, friends, coworkers, or HCWs that they have AIDS. Such rejection may occur because of the disease itself, or because of the high-risk behaviors known to be associated with transmission of the disease. HCWs can help patients determine the best ways of telling family and friends about the diagnosis. Educating family and friends about AIDS can turn rejection into acceptance. HCWs can help patients identify and seek out people who can form a good support system.

The final crisis a PWA experiences is facing the realization of impending death. Many PWAs are in their prime of life. They may be unprepared to face dying. Grief counseling and spiritual counseling are appropriate (see Chapter 5). Trained hospice volunteers or volunteers from AIDS projects can be very helpful to patients, significant others, family, and friends during this time.

NEEDS OF FAMILIES, FRIENDS, AND SIGNIFICANT OTHERS

As knowledge about AIDS becomes more widespread, family members, friends, and coworkers may change their attitudes towards PWAs. Frequently, an AIDS diagnosis has labeled someone as unclean. The parallel with a diagnosis of cancer 50 years ago is striking. Today, it is difficult to recall a time when people hid a diagnosis of cancer, and feared that it was contagious. Increased education and the work of public figures willing to speak openly about having cancer and about its treatment have changed the way people respond to the disease. Changes in attitudes toward AIDS will come, but perhaps not for several years.

Parents of gay men often have a double problem: learning simultaneously that their son is gay and that he has AIDS. If they did not know about his homosexuality, they have no time to face this issue before facing the AIDS diagnosis. They may feel loss of control and be angry that they have been deprived of information. Now their gay son is dying.

Similar problems face the gay man. "Should I tell my parents now, or wait until later?" This question may revolve relentlessly in his mind. He realizes that disclosing his homosexuality and his diagnosis could move him farther away from the people whose love and support he most needs.

Parents may feel they have to hide the fact that their son has AIDS. They are reluctant to tell their clergyman, coworkers, or even other family members, believing everyone "will know he's gay." They may believe others will judge them and blame their son or themselves for the situation. They may have heard many sermons about gay people. In this society, they must realistically fear losing the support of many persons whom they would otherwise trust.

Persons who learn that their spouses or sexual partners are infected with the HIV find themselves in a similar situation, and must also worry about their own HIV status. Women may also be concerned about their children's health, or about a present or future pregnancy. They may wonder who it is safe to tell, "This person I married has AIDS." Should they tell their parents? Can they still invite family members to their home? Can their children still attend school? Often, spouses feel there is no one to whom they can turn. They stand alone.

HCWs can help AIDS patients and their significant others, family members, and friends to address these questions. Deal only with the present, the "here and now." Do not cross future bridges or attempt to deal with "what if" situations. Provide information about the disease, methods of treatment, local support groups, and AIDS organizations.

Abraham Maslow[1] commented that, "Sure knowledge means sure ethical decisions." Acquire and maintain current knowledge, and discuss your knowledge with other health professionals. The possibility of exchanging information is one of the strongest reasons for forming an interdisciplinary team to treat persons at any stage of HIV infection and to assist their families. Discussing situations with other HCWs will help to secure the best counsel for patients. Sharing experiences can be beneficial to both HCWs and patients.

SUPPORTIVE MEASURES

Support Groups

Support groups may already exist in the community. Use the resource list in the Appendix to locate the support group nearest you. If none exists, one can be started. Persons working with AIDS projects are usually very willing to share their experience and knowledge in setting up support groups. A support group needs a facilitator, who may be a social worker, community health nurse, or teacher, or any interested individual (not necessarily a professional) who is knowledgeable about AIDS and wants to express concern in a tangible way.

Whatever their background, facilitators should be nonjudgmental. PWAs have usually already faced questions about how they acquired the disease. They may be asking themselves, "What did I do to deserve this? Why me?" They come to support groups for validation as individuals and to learn ways to cope with the devastating diagnosis of AIDS. Facilitators lead support groups in sharing the knowledge and experience of PWAs. Experience has shown that it is best to offer separate support groups for families and partners or significant others, rather than to combine these groups.

Support groups should be listed in telephone directories as well as in community resource listings. "Hot lines," staffed on a 24-hour basis, can be helpful. Support groups can prepare publications listing local community sources to meet specific needs (for example, dentists who are willing to care for AIDS patients).

Health Promotion Measures

Altering lifestyle, reducing high–risk behaviors, and using health promotion measures such as good nutrition, exercise, and stress management, do appear to affect the course of the disease for a PWA.

Sexual Counseling

Continued sexual activity is an important issue. HCWs should not allow their values to cloud their counsel, but should provide essential information on measures to prevent spreading infection to sexual partners. Appendix C provides guidelines for such counseling.

Nutrition

Infections and fever cause an increased need for calories and protein, but loss of appetite and diarrhea make it difficult for the person to meet these needs. Poor nutritional status can further depress the immune system. Maintaining good nutrition will not provide a cure for AIDS, but it can help combat the diseases that result from AIDS.

Exercise

Exercise suited to the person's capabilities, and planned to increase as tolerance develops, may also help PWAs recover from diseases associated with AIDS. Specific exercises that address neuromuscular deficits should be included in the care plan if applicable. Walking is good exercise, needing little special equipment other than supportive aids, when necessary.

Stress Management

Stress management can be a positive force for recovery. Principles of stress management applicable to PWAs are as follows:

1. Recognize that stress always accompanies a serious illness such as AIDS, so plan for stress management with every patient.
2. Identify stressors in the person's environment. Stressors may include, but are not limited to: dealing with reactions of friends, family, community, coworkers; loss or potential loss of ability to work or to carry on activities of daily living; fear of death; loss of housing; lack of financial support. For children with AIDS, loss of friends; problems with school attendance. For parents with AIDS, inability to care for or to support family; feelings of guilt.
3. List in order of priority the stressors to manage. Listing them may prevent stressors from seeming overwhelming.
4. Plan ways of coping with specific stressors. For instance, enlist a social worker's help in planning ways the person can maintain financial support for self and family, or outline and practice in advance ways of discussing feelings of rejection or guilt with family, partners, and friends.
5. Emcourage the patient to seek out and use the support of others, informally through friends or formally through support groups.
6. Traditionally, many people have been assisted through crises in their lives by their religious faith; with the AIDS crisis, however, this source is frequently denied because it may increase feelings of guilt. Increasingly, religious organizations are recognizing that they should support rather than condemn PWAs.
7. Additional methods of stress management that may be helpful are guided imagery, relaxation techniques, and meditation.

Alternative Therapies

Persons suffering from chronic or incurable diseases may become desperate and turn to alternative therapies that "promise" cure or relief. HCWs should consider it their responsibility to educate AIDS patients and their families and significant others about the potential harm of following questionable nutritional practices or using devices that are touted as cures for AIDS. AIDS patients are frequently already under a financial burden and should not waste their money on products purported to prevent or cure AIDS. Not only is money wasted on useless health promotion measures, but actual harm can result. For instance, large doses of vitamin C can result in kidney damage;[2] use of butylated hydroxytoluene (BHT) can result in liver damage.[3] Opportunistic infections, such as *Salmonella bacteremia,* can result from ingesting raw milk and raw eggs.[4] To date, no nutritional regimens have been demonstrated to prevent or cure AIDS. Maintaining good nutritional status can enable a person to survive bouts with opportunistic infections and promote a higher quality of life, but cannot provide a magic cure.

When counseling an AIDS patient, use the following guidelines about alternate therapies:

1. The therapy should not replace health care that is generally considered effective.
2. The therapy should not advocate ingesting substances in quantities that will be physically harmful.
3. The therapy should not place the individual at increased risk for opportunistic infections.
4. The therapy should not encourage unnecessary expenditures of limited financial resources.

Many PWAs volunteer to participate in clinical drug trials and form partnerships with physicians and other researchers searching for ways to combat HIV infection. Participation in such trials can provide meaning and quality to life, even though the outcome may not be all the person hopes.

HOME CARE

Most AIDS patients can be adequately cared for in their homes, and need hospital care only during critical stages and hospice, if necessary, only during the terminal stage. Caregivers in the home can be taught to provide most of the patient's care, with assistance from community health workers for special procedures.

Daily Care

Maintaining *good hygiene* and a safe environment for the patient includes the following practices:

1. Maintain good oral hygiene, especially if the patient has a candidal infection. Use swabs because gums may bleed easily. Use mouth rinses, such as warm salt water ($1/2$ teaspoon in a glass of water), or hydrogen peroxide ($1/2$ hydrogen peroxide and $1/2$ water). Do not allow the person to gargle if he or she is weak and may choke.
2. Ensure that the patient bathes regularly. If the patient is too weak to stand in the shower, place a stable stool for him or her to sit on while showering. If the patient is unable to shower or bathe, give a bed bath. Wash and dry each part of the body separately to avoid chilling.
3. Prevent transmission of infection to the patient by maintaining a clean environment. Use a dishwasher with minimum 140°F water, or rinse dishes in a freshly prepared 1:10 chlorine bleach solution (1 cup bleach in 10 cups water). Caregivers and visitors should wear masks if they have colds. Keep children and others with communicable diseases away from the patient until they have passed the communicable period.
4. Persons with symptomatic HIV infection should not handle waste products or litter boxes of pets. Many opportunistic organisms live in animal waste.
5. Prevent transmission of the HIV from the patient to others by wearing dis-

posable gloves when handling any body fluid containing blood (sputum, feces, vomitus, urine), or when handling linens, bedclothes, dressings, utensils, or equipment contaminated by blood. Do not reuse gloves. Washing gloves will not remove microorganisms.

6. Clean surfaces, including the toilet, touched by blood, semen, or vaginal fluids with a 1:10 solution of chlorine bleach. Soak laundry contaminated with such fluids in a similar solution. Using cold water will help prevent the blood from staining the laundry. After soaking, wash laundry in the usual manner.

7. Wear a protective gown and a mask in addition to gloves only when expecting splash or splatter of blood.

8. Soak any used syringes in a 1:10 solution of chlorine bleach before discarding in a shatterproof, tightly sealed container. A coffee can with plastic lid can serve for this purpose.

9. Use disposable tissues and dressings whenever possible. After use, place in a sealed plastic or paper container for trash removal or incineration.

10. All members of the household who shave should use electric razors because they are less likely to cut. Do not share razors or toothbrushes.

The chlorine bleach solution should be prepared fresh daily. Precautions for handling undiluted bleach at home may be found in Table 7-1.

If the patient is unable to use the bathroom, secure a plastic bedpan or a urinal for this purpose. Wash it regularly with soapy water and rinse with the 1:10 bleach solution. Use paper underpads in the bed if the patient cannot control elimination; a condom catheter may also be used for a male patient.

"Fever sponging" can help a patient who is feverish and sweaty. Using lukewarm water and a washcloth, expose and bathe 1 part of the body at a time. Continue until each part of the body has been bathed. Replace bed linens with clean, dry ones.

Tables 7-2 through 7-5 provide sample home care plans that allied health professionals can use to guide patients and their home caregivers.

Respite Care

Burnout is a common phenomenon among persons caring for PWAs. One solution is respite care, occasional relief care (a few hours or 1 day a week), provided by a volunteer or paid aide. Respite care allows caregivers time to reenergize and temporarily escape the overwhelming challenge they face. Friends, neighbors, and other family members can be helpful during this time. Just stopping by with a special meal, tickets to a concert or show, or an offer to stay with the patient for a few hours, provides the respite needed.

In some areas volunteer groups such as the SHANTI ("peace") organization in San Francisco have organized to provide respite care on an emergency or regular basis. "The Chicken Soup Brigade" sponsored by another AIDS project provides a daily meal along with a friendly visit.

TABLE 7–1. **Precautions for Using Chlorine Bleach**

Hazards	Storage and Disposal	Treatment
Can cause substantial injury to the eye and skin when splashed Harmful if swallowed	Store in cool dry place Rinse empty container with water Recap and dispose	*Eyes:* Remove contact lenses or glasses, rinse with water for a minimum of 15 minutes *Skin:* Remove clothing and wash skin with running water *Mucus membranes of the throat:* Drink a full glass of water and immediately contact physician

TABLE 7–2. **Sample Home Care Plan: Nutrition**

Problem	Symptoms	Suggested Care Plan
Nausea/ vomiting	Regurgitation of food/fluid Inability to consume foods adequately	Liquids or soft foods are usually better tolerated than regular solids. Small frequent meals/snacks may be helpful. Bland foods are usually preferred over spicy foods. Cold foods are often preferred over hot foods. Serve carbohydrates that are easy to digest, such as dry toast, fruit/vegetable juices, carbonated beverages, applesauce, pasta, etc. Lactose (the sugar in milk) should be avoided, as should foods high in fat content.
Dehydration	Weight loss Sunken eyes Decreased skin fullness Low urinary output Weak/rapid pulse Declining state of consciousness	Fluids should be replaced. Frequent sips of vegetable/fruit juices or complete liquid oral supplements should be offered frequently, every 1–2 hours. Water should be offered. Foods should be pureed. Complete liquid supplements supply calories, protein, fat, electrolytes, vitamins, and minerals, and assist with hydration.
Diarrhea/ steatorrhea	Increase in frequency or softening of consistency "Floating" stools due to high fat content	A lactose-free diet is recommended. Water-soluble fiber found in fruits, oat bran, and legumes, can be beneficial in slowing intestinal transit time. Water-insoluble fiber found in wheat bran and most vegetables, may need

TABLE 7–2—**Continued**

Problem	Symptoms	Suggested Care Plan
		to be reduced because it tends to decrease intestinal transit time. If the stool is high in fat because of fat malabsorption, medium-chain-triglyceride (MCT) oil may benefit because it is readily absorbed. This requires a prescription and is expensive but may be used in place of regular cooking oils temporarily. In acute steatorrhea, minimize fat intake. If chronic, fat replacement per physician order may be necessary.
Weight loss	Loss of more than 10 pounds in 2 weeks, or loss resulting in body weight less than 80% of standard	High-calorie foods should be offered. Fat intake may need to be liberalized temporarily in order to promote weight gain without eating an overwhelming volume of food. Nutrient-dense foods should be offered, such as nuts, seeds, and foods from the four food groups, before pastries, ice cream, etc. Snacks should be offered between meals. Meal replacement oral liquid high-calorie, high-protein beverages are often beneficial.
Dry mouth Esophagitis Gastritis Thrush	Painful swallowing Stomach irritation Lesions in oral cavity and esophagus	Smooth liquids are better tolerated than are solids. Foods should be pureed. Cold foods are preferred over hot foods. Small frequent meals should be offered. If solids are consumed, copious liquids taken with each bite can make eating more tolerable. Spicy and acidic foods, such as citrus fruits and juices, should be avoided.
Fever	Body temperature over 98.6°F, or above the normal temperature	For every 1°-increase in temperature, calorie needs are increased by 7%. High-calorie, high-protein foods should be offered frequently.
Anorexia	Lack of appetite Inability or refusal to eat in adequate amounts to maintain nutritional status	Small frequent meals should be offered. Nutrient-dense foods and drinks should be offered rather than low- or no-calorie foods. Frozen dinners, canned foods, etc., that are easy to prepare quickly can be purchased. Offer favorite foods in comfortable surroundings with family or friends.

Table 7-2—**Continued**

Ways to Increase Calories and Protein

1. Use whole milk, cream, "half and half," or nondairy creamers on cereals and in cooking.
2. Bread and fry meats, fish, and chicken.
3. Add sauces or gravy to meat, pasta, potatoes, rice, etc.
4. Prepare foods with generous amounts of margarine, cream cheese, sour cream, cheese, and mayonnaise.
5. Add nonfat dry milk to foods to increase calories and protein, such as puddings, scrambled eggs, meat loaf, casseroles, hot cereals, etc.
6. Add raisins, other dried fruit, and nuts to hot or cold cereal, ice cream, and other deserts.

Commercial Calorie-Containing Supplements

If unable to consume adequate foods, a commercial supplement that contains calories as well as vitamins and minerals may be necessary. Products can be consumed in the form in which they are sold, mixed into milk or water, or added to recipes. The following products are available in grocery stores or pharmacies:

Ensure (lactose-free)
Ensure Plus (lactose-free)
Resource Crystals (lactose-free)
Carnation Instant Breakfast
Nutrament
Slender
Alba
Meritene Powder
Sustacal
Citrotein
Nutri 1000

REHABILITATION TEAM MEMBER CONTRIBUTIONS

With AIDS as well as with other chronic progressive diseases, the goal of rehabilitation is to lessen the impact of AIDS-related disability on the patient's everyday life. An AIDS patient may have restorative goals after recovering from a serious bout with an opportunistic infection. Although the patient should not be limited in setting restorative goals, it is not realistic for a person with a diagnosis of AIDS to expect to lead a completely normal life. During periods when the person feels well, the rehabilitation team should stress the importance of employing the health promotion measures previously discussed.

Different members of the health care team assume varying roles during the course of the patient's illness, from initial diagnosis through bouts with opportun-

TABLE 7–3. **Sample Home Care Plan:
Respiratory Therapy**

Problem	Potential Causes	Related Findings	Response
Shortness of breath	Pneumonia	Fever, cough, tachypnea, cyanosis	Contact physician Pentamidine aerosol treatment Oxygen
	Bronchitis	Loose cough, wheezing, rales	Contact physician Bronchodilator and aerosol therapy Postural drainage and percussion
Loose, nonproductive cough	Pneumonia, bronchitis, malnutrition, and reduced lung capacity	Course rales, rhonchi, dyspnea	Postural drainage and percussion Bland mist aerosol Cough training Hydration Note color and consistency of sputum
Coughing up blood (hemoptysis)	Pneumonia, post-bronchos-copy, harsh coughing	Fever, dyspnea, tachypnea	Observe color and quantity of blood and sputum Contact physician

istic infections to hospice care at the end of the patient's life. The advantages of the team approach are important to both patient and HCW.

The rehabilitation team should consist of 2 or more representatives from the disciplines involved in patient care and committed to evaluation, treatment, and education.[5] Physicians, nurses, social workers, psychologists, recreational therapists, physical therapists, occupational therapists, dietitians, respiratory therapists, and speech pathologists can serve on the team. Members of the first 3 disciplines usually serve as team leaders. Leadership varies according to the stage of the patient's illness. Team interaction and clear communication are vital throughout the course of the patient's illness.

Family members, lovers, or friends who are caregivers should also be included on the rehabilitation team. Goals should be mutually agreed upon by the patient and his or her caregivers. Caregivers should be willing to adjust goals downward as the patient's disease progresses.

TABLE 7–4. **Sample Home Care Plan:**
Occupational Therapy

Problem	Objective	Treatment Method
Low function in self-care: Toiletry and grooming takes until 10 AM	Be able to finish toiletry, bathing, teeth, hair, makeup by 9 AM.	Evaluate each task in terms of personal needs and more efficient ways of completing sooner, *e.g.*, placing grooming aids at hand and reacher for picking things up from floor, supplying toothpaste squeezer, and scheduling bowel and bladder functions.
Muscle weakness	Develop a plan enabling patient to accept varying levels of weakness.	Select activities that can be graded to altered functional levels, *e.g.*, pleasurable crafts/play for restoring self-worth and social interaction.
Low endurance, fatigue	Pace schedule and conserve energy, keeping tasks within energy level.	Rearrange furniture, appliances, etc., for easy reach; supply light handle on appliances/utensils, supply adaptive holders/handles, spread chores out at more convenient times, *e.g.*, 2 each morning when energy level is higher.
	Arrange home for accessibility and efficient use of space.	Remove barriers, *e.g.*, throw rugs, extra furniture; replace door knobs and faucets with level handles; add ramp steps and grab bars at transfer support areas.
Meal preparation and purchasing	Organize food purchase and preparation.	Arrange for meal service ("Meals-on-Wheels") and assistance with grocery shopping.
Depression, self-isolation, lack of self-assertiveness, reduced social interaction, poor family communication, changed role in work/play, alienation	Be more active and communicative in desired social group.	Increase confidence by promoting independence in self-care. Arrange individual social interactions with family/friends, *e.g.*, short visits, phone calls, offering to do phone chores for others, run answering service. Set up buddy system. Attend AIDS support group.
Cognitive dysfunction	Increase self-control.	Use verbal/visual cues. Plan daily routine. Use written/verbal reminders. Use medication reminder devices.

TABLE 7–4—**Continued**

Problem	Objective	Treatment Method
Lack of knowledge of services, devices, environmental control	Increase independence and self-confidence in control.	Select adaptive devices for efficiency in daily activities. Secure devices for assistance: cane, walker, speaker phone, handicapped parking, computer controls for home appliances, security.
Lack of avocational/ recreational activities	Identify activities that can be satisfying and involve others.	Participate in short-term crafts/arts/ games, etc. that include others. Examples: serve as advisor to sports activity group, sell subscriptions to sports magazines.

Rehabilitation team members should be flexible. Constant re-evaluation of the patient's status is required. The patient may be competently performing activities of daily living (ADL) one day and the next day be unable to perform them safely. Any team member—from social worker to physical therapist—may discover this change in status and communicate it to other team members, with a consequent change in short-term goals.

Occupational therapists can assist in modifying or make suggestions for modifying the home environment to enable the PWA to function as independently as possible. Adaptive or assistive devices may be needed, such as grab bars by toilets, hand rails by steps, lever openers for doors, and appropriate lighting, appliance, and phone controls. Occupational therapists may develop energy-conserving plans helpful to both patient and caregiver.

Physical or occupational therapists may teach caregivers how to assist the patient with passive range-of-motion exercises. Gentle massage may also be soothing to the patient. Home caregivers may need 24-hour-a-day assistance from an attendant assigned through a hospice or visiting nurse organization. Hospice buddies or volunteers from an AIDS organization can provide respite to the regular caretakers when the patient care needs become continuous.

THE CHILD WITH AIDS

Most children with AIDS acquire the virus from their infected mothers before or during birth, through either the placenta or the birth canal. Before the safety of the blood supply was ensured through screening, some children were infected

TABLE 7–5. **Sample Home Care Plan:**
Physical Therapy

Problem	Objective	Skilled Intervention
Generalized weakness, or decreased strength	Strength will increase from "fair minus" grade to "fair plus" grade in 4 weeks, or strength will increase from "fair plus" grade to "good minus" grade in 4 weeks.	Strengthening exercises Progressive resistive exercises (PREs)
Impaired independence in transfers	Patient will be independent in transfers, or patient will increase level of independence from minimal assistance to standby assistance in 2 weeks.	Transfer training: bed to commode, bed to toilet, toilet to shower, and return
Pain (localized)	Patient will be 90% free of pain, or patient will decrease from an 8 to a 5 (scale 1–10) in stated number of sessions.	Apply alternate warm/ cold treatments to affected area Gentle range of motion exercises Massage
Loss of safety awareness	Patient will be aware of safety measures in the home.	Instruct patient and caregiver on safety awareness (*e.g.*, removing throw rugs)
Decreased range of motion (ROM)	Patient will gain 25% in range of motion in 3 weeks, or patient will be functionally within normal limits in 4 weeks.	Range of motion exercise for upper extremities: use dowel, shoulder flexion, elbow abduction, and wrist flexion/extension Active exercise of hip flexors, knee flexors/ extensors, and ankle dorsi/plantar flexors Neck and back flexion/ extension and rotation
Impaired balance and coordination in standing, or during ambulation	Patient will maintain sitting balance 2 minutes, or patient will stand independently for 30 seconds or 1 minute.	Balance activities in sitting, "all fours" Sitting: maintain sitting for 2 minutes Supine to sit, sit to supine

TABLE 7–5—**Continued**

Problem	Objective	Skilled Intervention
		Hands and knees: maintain 1 minute, lift 1 extremity, assume position Kneeling: maintain position, assume position Standing: maintain standing 30 seconds, stand on one leg 10 seconds
Impaired independence in ambulation	Patient will be independent in ambulation with pickup walker, or patient will require supervision or standby assistance during ambulation.	Gait-training (4-point gait with pickup walker or 2-point gait with crutches, depending on level of independence)
Skin breakdown (state site)	Skin will be checked twice daily and will be 99% free of breakdown. If ambulatory, check heels and toes before putting on shoes and when removing. If non-ambulatory, check all bony prominences, especially elbows, hips and heels.	Instruct patient and caregiver about skin care.

through transfusion of blood or blood products. Less than 2% of the known cases of AIDS involve children, although the number of HIV-infected children is growing, especially in areas of high intravenous drug use. Most pediatric AIDS patients are preschool children who die before they begin school.[6]

Schools and Day Care Centers

Not one case of AIDS is known to have been transmitted in a school, day care, or foster care setting. The chief danger posed by an HIV-infected child attending school is to the infected child, because his or her immune system is damaged. Children with damaged immune systems risk suffering severe complications from infections commonly contracted in school or day care centers, such as chicken-pox, tuberculosis, herpes, measles, and other diseases.

The child's physician should evaluate the risk of infection, based on the child's immune status. The risk of acquiring some infections, such as chickenpox, may be reduced by prompt administration of specific immunoglobulin following exposure.

Fear of AIDS on the part of teachers, staff, and parents will probably cause the greatest trauma to the child with AIDS who attends a day care center or school. Administrators, teachers, and school nurses are responsible for ensuring the confidentiality of information about a child's HIV status or about a diagnosis of AIDS. Past inability to keep this type of information confidential concerns those charged with protecting confidentiality now. The "need to know" rule should apply, with only those staff members who are responsible for protection of both the infected child and of other students being informed.

Because AIDS has been classified as a handicapping condition, entry into school may not be denied a child with AIDS. Theoretically, transmission is possible through contact with body fluids known to be infective (blood, semen, and vaginal fluid), although there is no case on record of this type of transmission occurring in schools. A restricted environment within the school or day care center may have to be arranged for neurologically handicapped children who lack control of their body secretions, or who display behavior such as biting, and for children who have uncoverable, bleeding lesions. Staff should use the same precautions used in health care institutions in handling infectious body fluids (see Chapter 4).

Adoptive and foster care agencies may wish to consider adding HIV testing to their routine medical evaluations. Placement parents should be aware of the additional medical care such children will require. In some areas of the country, caring and compassionate people have established homes that serve such children exclusively. This arrangement is preferable to allowing infected infants to be reared in hospitals.

The chief responsibility of school and day care staff is *education* about ways the HIV is transmitted and ways it is not. Misinformation must be replaced with accurate information. School nurses and other health personnel who work in schools must serve as reliable sources of information for students, parents, and staff members.

DISCUSSION QUESTIONS

1. Why should AIDS patients focus on quality living?
2. What may influence the way an HCW counsels an AIDS patient about sexual activity?
3. What are the pressures facing a person with an HIV-positive status? A person

experiencing the first recognizable symptoms of AIDS? A person with a diagnosis of AIDS?

4. What support groups serve PWAs in your community?
5. What benefits may a PWA realize from using health promotion measures?
6. What concerns are home caregivers most likely to express?
7. In what areas can your profession help a patient achieve quality living with AIDS?
8. What topics would you discuss if invited to speak to a group of elementary and/or secondary teachers about HIV-infected students in schools?

REFERENCES

1. Maslow, A: Fusion of facts and values. Am J Psychoanal 23:117, 1963.
2. Wollingscrift, J (quoted by Wolfsy, C.): Diseases-a-month. The Nation's Health, September 1988:18.
3. Llaurado, J: The saga of BHT and BHA in life extension myths. J Am Coll Nutr 4:481, 1985.
4. California Medical Association: Health tips: Raw milk: Is it really better for you? California Medical Association, Index 430, San Francisco, 1983.
5. Anderson, TP: Rehabilitation management and the rehabilitation team. In Basmajan, JV and Kirby, RL (eds): Medical Rehabilitation. Williams & Wilkins, Baltimore, 1984.
6. Black, JL: AIDS: Preschool and school issues. J Sch Health 56(3):93, 1986.

EIGHT

ECONOMIC IMPACT OF AIDS ON THE HEALTH CARE SYSTEM

Elizabeth A. Rogers

OUTLINE

OBJECTIVES

By the close of this chapter, the reader will be able to:
1. Describe the national economic impact of AIDS.
2. Cite and summarize studies about hospital costs of treating AIDS patients.
3. List and describe factors contributing to the costs of treating AIDS patients.
4. Describe types of indirect costs of caring for persons with AIDS.

171

5. Compare and contrast costs by area of the country.
6. Identify and describe various sources for financing care.
7. Identify some of the problems faced by uninsured patients.
8. Explore alternative ways of lowering costs of care.
9. Assess current studies on the costs of HIV infection.
10. Consider the effect of the AIDS epidemic on worldwide economics.
11. Project the economic impact of AIDS in the next decade.

CHALLENGE TO THE HEALTH PROFESSIONS

The economic impact of AIDS creates a challenge to health care institutions in the present climate of cost containment. How society responds to the AIDS epidemic will influence the future of health care for all Americans.

Today hospital boards and trustees fulfill the role of business managers. A health care institution that is not operated in a cost-effective manner faces possible closure, merger, sell-out, or give-away to a corporation that will attempt to make it profitable.

"AIDS will bring us face to face with many issues including equality of access to care, the ability of the providers to maintain their caring traditions in the face of infection dangers for the health care worker, burnout of employees, and potential bankruptcy for those shouldering the burden of what will probably be substantial uncompensated care," states Barbara McCool,[1] associate editor of the Health Care Management Review and president of Strategic Management Services in Shawnee Mission, Kansas. She asks, "Will the danger and harsh outcome of this disease put us in danger of losing our primary focus of compassion for the poor and the suffering?"

The confrontation of moral, ethical, and professional codes with the pressures of technology and the AIDS epidemic will truly test the individual and collective mettle of health care providers and managers.

The national economic impact of AIDS has barely been felt. The costs associated with infectious diseases make up less than 5% of the costs associated with all diseases in the United States. In certain geographic locations, however, the effects have already been felt; cities with high numbers of cases are straining their resources to meet the needs. As the epidemic spreads, both large and small communities will face mounting economic pressure.

COSTS ASSOCIATED WITH THE AIDS EPIDEMIC

Studies evaluating the actual costs of care for persons with AIDS (PWAs) are limited by the difficulty of identifying AIDS patients through studying medical records. The allocation of costs to other diagnoses may hide the real number of

AIDS cases. Costs of care also vary by area and according to the characteristics of PWAs treated.

Scitovsky[33] describes the characteristics of PWAs. In the United States, 99% of PWAs are adults or adolescents. Pediatric cases equal less than 1% of the total. By gender, 93% of the adults or adolescents are male. By age, 90% fall into the 20- to 49-year-old group. Seventy-three percent of these individuals are homosexual or bisexual, including 8% who are intravenous drug users. An additional 17% are intravenous drug users but are not homosexual or bisexual males. Four percent of PWAs are heterosexual. Hemophiliacs or persons who received blood transfusions or blood products comprise 3% of PWAs.

Minorities are disproportionately represented in the PWA total (see Chapter 5). Comparing risk behaviors with ethnicity, 74% of the homosexual and bisexual males with AIDS are white, while 80% of the intravenous drug users with AIDS are black or Hispanic.

To date, the AIDS epidemic has been concentrated in a number of metropolitan centers: New York City (23%), San Francisco (9%), Los Angeles (8%), Houston, Washington, DC, and Miami (each 3%). A shift is occurring from these 6 centers. In 1984, 43% of new cases reported were outside these centers, and this had increased to 58% by 1987. By 1991, the Centers for Disease Control (CDC) expect that 63% of all new cases will be outside of these 6 locations.

Distribution by risk group or risk behavior differs across the United States. In New York City, 61% of PWAs are homosexual or bisexual males and 31% are intravenous drug users. San Francisco reports 97% of PWAs are homosexual or bisexual males.

The major cost factor for a PWA is the number of days per admission. The number of days per admission is lowest in San Francisco (11 days), as compared with Los Angeles (19 days), Boston (21 days), and New York City (20–25 days). Two other factors are much less variable in different geographic regions: (1) the average number of admissions per year or per PWA's lifetime and (2) the average costs of charges per hospital day. Patients with the diagnosis of Kaposi's sarcoma are slightly more expensive to treat than patients with *Pneumocystis carinii* pneumonia or other infectious diseases associated with AIDS.

In 1986, Hardy and colleagues[2] estimated the economic impact of the first 10,000 cases of AIDS in the United States. Three factors were considered: cost of hospitalizations, resources lost because of disability, and resources lost because of premature death. This study determined the national average for patients' "length-of-stay" by surveying hospitals in 3 cities: New York City, Philadelphia, and San Francisco. According to the CDC, surveillance files indicated that AIDS patients in New York City and San Francisco each accounted for 11% of the national AIDS population, and AIDS patients in Philadelphia accounted for 2%. Average length of initial hospitalization was 31 days. No data on rehospitalizations were obtained. Hospital charges for 35 hospitalizations over a 17-month period were determined. Using a mean cost of $828/day in an acute care facility, the researchers calculated that the overall cost per patient was $147,000.

Hardy and colleagues[3] also calculated earnings lost because of disability at an 86% rate. This figure was based on information available from New York City indicating that 14% of AIDS patients worked during the 3 months before follow-up or death. Using age- and gender-specific employment rates, they calculated that potential earnings lost because of disability were $189 million. At approximately 2 years after the diagnosis of AIDS, the mortality of PWAs approaches 100%. The researchers discounted expected lifetime earnings by 4% to convert future earnings into their present day value. They calculated the cost of early death for the 10,000 persons to be $4.6 billion. The grand total of expenditures for hospitalization, loss of income because of disability, and loss of income because of premature death for these first 10,000 cases of AIDS in the United States was calculated to be $6.3 billion.

Factors Contributing to the Higher Cost of Treating AIDS Patients

The cost of acute care for an AIDS patient is above the average cost of care for other patients. Several factors contribute to this situation. A major expense in caring for PWAs is the extra nursing requirements. Green and colleagues[4] estimate the nursing requirements of AIDS patients to be 40% higher than requirements of other patients. Nursing accounts for 25% of hospital costs for PWAs.

Inservice and continuing education about universal precautions for infection control add to indirect health care costs. Physicians, nurses, and allied health professionals must be kept abreast of the latest information on AIDS. Nonprofessional staff, such as patient transporters, meal deliverers, and housekeepers, must be trained. The cost of training them is high because there is often a high turnover of staff in these areas.

Implementation of universal precautions is also costly. The cost of using supplies such as gloves, gowns, masks, and eye coverings mounts. Appropriate disposal of contaminated articles and infectious wastes adds to costs. Some institutions make it a policy to double-bag nondisposable items. This practice is another cost factor.

Hospital costs are also higher when a patient needs a private room. The CDC states that placing an AIDS patient in a private room is not necessary unless the patient has a communicable disease necessitating isolation. Generally, this additional cost is not borne by third-party payers.

Drugs for treating AIDS are major contributors to the high cost of care. Zidovudine (azidothymidine, or AZT) and aerosol pentamidine are apparently effective life extenders for many patients but are expensive; AZT costs approximately $8000/year and causes side-effects that may require the patient to have blood transfusions to combat anemia. No studies are yet available on the costs and benefits of these drugs. Future developments in treatment make it impossible to project costs for the next decade.

Two estimates of the indirect costs of the AIDS epidemic in the United States were available at the time of publication in 1989. These indirect costs were calculated in terms of loss of productivity resulting from the illness and especially from premature death. Both Hardy[34] and Scitovsky[35] used the human capital method to make estimates. With this method, morbidity costs are wages lost by people who are unable to work because of illness and disability, and mortality costs are the present value of future earnings lost by people who die prematurely.

Hardy[36] estimated the indirect costs of the first 10,000 cases at $4.8 billion or 3 1/2 times her estimate of the hospital costs of PWAs. Scitovsky[37] estimated indirect costs in current dollars at $3.9 billion in 1985, $7 billion 1986, and $55.6 billion in 1991—or almost 7 times the direct medical care costs. In that same study, mortality costs represented about 94% of indirect costs. Mortality costs are high because PWAs are concentrated among males in their most productive years.

Care Costs

Scitovsky and Rice[5] provide the most comprehensive study to date on the costs associated with AIDS, both direct and indirect. They reviewed costs for 1985 and 1986 and made estimates for 1991. Direct costs include expenditures not only for acute care hospital services but also for physician inpatient and outpatient services, other outpatient ancillary services, nursing home care, home health services, and hospice. Nonpersonal costs such as costs associated with research, blood screening, replacement of blood, health education and support services were also estimated. Morbidity costs (costs associated with loss of productivity because of disability) and mortality costs (potential future earnings lost because of premature death from AIDS), both of which are indirect costs, were also calculated.

No attempt was made to estimate the dollar value of services provided by community-based volunteer organizations. Also, there was no estimate made of the psychological costs of AIDS for patients and their families.

Estimates for health care costs were obtained by a retrospective study of AIDS patients treated at San Francisco General Hospital (SFGH) in 1984.[6] Costs associated with treating 3 types of AIDS patients were studied. The 3 types were patients admitted to SFGH in 1984 with an AIDS diagnosis (n = 445); AIDS patients who received both inpatient and outpatient care at SFGH in 1984 (n = 201); and AIDS patients who died in 1984 and who had received all their hospital and inpatient professional services at SFGH from diagnosis to death (n = 85). Monthly medical expenses were lowest ($586) for patients who were alive during this 12-month period; highest ($3660) for those who died during the 12-month period, who had lived an average of 6.4 months of the year; and between these extremes ($2617) for patients newly diagnosed in 1984, who had expenses for an average of 4.6 months. Within these 3 categories patients were also classified into 3 diagnostic groups: patients suffering *Pneumocystis carinii* pneumonia (PCP), pa-

TABLE 8–1. **Length of Stay, Daily Hospital Costs, and Outpatient Costs for Persons With AIDS in the United States**

	Range		
	Low	*Medium*	*High*
Length of stay	13 days	20 days	25 days
Daily cost	$740.00	$850.00	$950.00
Outpatient cost*	$4,000.00	$3,000.00	$2,000.00

*The researchers assumed that patients receiving inpatient care would receive less outpatient services.

Data from Seage, GR III, et al: Medical costs of ambulatory patients with AIDS-related complex (ARC) and/or generalized lymphadenopathy (GLS) related to HIV infection. Am J Public Health 78:969, 1988.

tients suffering Kaposi's sarcoma (KS), and patients suffering other infectious diseases. Patients with KS were slightly less expensive to treat than patients in the other 2 diagnostic groups.

Average number of hospital admissions was 1.7–2.2 admissions per patient. Table 8–1 shows the range of costs for inpatient and outpatient care.

Direct costs include both direct costs and nonpersonal costs. *Direct Costs:* hospital services, physician inpatient and outpatient services, outpatient ancillary services, nursing home, home care, and hospice. *Nonpersonal Costs:* research, blood screening and testing, replacement of blood, health education, and support services.

Indirect costs include both morbidity costs and mortality costs. *Morbidity Costs:* value of productivity losses due to illness and disability. *Mortality Costs:* present value of future earnings lost for those who die prematurely as a result of AIDS.

Direct Costs

Scitovsky and Rice[7] found it difficult to estimate nonpersonal costs. They classified the following items as nonpersonal services that are direct costs of AIDS: research projects funded by federal and state agencies, blood screening services, and support services provided by local governments and community-based organizations. Examples of support services included: counseling; emotional and spiritual care of patients and their families and friends; housing; and assistance with shopping and transportation. Table 8–2 provides estimates of cost for nonpersonal services.

TABLE 8-2. **Estimated Nonpersonal Services Cost of AIDS* in the United States**

Year	
1985	$232 million to $303 million
1986	$405 million to $486 million
1991	$900 million to $2.5 billion

*Estimated using 27% of health care costs and calculated using 1984 dollars.
Data from Scitovsky, AA, and Rice, DP: Estimates of the direct and indirect costs of Acquired Immunodeficiency Syndrome in the United States: 1985, 1986 and 1991. Public Health Rep 102:5, 1987.

The best estimate of 1985 personal health care expenditures in the United States indicates the $630 million (estimated yearly cost of AIDS) represents 0.2% of total national health care expenditures. The estimate for 1991—$8.5 billion—represents 1.4% of estimated 1991 personal health care expenditures. These costs are relatively low when compared with costs associated with other illnesses, such as cancer, kidneys and heart disease.

Scitovsky[8] acknowledges that there are no hard data on the number of persons with HIV infection but not diagnosed with full-blown AIDS. However, it is estimated that 2–10 times the number of persons with AIDS are seeking medical care because of HIV infection or they are worried about HIV infection. Estimates of persons infected range from 0.5 to 1.5 million. Scitovsky states that it is clear that the total direct costs of HIV epidemic will far exceed the $8.5 billion in 1991. She thinks this estimate may be doubled or even more than twice as high.

Bloom and Carliner[9] analysed 7 previous studies on the costs of AIDS. All personal health care costs were translated to 1986 dollars. The cost per AIDS patient ranged from $23,000[10] to $168,000.[11] Individual case costs estimated by Scitovsky[12] were as follows: low range $43,000, medium range $68,000, and high range $115,000.

Bloom and Carliner suggest that the lifetime cost of health care per AIDS patient should not exceed $80,000. Using this figure they project that the total costs for the 270,000 AIDS cases that experts predict will be diagnosed by the end of 1991 will not exceed $22 billion. They believe this expense should not have a major impact on total health care expenditures in the United States. They do warn that an economic impact is to be expected in places such as San Francisco and New York City. A comparison of 1986 AIDS patients in 1986 with projected figures for 1991 is found in Table 8-3.

Taxes to support such care will rise. If the CDC's predictions are correct, 8700 new cases of AIDS will be diagnosed in New York City in 1991. Based on Bloom's lifetime treatment figure of $80,000 per case, New York City residents would have

TABLE 8–3. **Percent of Medical/Surgical Beds Filled by AIDS Patients and Percent of Health Care Cost for Persons With AIDS in the United States**

Area	Bed Utilization (%)		Health Care Cost (%)
	1986	1991	1991
San Francisco	2.7	12.4	16.2
New York City	3.0	8.1	8.4
Nationally	0.4	1.9	3.0

Data from Bloom, DE and Carliner, G: The economic impact of AIDS in the United States. Science 239:604, 1988.

to share a tax increase of $100 per resident each year to care for persons with newly diagnosed AIDS. The CDC projects that 5900 new AIDS cases will be diagnosed in San Francisco during 1991. Based on a $40,000 lifetime treatment figure, local residents would have to contribute $350 apiece annually. Other groups that will share the costs of care for AIDS patients are insurance companies, government agencies, and patients themselves. In 1987 local taxes in New York City paid 27% of the total costs associated with AIDS.

Bloom and Carliner's[13] comparative study indicates that cumulative medical costs will range from $6.3 billion to $45.5 billion by 1991. Total cost was affected by the wide variation in estimates of lifetime number of inpatient days, from 34 to 168 days. Inpatient hospital costs ranged from $683 to $1003.

Indirect Costs

Morbidity costs, calculated in 1984 dollars, are presented in Table 8–4. Scitovsky and Rice[8] calculated mortality costs using a 4% and a 6% discount rate. Table 8–5 presents the estimated mortality costs of AIDS, in lifetime earnings calculated in 1984 dollars.

Nonpersonal Costs

Nonpersonal costs of AIDS are substantial. The federal government currently spends more on research and education about AIDS than on treatment of AIDS. State and local agencies, universities, and drug companies also spend money on AIDS. The total amount that has been spent is unknown.

Blood testing for the human immunodeficiency virus (HIV) is also expensive; figures reflecting the expenses of private firms that do this testing are not avail-

TABLE 8-4. **Estimated Morbidity Cost of AIDS in the United States***

Year	
1985	$251 million
1986	$421 million
1991	$2.3 billion

*Calculated in 1984 dollars.

Data from Scitovsky, AA and Rice, DP: Estimates of the direct and indirect costs of Acquired Immunodeficiency Syndrome in the United States: 1985, 1986 and 1991. Public Health Rep 102:5, 1987.

able. The federal government alone spent $79 million in 1986 and $76 million in 1987, and projected it would spend $55 million in 1988 for HIV testing. Most of this money was spent on testing military personnel and new recruits. In 1986, $50 million was spent on testing 12 pints of blood collected in the United States. How much private firms and individuals spend on testing is not known.[39]

Scitovsky and Rice[14] estimate that nonpersonal direct costs of AIDS accounted for 33% of all AIDS-related costs in 1986. They predict those costs will decrease to 21% of total costs in 1991.

Presently AIDS most often affects people who are young and in their most productive years. Bloom and Carliner[15] estimate that lost earnings are 6–8 times more than the $80,000 per AIDs patient in health care costs. This loss will be the most dramatic economic impact.

TABLE 8-5. **Estimated Mortality Cost of AIDS in the United States***

Year	6% Discount Rate	4% Discount Rate
1985	$2.8 billion	$3.5 billion
1986	$4.8 billion	$6.0 billion
1991	$28.6 billion	$36.3 billion

*Based on lifetime earnings calculated in 1984 dollars.

Data from Scitovsky, AA and Rice, DP: Estimates of the direct and indirect costs of Acquired Immunodeficiency Syndrome in the United States: 1985, 1986 and 1991. Public Health Rep 102:5, 1987.

METHODS OF FINANCING CARE

Responsibility for financing direct costs of care for PWAs falls upon a variety of persons and groups: AIDS patients and their families, employers of PWAs, insurance companies, public and private hospitals, and federal, state, and local governments.

A federal taskforce endorses an AIDS federal grant program as an interim measure to ensure that PWAs and those with HIV-related conditions have access to appropriate and cost-effective care. Furthermore, the taskforce recommends that Medicare and private insurers consider reimbursement, but with cost-sharing provisions to limit the burden on public funds, for costly AIDS therapies and treatments. The taskforce acknowledges that priorities may need to be established among potential treatments. Directing monies to states and reimbursement for costly therapies would be temporary solutions. The federal government is being urged to provide leadership in developing a comprehensive national plan for delivering and financing care for the entire spectrum of HIV-infected persons. The taskforce recommends the following: coverage be from the onset of HIV infection, relief be extended to communities hardest hit by HIV infection, shared financial responsibility occurs between the public and private sector, and the payment mechanisms encourage cost-effective care of HIV-infected persons.[40]

Third-Party Payers

In today's health care market both the public and private sector have adopted the "prudent buyer" approach to the purchase of health care. Health care purchasers are shopping prudently and demanding more for their dollar. This approach is very reasonable, but it has brought the problems of uninsured persons into the limelight. Traditionally, health care institutions have financed care for uninsured persons by including these charges in the private-paying patient's bill. This practice has been discontinued in the present competitive health care market.

Private insurance typically pays health care costs associated with the onset of AIDS symptoms and hospitalizations. Patients without insurance must pay for health care themselves until they have spent nearly all of their assets and are declared disabled. Then they become eligible for Medicaid coverage in most states. Limits on income as an asset vary from state to state. The percentage of costs that can be reimbursed varies from region to region. The United States Veterans Administration pays some costs for AIDs patients who qualify. Private and public hospitals absorb a share of the costs because reimbursement from the previously mentioned sources usually does not cover 100% of costs. Generally, the patient is not capable of making up the difference. Figure 8–1 shows the types of medical coverage for patients with AIDs in 1988.

Before 1986, when an employee left employment, generally his or her health insurance coverage was discontinued. Federal regulations now stipulate that a

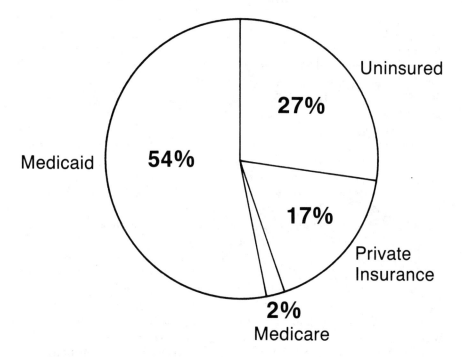

FIGURE 8-1. Types of medical coverage for patients with AIDS in 1988. (Data from Wilensky, GR.[16])

person may continue to pay for these benefits for up to 18 months, at a premium not to exceed 102% of the employer's costs. If AIDS patients can afford to continue coverage, this change will shift some of the burden back to private insurance.

Wilensky[16] suggests that there are at least 2 fundamental problems with the Medicaid system. The first is that eligibility is tied to the receipt of cash assistance. Secondly, each state can set the income level that it deems appropriate for cash assistance. Therefore, Wilensky suggests that 2 changes occur. Minimum federal standards for Medicaid income eligibility should be established. There also should be a severing of the link between the receipt of cash assistance and eligibility for Medicaid.

Caring for Uninsured Persons

Many persons with AIDS are young, minorities, poor, jobless, or homeless. These people frequently have no insurance and few personal resources. According to

Wilensky,[17] it is difficult to determine the exact number of uninsured Americans; the number is approximately 35 million. The following characteristics of uninsured persons, however, remain stable: about half of uninsured persons are employed; most employed uninsured persons (75%–80%) are low-wage earners, some of whom support dependents on an annual income of less than $10,000; despite low wages, only about 35% of uninsured families are below the poverty line; another 35%, however, have incomes less than half that required to live at the poverty line.

Two sources[18,19] suggest that health insurance risk pools for medically uninsurable perons be established. A combination of private and public sector funds should be used. With a shared commitment, there will be a great incentive to broaden support for AIDs treatment and research. It has been suggested that the burden for risk pools be shouldered in the private sector not only by group insurers but also by companies that provide individual coverage, self-insured employers, charities, churches, and private foundations.

The problem of "patient dumping" has become more acute because of increasing financial pressures on health care institutions as a result of cost-containment efforts by third-party payers (Medicare, Medicaid, and health insurance companies). The United States Department of Health and Human Services (DHHS)[20] regulations require that hospitals treat and stabilize any emergency room patient "until the condition ceases to be an emergency or until the patient is properly transferred to another facility." In case of violation, the regulations provide for a period of suspension of Medicare and Medicaid payments and possible civil penalties of up to $50,000 for the institution and each responsible physician. But the "anti-dumping" regulations have been criticized on the ground that they are too vague to be effective. Even the idea of "stabilizing" an acutely ill patient has been challenged as a dangerous means by which hospitals endeavor to transfer uninsured emergency patients to other institutions. To be medically sound, "stabilizing" a patient might involve surgery or several days of intensive care.[21]

In principle, patients with AIDS are no different from other patients except for the fact that they are often no longer employed and therefore without health insurance. Often they are medically indigent and dependent on Medicaid assistance, and thus vulnerable to "dumping" practices.

Alternative Ways to Lower Costs

When searching for alternative ways to lower costs, it is appropriate to consider the San Francisco model. Most metropolitan areas do not have the multisystem, multisource approach to patient care that this community does. Care in most communities for a PWA is provided in the acute care hospital. Patients often remain hospitalized longer than necessary because there is no plan for care outside the hospital setting. This is especially true for intravenous drug users and children with AIDS. In fact, many babies with AIDS are abandoned in the acute care hospital setting.

In San Francisco, there is a well-established health, political, and social system of care for persons who are HIV-infected. Dr. Don Abrams,[22] assistant director of the AIDS Clinic at San Francisco General Hospital [SFGH], states that "AIDS is essentially an outpatient disease." The length of stay in SFGH has dropped from 18 to 11 days because of outpatient services.

A multisystem and multiservice coordinated team approach has helped to reduce costs for treating PWAs. The San Francisco program depends heavily on volunteer agencies to help with transportation, cooking, cleaning of AIDS patients' homes, legal assistance, counseling services for patients, and their friends and family, and financial support. Included in outpatient services are home health visits by professionals, hospice care, and a variety of ancillary services formerly provided in the acute care setting. The efforts are coordinated by a case manager.

In 1987, the director of the AIDS Home Care and Hospice Program of San Francisco said that approximately 15% of the patients in the home care program needed 24-hour attendant care because of severe neurologic and physical status changes.[23] Treatment cost estimates from San Francisco for patients in skilled nursing care, intermediate care, and ambulatory care settings for AIDS patients range from $120–$300/day. In the AIDS Home Care and Hospice Program the cost is $94/day. The average cost at San Francisco General Hospital is $698/day.

There is some question about the appropriateness of placing AIDS patients in skilled nursing facilities. Occupancy rates are high and many centers have a waiting list. AIDS patients need more direct care than nursing homes can provide given present staffing patterns. Additionally, an AIDS patient might feel out of place with the geriatric clientele. There also could be fear on the part of nursing home residents and staff about the communicability of AIDS.

ALLOCATION OF RESOURCES

The issue of how much will be spent on AIDS research, prevention, and treatment must be addressed by both government and private agencies. Where should monies be targeted? Should certain groups be targeted to receive education and prevention information? For example, because there is a disproportionate number of black and Hispanic PWAs, should more funds be targeted for these groups? Will special funding for educating intravenous drug users yield adequate benefits for the costs?

Much education has been targeted to the gay male community in the United States, with apparent success in reducing high-risk behaviors.[24] Should education be targeted to reach individuals that do not self-identify as gay or bisexual but who participate in high-risk sexual activities? Education for so many diverse groups will be costly, and may yield poor results if persons in those groups do not perceive themselves as being at risk.

The major focus of this chapter has been on persons with full-blown AIDS. It is appropriate, however, to consider the care of all individuals who are infected with the HIV. At the time of this writing, there is very little information on the economic impact of HIV infection. No cost studies have been done since the definition of AIDS was expanded to include the "wasting syndrome" and AIDS dementia complex. Because the latency period for HIV infection keeps lengthening, it may be several years before an analysis covering the period from HIV infection to symptomatic AIDS can be completed.

Present economic impact studies indicate that AIDS probably will not have a great effect on the nation's attitudes toward health care insurance. Each study has been based on the assumption that risk factors and at-risk populations would remain stable. If the disease continues to spread to the heterosexual population then there will be a much greater economic threat. Also, it appears that none of the studies have dealt with the CDC's[25] prediction that 80% of PWAs in 1991 will reside outside of the current high-concentration areas of New York City and San Francisco. This switch in distribution of AIDS patients will have a direct economic effect on these areas.

INTERNATIONAL ECONOMIC IMPACT OF AIDS

Because the AIDS pandemic is still in its early stages, it is difficult to project the global effect of the disease. Dr. Jonathan Mann,[26] director of the World Health Organization (WHO) Special Programme on AIDS, stated that the global epidemic in 1988 would include 300,000 cases. This number equals the number of cases that have occurred since the 1970s. WHO[27] predicts there will be 1 million new cases of AIDS by 1992 among persons who are already infected. As of January 1989, AIDS is known to occur in 138 of the 175 countries that report to WHO[28] (Fig. 8–2).

Because the disease most commonly affects persons in the most productive age groups, AIDS will have a significant economic and social effect. Many patients are young and middle-aged adults who are employed in business and government. The Harvard Institute of International Development estimates that by 1995 the annual loss to Zaire from AIDS deaths will be $350 million, or 8% of the country's gross national product. Extrapolating to the rest of central Africa, a loss of $980 million by 1995 is estimated. It is conceivable that the social and economic impact of AIDS could lead to political destabilization of the countries involved.

Preliminary results of studies in 2 developing countries were given at the First International Conference on the Global Impact of AIDS. Zaire and Tanzania were studied by a cooperative team from the World Bank, Global Programme of AIDS, WHO, and the National AIDS Control Programme in Zaire and Tanzania.[41] Both

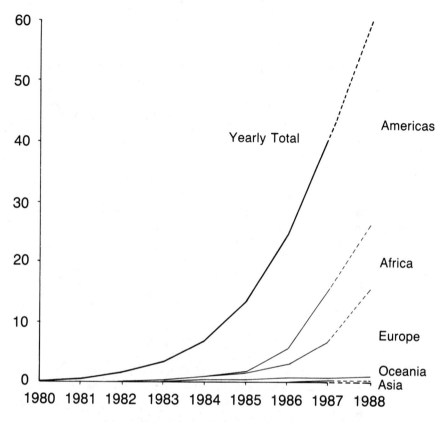

FIGURE 8-2. Worldwide cases of AIDS.

direct and indirect costs of AIDS were studied. The goals of the team were to propose an approach to estimate the costs of HIV infection in a developing country and to present estimates of the indirect costs as the value of the healthy years of life that are taken from society because of AIDS. In both cases studies of the direct costs per patient varied within a single country depending on clinical symptoms of the HIV infection, socioeconomic characteristics of the patient, and characteristics of health care options available. Range of estimates for direct care in Zaire were $132 to $1585 and in Tanzania were $104 to $6311.[42] Indirect cost estimates ranged from $890 ot $2,663 in Zaire and from $2,425 to $5,053 in Tanzania.[43]

In doing the calculations on direct and indirect costs, no attempt was made at calculations of AIDS prevention and its effect on costs. If this calculation is attempted, it must account for the fact that for each primary case prevented, secondary and tertiary cases also are prevented.[44]

Nearly half of all hospital beds in affected central African countries are occupied by PWAs. It is predicted that total adult mortality will have been doubled or tripled by the 1990s. Additionally, because between 10%–25% of the women of childbearing age in central Africa are HIV-infected, an increase in child mortality of at least 25% is expected. This rate will nullify gains that have been made in the last 20 years by child survival programs.

The health care systems of these countries are unable to cope with the present 100,000 patients with AIDS. Projections for another 400,000 cases by 1993 present a serious challenge to national governments and external assistance groups.

Brazil, which has the third largest number of AIDS cases in the world (the United States reported the largest number, France the second largest number), has identified AIDS as a disease needing priority attention.[29] Until recently, other diseases such as malaria, tuberculosis, schistosomiasis, and yellow fever were priority diseases because of the number of deaths they caused each year. Brazil has a massive foreign debt, and approximately 60% of the population lives in "absolute poverty." The government of Brazil currently invests only 4% of its gross national product on its health care system, as compared with 10% in some European countries and in the United States.

Seventy-eight percent of the AIDS cases reside in Brazil's 2 principal cities, Rio de Janeiro and São Paulo. Treatment of AIDS patients has occurred mainly in university hospitals. The national health care system pays these hospitals about $200 per patient for lifetime treatment. Hospitals are expected to absorb the difference between the $200 and the actual cost of care. Large corporations are working with the government to fund blood screening and patient care. The Ministries of Health and Education are working together in this, the world's largest Catholic nation, to place AIDS and sex education in public school curricula for the first time.

In Asia and the Pacific, 4 countries had reported cases of AIDS as of June 1988. Of the 892 cases reported, 890 were in Australia and New Zealand. Other countries in Asia and the Pacific have generally low rates of reported HIV infection and few AIDS patients. In China and Japan the largest number of documented HIV infections are among people to whom imported blood or blood products were administered before 1986. In absolute and relative terms the number of AIDS patients is very low. Also, very few female prostitutes are infected. Two exceptions should be mentioned: in the Philippines, the prostitute infection rate is 0.5%, and in India 6%.[30] Bangkok, Thailand has approximately 60,000 intravenous drug users; approximately 16% of these persons are infected. These infected persons may provide a major source of sexual transmission to other members of the community.

Rothermel,[45] of the United Nations Development Programme, reported at the first International Conference on the Global Impact of AIDS in March 1988 that the prospect in some of the poorest developing countries, based on present HIV infection levels, is that the death rate from AIDS could equal or exceed the number of deaths from all other causes by the early 1990s. Excluding the pediatric population who will die of AIDS, the men and women who will die are generally in the 20- to 40-year-old age bracket, depriving countries already lacking in human resources their most productive citizens. At the same Conference, Rothermel[46] indicated the necessity of rethinking development priorities and programs for developing countries just to cope with the AIDS crisis.

The United Nations has responded to the AIDS epidemic, especially in developing countries.[47] There are 2 objectives: (1) development and implementation of AIDS prevention and control, and (2) international leadership for coordination and cooperation through the WHO Global Programme on AIDS. Also, the United Nations (U.N.) is working with UNICEF on the impact of AIDS on mothers, children, and family life. The World Bank has begun studies on the direct and indirect costs of AIDS in developing countries. Another global project being directed by the U.N. is the Global Blood Safety Initiative. The purpose of the project is to make blood supplies safe throughout the world and thus stop the spread of AIDS and other diseases.[48]

The goals of the WHO Special Programme on AIDS[31] are threefold: (1) prevent new HIV infections, (2) provide care for persons already infected, and (3) develop national and international AIDS networks. The first 2 goals will consume considerable resources. For example, screening the blood supply is costly. Providing education and protective supplies for all health care institutions and workers is costly. Education about sexual and perinatal transmission of the HIV is costly and difficult given cultural values in many countries.

Most developing countries have limited financial resources. Volunteer organizations, churches, and other international aid groups are needed to assist not only financially, but also with personnel, supplies, and education.

WHO is pursuing its third goal by establishing national AIDs committees. WHO has already received requests for technical assessments and evaluations from 151 countries, of whom 137 had received that assistance by 1988.[32] Historically, there seems to be no record of public health efforts ever having been mobilized so quickly and with such intensity.

CHALLENGE OF THE FUTURE

As of 1989, the cost estimates for care of a PWA are uncertain for several reasons. Data sources for cost studies vary. Methods used to estimate direct health care costs attributable to AIDS also vary. The geographic specificity of research studies may limit the generalizability of findings to other locales. Some of the studies excluded nonhospital costs such as drugs, ambulatory services, long-term care, hospice, home health, and counseling services. Apparently, no studies estimated the cost of community services provided to AIDS patients.

The trend in treatment for PWAs is toward fewer hospitalizations per patient and shorter lengths of stay. There seems to be greater reliance on outpatient care and community support services that allow the patient to leave the hospital sooner or to avoid hospitalization altogether. This shift in care will directly affect costs.

New treatment regimens will influence health care costs. It is not clear if these protocols will increase or decrease overall cost of health care for PWAs. Will possible decreases in expense by using new treatments be offset by the need for closer monitoring? Will the increase in life expectancy (and hope of lowered costs) be negated by the fact that patients may die from other AIDS-related disorders?

How will the expansion of the definition of AIDS to include dementia and wasting syndrome affect costs? Treatment of the patient with AIDS dementia may be more expensive than any of the previous studies reflect.

According to *Confronting AIDS: Update 1988,* some headway is being made gathering information on all aspects of the costs of care for persons with HIV-related conditions. Proposed studies are expected to examine:

1. The total costs of health, social, and support services for AIDS patients and patients with HIV-related conditions
2. The cost of treating AIDS compared with the cost of treating other types of conditions in general
3. The costs of treating AIDS at various stages of the disease
4. The cost-effectiveness of various treatment protocols
5. The costs and benefits of various methods of organizing, delivering, and managing services in institutional and noninstitutional settings
6. The costs associated with HIV testing using current methods and current utilization levels, as well as under circumstances of expanded use
7. The costs associated with the introduction of different HIV testing methods
8. The costs of providing additional training for health care professionals in a wide variety of health care settings

As time passes, the economic impact of AIDS will become clearer. Such information will assist policy makers to make appropriate decisions so that all PWAs can receive adequate health care.

DISCUSSION QUESTIONS

1. What are alternative ways of financing the costs of treating persons with HIV infection or symptomatic AIDS?
2. If a PWA can "buy into" private health insurance policies for up to 18 months after being forced to stop working because of health problems, will the financial burden of treating AIDS patients shift from government assistance to private insurance in a significant way?
3. What can communities learn from the San Francisco General Hospital model of care for AIDS patients?

4. In what ways may AIDS cause political destabilization in developing countries?
5. Should an international organization, such as the Red Cross, adopt a special set of goals to assist developing countries with the AIDS pandemic?
6. What kind of services that require funds must a PWA be expected to need?

REFERENCES

1. Brown, M: The 1990's: Just around the corner. Health Care Manage Rev 13:81, 1988.
2. Hardy, AM, et al: The economic impact of the first 10,000 cases of Acquired Immunodeficiency Syndrome in the United States. JAMA 255:209, 1986.
3. Hardy, AM, et al: Ibid.
4. Green, J, et al: Projecting the impact of AIDS on hospitals. Health Aff Fall: 19, 1987.
5. Scitovsky, AA and Rice, DP: Estimates of the direct and indirect costs of Acquired Immunodeficiency Syndrome in the United States: 1985, 1986 and 1991. Public Health Rep 102:5, 1987.
6. Scitovsky, AA and Rice, DP: Ibid.
7. Scitovsky, AA and Rice, DP: Ibid.
8. Scitovksy, AA and Rice, DP: Ibid.
9. Bloom, DE and Carliner, G: The economic impact of AIDS in the United States. Science 239:604, 1988.
10. Andrulis, DP, et al: The provision and financing of medical care for AIDS patients in U.S. public and private teaching hospitals. JAMA 258:1343, 1987.
11. Hardy, AM, et al: Ibid.
12. Scitovsky, AA and Rice, DP: Ibid.
13. Bloom, DE and Carliner, G: Ibid.
14. Scitovsky, AA and Rice, DP: Ibid.
15. Bloom, DE and Carliner, G: Ibid.
16. Wilensky, GR: Filling the gap in health insurance: Impact on competition. Health Aff Summer: 133, 1988.
17. Wilensky, GR: Ibid.
18. Wilensky, GR: Ibid.
19. Roper, WL and Winkerwerder, W: Making fair decisions about financing care for persons with AIDS. Public Health Rep 103:305, 1988.
20. Anti-dumping regulations proposed and criticized. The Nation's Health, August 1988:1.
21. Ansell, DA and Schiff, RL: Patient dumping: Status, implications and policy recommendations. JAMA 257:1500, 1987.
22. Roper, WL and Winkerwerder, W: Ibid, p 313.
23. Iglehart, JK, Read, JL, and Wells, JA: The socioeconomic impact of AIDS on health care systems. Health Aff 6:137, 1987.
24. Office of Technology Assessment: Effectiveness of Educational Interventions to Change Risky Behaviors: How Effective is AIDS Education? Staff paper no. 3, Office of Technology Assessment, United States Congress. US Government Printing Office, Washington, DC, May 1988.
25. Green, J, et al: Ibid.

26. Mann, JM: WHO estimates 300,000 AIDS cases by year's end. Public Health Rep 103:207, 1988.
27. Mann, JM, et al: The international epidemiology of AIDS. Sci Am 259:82, 1988.
28. Mann, JM, et al: Ibid.
29. Genasci, L: Brazil steps up AIDS campaign. AIDS Watch 2(2):5, 1988.
30. Mann, JM, et al: Ibid.
31. Mann, JM, et al: Ibid.
32. Mann, JM, et al: Ibid.
33. Scitovsky, AA: Estimates of the direct and indirect costs of AIDS in the United States. In Fleming, AF, et al (eds): The Global Impact of AIDS. Alan R. Liss, New York, 1988.
34. Hardy, AM, et al: Ibid.
35. Scitovsky, AA: Ibid.
36. Hardy, AM, et al: Ibid.
37. Scitovsky, AA: Ibid.
38. Scitovsky, AA: Ibid.
39. Bloom, DE and Carliner, G; Ibid.
40. Confronting AIDS: Update 198, Executive summary, Institute of Medicine/National Academy of Sciences. Journal of Acquired Immune Deficiency Syndromes 1:181–182, Raven Press, New York, 1988.
41. Over, M, et al: The direct and indirect cost of HIV infection in developing countries. In Fleming, AF, et al (eds): The Global Impact of AIDS. Alan R. Liss, New York, 1988.
42. Over, M, et al: Ibid.
43. Over, M, et al: Ibid.
44. Over, M, et al: Ibid.
45. Rothermel, TS: AIDS: Its impact on development programmes. In Fleming, AF, et al (eds): The Global Impact of AIDS. Alan R. Liss, New York, 1988.
46. Rothermel, TS: Ibid.
47. Rothermel, TS: Ibid.
48. Rothermel, TS: Ibid.

NINE

ETHICAL AND LEGAL DIMENSIONS OF AIDS FOR THE HEALTH PROFESSIONS

Fritz Guy

OUTLINE

OBJECTIVES

By the close of this chapter, the reader will be able to:
1. Explain why AIDS presents an ethical challenge.

2. Explore the ethical dilemmas many health personnel face.
3. Cite historical examples of similar challenges to the health professions.
4. Review the level of risk to individual health care workers.
5. Analyze your own feelings about the responsibility to provide care.
6. Clarify your own ideals of service.
7. Locate and review your profession's code of ethics.
8. Rate your own level of risk.
9. Recognize the level of your obligation to treat.
10. Evaluate the effect of designating AIDS patients and people who are HIV-positive as protected under the Rehabilitation Act.
11. Assess a health professional's duty to warn.
12. Explain issues in confidentiality.
13. Cite additional responsibilities of health professionals in confronting AIDS.
14. Describe current trends in public policy development.
15. State pros and cons of mandatory HIV testing.

THE ETHICAL CHALLENGE OF AIDS

AIDS is an ethical challenge for the health professions for 2 principal reasons. One reason is the increasing *severity of the epidemic.* By October 1988, 7 years after AIDS was identified, nearly 75,000 persons in the United States were known to have developed the disease and more than 42,000 had died. It was projected that the rate of new cases would increase to 80,000/year in 1992 and that by the end of that year the cumulative total of persons with AIDS (PWAs) in the United States would reach 365,000, with a cumulative total of 263,000 deaths.[2] It was also estimated, on the basis of epidemiologic studies reported to the World Health Organization (WHO), that more than 250,000 persons worldwide already had AIDS, that between 5 and 10 million people worldwide were HIV-infected, and that within 5 years about 1 million new AIDS cases would develop.[3] In short, the situation is going to get worse before it gets better, and for at least a decade AIDS will be an increasingly common fact of life for an increasing number of health professionals as well as for society as a whole.

The other reason why AIDS is an ethical challenge for the health professions is less empirically verifiable but just as significant: the *widespread* (and perhaps increasing) *reluctance to provide competent, compassionate care* for PWAs. Such persons are sometimes unnecessarily isolated, sometimes receive substandard care, and sometimes are refused treatment altogether. As one dentist responded when asked about caring for patients with AIDS, "I just tell them that my office is not equipped to take care of them." In many communities persons who have AIDS or who are HIV-positive find that good professional health care is difficult to obtain even for conditions unrelated to their HIV infection.[4,5]

AIDS, then, is a major ethical challenge to the health professions because of the increasing severity of the epidemic and because of the understandable reluctance of health professionals to provide competent, compassionate care. To this challenge, health professionals can respond individually and collectively. It is the purpose of this chapter to explore the nature of the challenge and the possibilities of response.

The ethical challenge of AIDS was unexpected and unwanted, but it is not qualitatively unique. The challenge was unexpected because for at least 3 decades health professionals were largely free from concern about occupational exposure to disease. In 1847, the first general meeting of the American Medical Association adopted a code of ethics declaring that "when pestilence prevails" it is the duty of physicians to "face the danger, and to continue their labors for the alleviation of the suffering, even at the jeopardy of their own lives"; but in 1957 this kind of language was dropped because of the conquest of pestilential diseases by the health professions.[6] To be sure, these diseases had not been completely eliminated from the human population, but antiseptic techniques, treatment by antibiotics, and vaccines had drastically curtailed their devastating potential, so that in recent years health personnel had let down their guard about the occupational hazards of caring for infectious diseases. They had "come to believe (with some justification) that they are exempt from the riskier aspects of medicine that had claimed the lives of so many of their predecessors."[7] But now the sense of invulnerability has been shattered by the possibility of HIV infection.

The Need for a New Sense of Vocation Among Health Care Professionals

The ethical challenge of AIDS was unwanted because the earlier sense of vocation among health professionals has eroded. Perhaps related to the decreased sense of personal risk and awareness of the need for self-sacrifice, an increasingly entrepreneurial spirit in the health professions encourages professionals to view health care largely in economic terms rather than as ministry to human need. Many professionals feel they are free to choose the matters in which they become involved on purely personal or financial grounds. Thus the ethical challenge of AIDS is a challenge to health professionals to reconsider the values and goals by which they are individually and collectively motivated.

But the challenge is not new, nor is the diversity of views regarding the proper response to the threat of contagious disease. On the one hand, "during most epidemics for which records survive, most physicians seem to have treated most of the patients who sought their help, though they frequently charged higher fees," and one of the best-known episodes in American medical history is the story of Benjamin Rush "racing about Philadelphia" during the outbreak of yellow fever in 1873, "trying to bleed patients back to health."[8]

On the other hand, however, from Galen (Rome, 2nd century) on, many people who could have provided health care instead fled to safer places, and many who did not flee refused to treat patients who were severely ill.[9] Furthermore, many of those who stayed to treat the sick were motivated either by fear of social disgrace (like the 16th century physician who wrote, "To avoid infamy [I] dared not absent myself but with continual fear preserved myself as best I could") or by desire for financial benefit (like the physician in Chaucer's *Canterbury Tales,* who is described as pleased by the "gold he kept from pestilence").[10]

Occupational Risk of HIV Infection

Sound ethical reasoning requires not only the recognition and application of ethical principles but also the recognition and interpretation of relevant facts. Ethical decision making always involves the application of principles to specific situations. In regard to AIDS, it is useful to look first at the available facts regarding the occupational risk of HIV infection (see Chapter 4).

The present situation is described in the opening paragraph of a report summarizing the research data currently available to the Centers for Disease Control (CDC):[11]

> *In the last decade, tens of thousands of persons with acquired immuno-deficiency syndrome (AIDS) have been treated in the health care system in the United States. Hundreds of thousands more infected with human immunodeficiency virus (HIV) but often not identified as such have also received medical, dental and nursing services. Although isolated cases of HIV infection in health care personnel have created a high level of anxiety about the risk of treating such patients, the actual probability of contracting infection is extremely small.*

An initial series of CDC studies of persons working with AIDS patients or exposed to the blood or body fluids of AIDS patients indicated that although the HIV can be transmitted to health care workers (HCWs), this kind of transmission is extremely infrequent and almost always results from accidental needle-stick injury. But in May 1987, a report of 3 health care workers who became HIV-positive after exposure to infected blood on their skin or mucous membranes[12] engendered a high level of concern. In contrast to this highly publicized anecdotal report, however, studies of employment data on 47,532 of the first 55,315 cases of AIDS in the United States show that 5.4% of AIDS cases occurred among HCWs, who represent 5.7% of the total labor force[13]—indicating no significantly increased risk of AIDS because of occupational exposure. Of the HCWs with AIDS, 94.7% had significant risk factors unrelated to their employment. Only 41 persons, including physicians and surgeons, a dentist, nurses and nursing assistants, laboratory technicians, therapists, housekeeping and maintenance workers, a respiratory therapist, a paramedic, a mortician and 2 others who had no known contact with patients or clinical specimens, were found to be without probable means of exposure.[14]

A seroprevalence study published early in 1988 reported that of 1,132 dentists, 131 dental hygienists, and 46 dental assistants, 47% practiced in geographic areas with a high incidence of AIDS; 15% had treated patients with AIDS; 72% had treated patients at risk of HIV infection; 94% had 1 or more injuries with sharp instruments in the preceding 5 years.[15] Of the total of 1309 dental personnel, 1 dentist with no other risk factors became infected. He reported that he frequently treated patients without wearing gloves, even though he had had breaks on the skin of his hands, and estimated having had 10 accidental needle-stick exposures during the previous 10 years.[16]

Available studies on HCWs accidentally exposed to potentially infectious blood or other body fluids were conveniently summarized early in 1988:[17]

> *The combined studies of almost 1,400 health care workers and 1,300 dental personnel suggest that the risk of HIV infection even after mucous membrane exposure or parenteral inoculation of infected blood, fluids, or secretions is extremely low—probably less than one per 200 incidents. This risk is probably a maximum estimate, since the denominator was selected only from those persons who had sustained one or more direct accidental exposures to potentially infectious blood or other fluids.*

In many csses of HIV transmission the CDC's[18] recommended blood and body fluid precautions were not used; and in some cases of infection after accidental inoculation of blood, the amount involved was significantly greater than the average of 1.4 microliters injected during a needle-stick injury.

It is worth noting the contrast between the observed 0.5% risk of HIV transmission after accidental exposure to infected blood or body fluids[19] and the 6%–30% risk of hepatitis B transmission after parenteral exposure to infected blood. According to the American Nurses' Association,[20] the risk ordinarily involved in giving nursing care to PWAs is "minimal."

Furthermore, "although the risk of HIV transmission in the health care setting is already low, it can be reduced even further if health care personnel are meticulous in following [infection control] guidelines and in avoiding accidental injuries with needles and other sharp instruments."[21] Unfortunately, "many health care workers seem to find it less threatening to deny that they are at risk (and therefore take no precautions) or to overstate vastly the risk (and refuse to provide care) than to accept a definite, albeit very low, risk and then to lower this risk still further through rigorous compliance with infection control guidelines."[22] The fact remains, nevertheless, that using appropriate control measures makes the risks "manageable, if not negligible."[23]

Responsibility to Provide Health Care

Opposite the reluctance of some health professionals to treat PWAs or persons with HIV infection is the responsibility to provide competent and compassionate care. This responsibility has 3 principal components: the nature of the relationship between the health professional and the patient, the indebtedness of the health professional to society, and the historic tradition of the health professions.[24,25] The responsibility to provide care is individual as well as collective; it is not met simply by referring a patient to another source of care.

Relationship of Power and Vulnerability. The relationship between the health professional and the patient is a relationship of power and vulnerability. On the one hand, the patient is a person in need of professional service that cannot be provided by oneself, because the patient does not have the requisite knowledge and skill. And the need is not trivial; it involves the patient's own person. The typical gratitude, often enormous and sometimes lifelong, of patients toward those who have given them compassionate care is evidence of the existential significance of that care. On the other hand, to the health professional belongs the power to meet the patient's need and provide the necessary care. While this power is not unique to any individual health professional, it is limited to a specific group of persons enabled, through education and licensure, to function in a particular way. The combination of the patient's deeply personal need and the professional's particular ability to help "generates a moral duty to *respond*—that is, a moral responsibility."[26]

Indebtedness of Professionals to Society. There is no self-made health professional; all professionals are indebted to society for the knowledge and skills that are requisite to professional health care. Educational and medical institutions, lecturers and mentors, laboratories and libraries—all are essential to the health professional's ability to function, and all are provided by someone else's resources of energy, expertise, and money. Most often the agency providing the funding is some level of government—municipal, county, state, or national—which means that the money comes ultimately from the public. Considering these facts of educational and professional life exposes the illusion that professional skills are one's own property, to be used solely according to one's own preferences.

Ideals of Service. Traditionally, the health professions have maintained high ideals of service that transcend self-interest. What is well said of medicine and physicians is true of all the health professions and their personnel:[27]

> . . . [I]f medicine is not a profession, if patients are accurately described as consumers, and if health care is a "marketplace product lines," then physicians have the same responsibilities as ordinary citizens, with no obligation to care for patients with AIDS. If society values medicine as a trade, subject to

the laws and policies of commerce, then it is hard to defend a unique obliga-
tion of physicians . . .

If [on the other hand] physicians have an obligation to treat such pa-
tients, it is derived from the concept of medicine as a profession and from the
physician's particular professional role. The objective of a commercial enter-
prise is the pursuit of wealth; the objective of the medical profession is devo-
tion to a moral ideal—in particular, healing the sick and rendering the ill
healthy and well. The physician is committed to the help and betterment of
other people . . . When a person joins the profession, he or she professes a
commitment to these ideals and accepts the obligation to serve the sick. It is
the profession that is chosen. The obligation is neither chosen nor transfer-
able; it is constitutive of the professional activity.

In other words, "Medicine is an inherently moral enterprise, the success and
future of which depend to a great extent on the integrity of individual professionals as they face the duties the calling of healer entails."[28]

The duties of health professionals include service even in the face of personal
risk. One is "no more free to flee from danger in performance of his or her duties
than the fireman, the policeman, or the soldier."[29] It is reasonable to hope that all
health professionals, "realizing that the risk is miniscule, will take ordinary precautions and treat those patients no differently from anyone else with an infectious disease."[30]

Ethical Statements

The American Nurses Association's Committee on Ethics[31] concludes that "in
most instances, it would be considered morally obligatory for a nurse to give care
to an AIDS patient." In the special case of a nurse who is immunosuppressed, "the
individual nurse must . . . choose whether or not to go beyond the requirement of
duty."

The American Dental Association (ADA)'s *Principles of Ethics* declares that
service to the public is a dentist's "primary professional obligation," and that
"competent and timely delivery of quality care within the bounds of clinical circumstances presented by the patient, shall be the most important aspect of that
obligation." Accordingly, a revised ADA policy statement on AIDS and HIV infection stated that dentists should not refuse treatment to any patient "whose condition falls within the dentist's current realm of competence solely because the
patient is HIV infected."[32]

Facing the Reality of Risk

This argument for the responsibility of health professionals to treat PWAs or
persons with HIV infection does not ignore the fact that there is some risk (from
needle-stick and similar injuries) to persons who care for patients with AIDS. It

also recognizes that there is a point at which a risk is so great in relation to the potential benefit to the patient that taking the risk is a matter not of duty but of heroism. And there is a further point at which taking the risk is not courageous or heroic but foolish. For example, one need not—indeed should not—take even a small risk of HIV infection if the patient is dead. But it is impossible to provide specific *a priori* criteria or rules for making such judgments.

Except for a few special groups (such as emergency room surgeons), the risk is ordinarily comparable to that of, say fire fighters.[33] No one is obligated to be a fire fighter, but to choose that role is to accept certain risks that are not faced by others. The same is true for those who choose to be professionally involved in health care. The history of the health professions shines with examples of persons for whom the risk of disease was recognized and transcended by a commitment to service, and who were therefore willing to take significant risks for the good of their patients.

The various health professions should work out guidelines for case-by-case evaluation of potential risks and benefits. The professions can reduce the risk to any one person by involving all the relevant personnel in caring for patients with AIDS or HIV infection. Determining these guidelines will not be an easy task, but it will reduce the likelihood that another group of people (such as politicians or bureaucrats) will take responsibility for determining such guidelines and in effect telling health care personnel what risks they must take. If the appropriate professional groups do not do this work, some government agency will do it for them.

LEGAL DIMENSIONS OF AIDS

Obligation to Treat

Under certain conditions, there are legal obligations to treat. These conditions include medical emergencies, prior patient–professional relationships, contractual obligations, and situations in which laws prohibiting specific kinds of discrimination would be violated if treatment were not rendered. These conditions are related in various ways to the care of PWAs and persons with HIV infection.

AIDS as a medical condition occasionally requires emergency treatment (for example, in connection with *Pneumocystis carinii* pneumonia ([PCP]), but this is not common. More often, if a PWA or a person with HIV infection needs emergency care it is because of unrelated circumstances, such as trauma from an automobile accident. In such situations emergency room personnel are obligated to provide appropriate treatment; the presence of HIV infection and the possibility of its transmission do not constitute an exception from the general obligation to treat. The professional personnel do, of course, have the right (and should be urged) to take appropriate precautions in terms of procedures and clothing, but they do not have the right to refuse treatment.

Apart from emergency care, a legal obligation to treat is created by a prior professional relationship with the patient. This is the principle of nonabandonment, according to which a professional provider–patient relationship continues until it is terminated by mutual consent or by the patient, or until professional services are no longer needed, or after reasonable notice to the patient. Thus a patient who becomes HIV-positive after the establishment of a professional health care relationship has a legal right to continued treatment. "Abandonment" in the technical legal sense is "a cause of action for professional liability."[34] The professional cannot refuse to treat a patient already under his or her care simply because of HIV infection, at least not without reasonable notice. In the case of patients with symptomatic AIDS, however, effective treatment may involve special knowledge or skills; then the professional may be legally able (or required) to refer the patient to an available person who is qualified to treat.[35]

An obligation to treat is also created by certain contractual relationships between professionals and insurance plans (such as health maintenance organizations) or health care institutions (such as hospitals). Many years ago it was not uncommon for hospitals to discriminate in the admissions process against certain categories of patients on racial or ethnic or other similar grounds. Today, such discrimination is prohibited by various legal authorities. Public hospitals must comply with the provisions of the federal constitution, which prohibits states from denying "equal protection of the laws" to all persons. As this language has been interpreted by the courts, discrimination based on race, national origin, ethnic group, or sex is prohibited. Discrimination on any other grounds must be rationally related to a legitimate stated purpose.

Various forms of discrimination by private hospitals are also prohibited. The Medicare conditions of participation prohibit discrimination based on race or ethnicity. The Hill-Burton regulations are broader, prohibiting discrimination based on race, color, national origin, creed, or any other ground unrelated to an individual's need for the service or the availability of the service in the facility.[36] Title VI of the Civil Rights Act of 1964 prohibits discrimination on the basis of race, color, or national origin by any facility receiving federal financial support.[37]

The Rehabilitation Act of 1973 prohibits exclusion based on handicap for all hospitals receiving federal funds, including Medicare and Medicaid.[38] The same prohibition applies to private practitioners receiving Medicare and Medicaid funding. In 1988, a Department of Justice[39] ruling applied this to PWAs and persons with HIV infection, stating "[they] are protected by the federal law barring discrimination against the handicapped in government jobs and federally funded programs."

In regard to the risk of HIV infection, the attitude of health professionals toward hepatitis B infection may be relevant:[40]

> *The risk of hepatitis B infection is real, and the disease is sometimes fatal, but this risk has never been seen as sufficiently high to justify discrimination against either infected patients or surgeons. Thus at least as long as scientific*

estimates place the chance of becoming infected with HIV and dying at less than the probability of becoming infected with hepatitis B and dying, there is no objective data to warrant discriminating against an HIV-infected individual.

Related to the obligation of individual health professionals to treat PWAs or persons with HIV infection is the corresponding obligation of medical institutions. This obligation involves the legal question of "patient dumping."[41,42] A federal "anti-dumping" law was passed in 1986, but only in 1988 did the United States Department of Health and Human Services (DHHS) propose actual regulations to prevent the transfer of "unstable, acutely ill" patients from 1 hospital to another because of the patients' inability to pay for hospital services. When a patient is transferred, treatment is delayed from 1–18 hours, with often serious and sometimes fatal results.

Duty to Warn

A legal obligation quite different from the obligation to treat is the duty to warn. Health professionals not only may but must disclose confidential patient information to a person who is in foreseeable danger of serious harm by a patient. In the much discussed case of *Tarasoff v. Regents of the University of California,* the California Supreme Court[43] held a psychologist liable for his failure to warn a woman that a patient intended to murder her. The court concluded that "the public policy favoring protection of the confidential character of patient–psychotherapist communications must yield to the extent to which disclosure is essential to avert danger to others. The protective privilege ends where the public peril begins." Even before that case, physicians were held to be obligated to warn specific persons in danger of being infected by particular patients, although not obligated to warn the general public of infectious diseases in the community. Thus there is a legal duty to warn in the case of AIDS:[44]

> *The duty to protect third parties from transmission of HIV arises in relation to specific persons who the physician knows are likely to have an intimate exchange of bodily fluids with the patient. The steps the physician must take to fulfill his "duty to protect" are unclear. But they at least include a threshold obligation to advise the patient of his responsibility to warn close contacts of his infection and to behave safely.*

DHHS[45,46] guidelines go further, recommending that if persons with HIV infection "are unwilling to notify their [sexual or IV drug] partners or if it cannot be assured that their partners will seek counseling, physicians or other health department personnel should use confidential procedures to assure that the partners are notified."

The duty to warn takes a somewhat different direction in the case of health professionals who are themselves HIV-positive and who continue to treat patients. It is obvious that such circumstances require scrupulous attention to and implementation of the CDC recommendations for universal precautions. Every patient has a right to freedom from the risk of HIV infection during treatment. (See Chapters 4 and 10 for further discussion of this point).

Confidentiality

The issue of confidentiality involves balancing individual rights to privacy against the public health need to protect others from HIV infection[47,48] and against the rights of others to know of the health risks to which they are exposed. In general, the privacy of persons who are HIV-positive is to be rigorously protected, but there are some exceptions. Not only do the partners of infected persons have a right to know the risk they are taking, but also certain particularly vulnerable health personnel—emergency room surgeons, for example—have a right to know the risks involved in treating particular patients. No one else has a right to information about a person's HIV status—not the medical profession in general, not a person's employer or landlord, and not the government.

The issue of confidentiality arises largely from the problem of discrimination[49] in such areas as housing, employment, and education. In general, it is unwise to depend on the law to provide strict protection of HIV-status information, because as has been noted above, the law itself excuses, justifies, and even compels the disclosure of such information in certain circumstances. Rather, there should be efforts toward the enactment of legislation prohibiting such discrimination.

ADDITIONAL WAYS HEALTH CARE PROFESSIONALS CAN HELP

The ethical challenge of AIDS for health professionals goes beyond treating persons who are HIV-infected and protecting others from infection. It includes enhancing community resources for such persons, educating the public about the means of transmission, and influencing public opinion and policy about AIDS.

Community Resources

Every health professional can be aware of and in touch with local community resources relevant to AIDS. In many cities there are "AIDS projects" and action committees, not-for-profit, community-based organizations that are funded by private donations and by city, county, state, and federal grants, and that specialize in providing various kinds of services to persons affected by AIDS. Typically, case managers evaluate individual needs and put patients and their families in touch with appropriate medical, social, financial, and legal resources. Often case managers can facilitate the provision of these services so that the needs are meet promptly and compassionately. Volunteers trained as "buddies" provide direct one-to-one emotional and practical support; they offer personal companionship and assistance. Professional therapists provide crisis intervention, individual and group counseling, and support groups for various persons affected by AIDS: patients, family members, and friends. Pastoral volunteers offer spiritual care, bereavement counseling for family and friends, and help in planning and conducting funeral services. AIDS educators speak to school, church, and community groups about the means of HIV transmission and prevention, advances in medical research, and psychosocial issues. Some AIDS projects and committees also maintain shelters to provide short-term housing for patients, and operate hospices for patients who are terminally ill. All AIDS organizations have copies of the Surgeon General's Report,[50] posters, pamphlets, and other educational materials that are available free to anyone who is interested.

County health departments are another source of valuable help. Besides educational materials, they often provide free, anonymous testing for persons who may be infected with the HIV. For persons who are HIV positive, confidential counseling is usually available at the testing site.

Health professionals can enhance the usefulness of such community resources by making appropriate referrals They can also encourage people to volunteer at a local AIDS organization—as a "buddy," an office worker, a board member, a fundraiser, or a person answering a telephone hot line. They can volunteer some of their own time and skills, either indirect client services or training programs. At the very least, every health professional should have the telephone numbers of the nearest AIDS organization office and the county health department, and make them available to anyone who needs help or would like to be of help.

Education

Health professionals have a responsibility to help educate the public, especially children and teenagers, about AIDS. Nothing can be done to prevent the development of AIDS in persons already infected, but much can be done to prevent the transmission of the virus,[51] and to reduce the irrational fears that are often generated by the virus.

In their offices, in schools, in service clubs, and elsewhere health professionals can emphasize the fact that the AIDS virus is comparatively hard to contract, and that there is no need to panic. It must enter one's own blood stream from infected blood or semen; it is not "caught" from mosquito bites, restaurant dishes, toilet seats, hugs, or handshakes. Because donated blood is now screened for the virus and blood products are treated to inactivate it, the primary ways in which a person becomes infected with the HIV is through sexual activity, parenterally, or perinatally.

People should be encouraged to understand AIDS the same way they understand crossing a busy street: they can recognize the danger and deliberately avoid it. Heavy traffic is dangerous; if ignored, it is likely to be fatal. But it need not cause anxiety, much less panic, because being hit by a car can be avoided by careful, intelligent behavior. So can the danger of HIV infection. It is personal behavior, in most instances, that invites or avoids transmission of the virus.

Health professionals can emphasize the fact that the AIDS virus does not care at all about a person's social reputation, economic status, or sexual orientation. AIDS is not a "gay disease" or a "junkie disease"; it is a viral disease that is transmitted primarily through a very small number of very high-risk behaviors.

Education must remain an ongoing activity, because of the widely known and well documented gap between personal knowledge and behavior change. Sexual activity is popular but condoms are not, and people tend to be optimistic. Success in getting large numbers of people to alter their sexual practices does not come easily.[52]

Public Policy

The time and energy of health professionals may also be directed toward influencing public opinion and policy about such AIDS-related matters as the funding of research, patient care, and preventive education; the mandatory testing of selected groups for HIV status; the privacy of patient information; and the prohibition of discrimination against PWAs or persons with HIV infection. Nearly 600 varied (and sometime contradictory) recommendations in these and other areas of public policy are contained in the *Report of the Presidential Commission on the Human Immunodeficiency Virus Epidemic,** issued in June 1988. An almost simultaneous and remarkably similar report came from a committee of scientists organized by the National Academy of Sciences and the Institute of Medicine under the title *Confronting AIDS: Update 1988.**

The progress of biomedical research in relation to AIDS and the HIV is an astonishing achievement.[53]

> We now know more about HIV's structure, molecular composition, behavior and target cells than about those of any other virus in the world. The work, in short, is going well. But it is in its early stages, and there is an unknown distance still to go. . . .
> . . . The research done in the past few years has been elegant and highly productive, with results that tell us one sure thing: AIDS is a soluble problem, albeit an especially complex and difficult one. No one can predict at this stage how it will turn out or where the really decisive answers will be found, but the possibilities are abundant and the prospects are bright.

Among the most promising lines of investigation are the searches for new drugs that can kill viruses inside cells without killing the cells, for a vaccine that can prevent the spread of HIV infection, and for procedures that can repair damaged immune systems. But however bright the prospects for these approaches, "there is a conspicuous shortfall in the funds needed for each of them."[54]

Massive amounts of money are needed not only for research toward a vaccine to prevent AIDS but also for the care of patients, as the number of cases increases and the costs soar into billions of dollars. At an average of $80,000 per patient[55] the cumulative cost of caring for the 365,000 patients expected by the end of 1992 will be approximately $29.2 billion. That year alone the costs of caring for the expected 172,000 surviving patients is expected to range from $6.3 billion–$45.5 billion.[56] These expenditures are not a large percentage of the total national spending for medical care, but will disproportionately affect the areas where PWAs are already concentrated (see Chapter 8).

Funding is also needed for broad preventive education in all schools (public and private) and at all levels, as well as in the various information media. The government pamphlet *Understanding AIDS,*[57] which was mailed in 1988 to more than 100 million households in the United States, was a good beginning, but only a beginning. People—especially young people—need more information.

Funding for research, care, and education is more likely to be provided if citizens communicate vigorously and persistently with legislators and other public officials at state and national levels, and if there is positive discussion in public forums like letters to editors and radio talk shows. More effectively than many other people, health professionals can remind both politicians and the public that before it is conquered, AIDS will affect everyone. Fortunately, federal, state, and local governments have begun to move in the right direction. This movement needs and deserves encouragement.

Both individually and governmentally, however, caring for PWAs and educating people about AIDS will mean less money for other things. If the necessary funding is not taken from other programs and projects, there will certainly be higher taxes and higher premiums on health insurance.[58] Compassion is always costly, to persons and to society, and therefore it is not always popular. But it is always possible.

Health professionals can help society resist panic in the face of the AIDS epidemic. Health education, for example, "must go beyond explicit sex education; it must seek to educate the public on upholding the civil liberties of people with AIDS or who test HIV seropositive."[59] Beyond the simple wrongheadedness of legislative proposals and ballot initiatives to identify and quarantine all people who are HIV-positive, there are questions that are more difficult and complicated.

Public concerns about AIDS continually produce proposals to require the mandatory testing of certain groups and the reporting of test results. It has been suggested, for example, that everyone who applies for a marriage license be required to take a test for HIV infection. But such a test would cost $100 million/ year, and would detect fewer than 0.1% of infected persons in the United States. Furthermore, for more than 100 of the people tested annually, the test would produce false-negative results (telling them they were not infected when they actually were. And for more than 350 people, the test would produce false-positive results (telling them they were infected when they actually were not).[60] The Surgeon General and almost all other public health officials agree that mandatory testing of large groups is not a good use of time, effort, and money, because the effectiveness of any testing program depends on the cooperation of the groups to be tested. These resources are better invested in education for prevention and voluntary testing.

In relation to these and other public issues regarding AIDS, health professionals are in a privileged position to be informed, to establish responsible positions, and to influence public policy.

INEVITABILITY OF RESPONSE

The dean of Harvard University's School of Public Health has described the challenge of AIDS to the world at present:[61]

> *The AIDS epidemic exposes hidden vulnerabilities in the human condition that are both biological and social. AIDS prompts courageous and generous acts, and it provokes mean-spirited and irrational responses. AIDS throws new light on the traditional questions of value, compels a fresh look at the performance of the institutions we depend on and brings society to a crossroads for collective action that may, with the passage of years, mark a key measure of our time.*

In one way or another the allied health professions will respond to the ethical challenge of AIDS. They cannot escape it. It is the kind of situation that William James called a "forced option."[62] They can choose *how* to respond, but not *whether* to respond, for they cannot choose *not* to respond. Even a denial of their responsibility, or a denial of the ethical challenge of AIDS itself, is a response.

The response to the ethical challenge of AIDS will be made individually as well as collectively. A profession is not an impersonal establishment governed by an administrative structure, but a collegium of persons united by similar interests, functions, and commitments. So one by one health professionals will decide what they are going to do about providing appropriate care for PWAs and persons with HIV infection.

DISCUSSION QUESTIONS

1. To what lengths should HCWs go to protect an HIV-infected person's right to confidentiality?

2. Why is confidentiality more important with HIV infection and/or a diagnosis of AIDS than it is with other viral infections, such as hepatitis B?
3. What obligation does being a profession impose on your particular specialty?
4. Why does the law often follow practice rather than lead in developing it?
5. What role do you believe health professionals should play in developing public policy? Community resources? Lobbying for funding?
6. To whom would you turn for advice and/or discussion when faced by an ethical decision in rendering health care?

REFERENCES

1. Ostrow, RJ and Cimons, M: AID covered under anti-bias law: U.S. rules. The Los Angeles Times, October 7, 1988.
2. Centers for Disease Control: Quarterly report to the domestic policy council on the prevalence and rate of spread of HIV and AIDS: United States. MMWR 37:552, 1988.
3. Mann, JM, et al: The international epidemiology of AIDS. Sci Am 259:82, 1988.
4. Kelly, JA, et al: Stigmatization of AIDS patients by physicians. Am J Public Health 77:789, 1987.
5. Lewis, CE, Freeman, HE, Corey, CR: Aids-related competence of California's primary care physicians. Am J Public Health 77:795, 1987.
6. Arras, JD: The fragile web of responsibility: AIDS and the duty to treat. In Nolan, K and Bayer, R (eds): AIDS: The responsibilities of health professionals. Supplement to Hastings Center Report 18:14, 1988.
7. Arras, JD: Ibid, p 10.
8. Fox, DM: The politics of physicians' responsibility in epidemics: A note on history. In Nolan, K and Bayer, R (eds): AIDS: the responsibilities of health professionals. Supplement to Hastings Center Report 18:5, 7, 1988.
9. Zuger, A and Miles, SH: Physicians, AIDS, and occupational risk: Historic traditions and ethical obligations. JAMA 258:1924, 1987.
10. Fox, DM: Ibid pp 7 and 9.
11. Allen, JR: Health care workers and the risk of HIV transmission. In Nolan, K and Bayer, R (eds): AIDS: The responsibilities of health professionals. Supplement to Hastings Center Report 18:2, 1988.
12. Centers for Disease Control: Acquired immunodeficiency syndrome and human immunodeficiency virus infection among health-care workers. MMWR 36:285, 1987.
13. Centers for Disease Control: Update: Acquired immunodeficiency syndrome and human immunodeficiency virus infection among health care workers. MMWR 37:229, 1988.
14. Centers for Disease Control (1988): Ibid, p 230.
15. Klein, RS, et al: Low occupational risk of human immunodeficiency virus infection among dental professionals. N Engl J Med 318:86, 1988.
16. Jakush, J: AIDS: The disease and its implications for dentistry. J Am Dent Assoc 115:395, 1987.
17. Allen, JR: Ibid, p 4.

18. Centers for Disease Control: Recommendations for prevention of HIV transmission in health-care settings. MMWR 36:3S, 1987.
19. Centers for Disease Control: (1988): Ibid, p 15.
20. American Nurses' Association Committee on Ethics: Statement regarding risk v. responsibility in providing nursing care. Cited by Freedman, B: Health professions, codes, and the right to refuse to treat HIV-infectious patients. In Nolan, K and Bayer, R (eds): AIDS: The responsibilities of health professionals. Supplement to Hastings Center Report 18:21, 1988.
21. Allen JM: Protecting yourself from infection. Nursing Life 8:39, March, 1988.
22. Cotton, DJ: The impact of AIDS on the medical care system. JAMA 260:521, 1988.
23. Zuger, A and Miles, SH: Ibid, p 1928.
24. Arras, JD: Ibid, p 15.
25. Pellegrino, ED: Altruism, self-interest and medical ethics. JAMA 258:1939, 1987.
26. Arras, JD: Ibid, p 15.
27. Emmanuel, EJ: Do physicians have an obligation to treat patients with AIDS? N Engl J Med 318:1686, 1988.
28. Zuger, A and Miles, SH: Ibid, p 1928.
29. Pellegrino, ED: Ibid, p 1939.
30. Dan, BB: Patients without physicians: The new risk of AIDS. JAMA 258:1940, 1987.
31. Freedman, B: Health professions, codes, and the right to refuse to treat HIV-infectious patients. In Nolan, K and Bayer, R (eds): AIDS: The responsibilities of health professionals. Supplement to Hastings Center Report 18:21, 1988.
32. House to review news AIDS policy in October. American Dental Association News 19:1, 1988.
33. Emanuel, EJ: Ibid, p 1688.
34. Logan, MK: Legal, ethical issues for dentists. J Am Dent Assoc 115:402, 1987.
35. Annas, GJ: Legal risks and responsibilities of physicians in the AIDS epidemic. In Nolan, K and Bayer, R (eds): AIDS: The Responsibilities of Health Professionals. Supplement to Hastings Center Report 18:27, 1988.
36. 42 C.F.R. 124.9 (1984).
37. 42 U.S.C.A. 2000d (1981).
38. 29 U.S.C.A. 701-709 (1975).
39. Ostrow, RJ and Cimons, M: Ibid.
40. Annas, GJ: Ibid, p 28.
41. Annas, GJ: Your money or your life: "Dumping" uninsured patients from hospital emergency wards. Am J Public Health 76:74, 1986.
42. Annas, GJ: Too poor to pay: The scandal of patient dumping. Am J Nurs 87:1447, November, 1987.
43. *Tarasoff v. Regents of the University of California* 551 P2d 347 (Cal 1976). Cited in Dickens, BM: Legal limits of AIDS confidentiality. JAMA 259:3449, 1988.
44. Gostin, L and Curran, WJ: AIDS screening, confidentiality, and the duty to warn. Am J Public Health 77:364, 1987.
45. Centers for Disease Control: Public Health Service guidelines for counseling and antibody testing to prevent HIV infection and AIDS. MMWR 36:509, 1987.
46. Centers for Disease Control: Partner notification for preventing human immunodeficiency virus (HIV) infection. Colorado, Idaho, South Carolina, Virginia. MMWR 37:393, 401, 1988.

47. Gostin, L and Curran, WJ: Ibid, p 361.
48. Mitchell, C and Smith, L: If it's AIDS, please don't tell. Am J Nurs 87:911, July, 1987.
49. Confidentiality and discrimination: Tough targets in AIDS strategies. Hospital Ethics 4:9, 1988.
50. Koop, CE: The Surgeon General's Report on Acquired Immune Deficiency Syndrome. U.S Public Health Service, Washington, n.d.
51. Fineberg, HV: Education to prevent AIDS: Prospects and obstacles. Science 239:592, 1988.
52. Fineberg, HV: The social dimensions of AIDS. Sci Am 259:130, 1988.
53. Thomas, L: AIDS: An unknown distance still to go. Sci Am 259:152, 1988.
54. Thomas, L: Ibid, p 152.
55. Bloom, DE and Carliner, G: The economic impact of AIDS in the United States. Science 239:604, 1988.
56. Bloom, DE and Carliner, G: Ibid.
57. Koop, E and the Centers for Disease Control, U.S. Public Health Service: Understanding AIDS. U.S. Government Printing office, Washington DC, 1988.
58. Bloom, DE and Carliner, G: Ibid, p 609.
59. Sheikh, HH: AIDS and the law. World Health, 29, June 1988.
60. Fineberg, HV, et al: Compulsory premarital screening for Human Immunodeficiency Virus. JAMA 258:1758–62, 1987.
61. Fineberg, HV: The social dimensions of AIDS. Scientific American 259:128, 1988.
62. James, W: The Will to Believe and Other Essays in Practical Philosophy. Dover, New York, 3, 1956.

TEN

HEALTH CARE PROFESSIONALS' ROLE IN THE TREATMENT OF AIDS

Leif Kristian Bakland, Sylvia A. Burlew, Mark J. Clements,
Mary Ann Frew, Marguerite McMillan Jackson,
George Edward Johnston, Cindy L. Kosch, John Edwin Lewis,
Edwinna May Marshall, Ann Elizabeth Ratcliff,
Elizabeth A. Rogers, Robert L. Wilkins

OUTLINE

OBJECTIVES

By the close of this chapter, the reader will be able to:
1. State the advantages of a health care team in the treatment of AIDS.

2. Identify contributions of your profession in treatment and prevention of HIV infection and AIDS.
3. State precautions specific to your profession that can be used to limit the spread of the HIV.

The allied health professions comstitute the largest group of health professionals in the United States. Depending on which professions are included in the count, health care workers (HCWs) number between 3 and 4 million.[1] These professionals, whether working in acute care, long-term care, community health, schools, or the military, must all care for persons with AIDS (PWAs) or persons with HIV infection, and their families and friends. Members of each profession have different contributions to make.

In this chapter we present an application of knowledge about AIDS to the major fields of allied health. From over 300 allied health professional specialties, we have selected those with broadest application. Subspecialties or related professions can determine applications for their own fields. Depth of coverage in this text reflects, in most instances, the level of involvement that members of a given specialty generally have with AIDS patients. Because nursing is one of the major professions rendering preventive and primary care to HIV-infected persons, nurses have developed other texts specific to their involvement with AIDS patients.

The importance of allied health professionals working as a team, in diagnosis, treatment, and prevention of HIV infection has been emphasized in chapters 3, 5, and 7. Although this chapter presents information according to discipline, we do not intend to underemphasize the teamwork concept. In fact, teamwork is essential to a coordinated and effective response to this epidemic.

PRECAUTIONS FOR HEALTH CARE WORKERS AND IMMUNOSUPPRESSED PATIENTS

Protection for HCWs (described in Chapter 4) varies according to the risk of exposure to the HIV different workers face. Current data continue to indicate that HCWs run a low risk of occupationally acquired HIV infection.[2,3]

Because persons with HIV infections are at higher risk of illness than persons with normal immune systems, it is also important to minimize their risk of becoming infected with other diseases by cross-contamination from other patients. Following a strict protocol for aseptic management of instruments and equipment will reduce these risks.

DIETETICS AND NUTRITION

Because the interaction between nutritional disorders and immunodeficiency states is well-documented, the relationship of nutritional status to AIDS has been investigated.[4-6] The complications of this disease place patients in a high nutritional risk category. Studies indicate that the ability of a human being to withstand the consequences of infection is generally decreased by malnutrition. Patients with AIDS may experience a severe loss of their natural immunity against disease. For instance, vomiting and diarrhea may cause changes in the acidity and alkalinity of body fluids. These changes can leave patients vulnerable to illnesses that might not otherwise be a threat.[7] Protein–calorie malnutrition is a well-established cause of immune aberrations, with great effect on cell-mediated immunities.[8] Impaired phagocyte function can be caused by malnutrition. This condition alone may explain the increased incidence of infection in malnourished persons. Single vitamin deficiencies can also impair the immune response. Because weight loss and malnutrition are common problems of AIDS patients, it is essential to direct attention to their nutritional status. Some nutritional issues associated with AIDS are reviewed here.

Anorexia and Complications From Therapy

Suppression or lack of appetite can exist independently, as a result of depression associated with AIDS.[9] Often, however, it is secondary to the various forms of therapy. For example, chemotherapy for Kaposi's sarcoma (KS) may cause stomatitis, loss of appetite, nausea, vomiting, and diarrhea. Some patients report taste alterations. Immunological agents such as aminoglycosides and trimethoprim/sulfamethoxazole may produce severe nausea and vomiting, and amphotericin B may cause a metallic taste and anorexia. Mouth pain, loss of appetite, and diarrhea may occur with use of rifampin. Pyrimethamine can cause vomiting, loss of appetite, and tongue tenderness. Isoniazid causes disruption in folate, niacin, pyridoxine, and vitamin B_{12} levels, along with epigastric pain, anorexia, and dry mouth.[10] Nutritional management of these problems is approached in the same manner as that of any other malignancy,[11] in that each particular symptom is treated individually. (Treatments are discussed later in this section.) Cases of KS involving the palate, larynx, trachea, and esophagus have resulted in extreme anorexia leading to exhaustion from lack of food.[12] Anorexia can result from depression, which often occurs immediately after diagnosis.[13] High-calorie, high-protein liquid nutritional supplements can play an important role in combatting anorexia, because it is often easier for a patient to drink a liquid than to consume a meal when the appetite is suppressed.

Nausea and Vomiting

Various forms of treatment can also lead to nausea and vomiting. KS lesions in the oropharyngeal and oral–esophageal areas may also decrease the patient's ability to keep food down.[14] Gastritis and esophagitis, diagnosed by endoscopy, have been found to aggravate this problem further.[15] When nausea and vomiting result from therapy, a conventional nutritional approach to the problem, such as restricting lactose and residue, combined with administering an effective antiemetic, may be feasible. However, when they are due to extensive KS lesions, oral feeding may be unsuccessful. In such cases, enteral or parenteral nutritional support should be considered.

Mucositis and Stomatitis

Herpes virus and KS lesions of the oral cavity can impede proper nutritional intake. The most common oral lesions, however, are secondary to candidiasis.[16] A soft, blended, or liquid diet with nutritional supplements is appropriate during this period. In the most severe stages of candidiasis, it is seemingly impossibly painful for a patient to drink any fluid. Alternative means of nutritional support such as enteral feedings or total parenteral nutrition should be considered.

Fever

Fevers are very common in AIDS patients, and may result from various opportunistic infections or occur as part of the syndrome itself.[17] When nutritional requirements are assessed, fever must be considered, because it causes a rise in basal energy expenditure by 7%/degree Fahrenheit above normal. Furthermore, fever exacerbates the problem of anorexia.

Diarrhea

Diarrhea and malabsorption are often major nutritional problems in AIDS patients. Often they occur before AIDS is diagnosed. The differential diagnosis of diarrhea includes a variety of organisms. Intestinal parasites appear to play a major role in causing diarrhea. Diarrhea may also be caused by antibiotic therapy, a fact that increases the difficulty of treating it. A low serum albumin level can also induce diarrhea. Low serum albumin levels resulting from malnutrition occur as the disease progresses.[18] This diagnosis should be considered in cases of diarrhea for which no causative organism can be identified.

Successful dietary therapy for AIDS-related diarrhea has yet to be identified. Occasional, low-volume diarrhea may respond to treatment with a low-fiber, low-fat, lactose-free diet, along with antidiarrheal agents. If steatorrhea is documented by means of a fecal fat test, a low-fiber, low-fat, lactose-free diet is appropriate. High-volume diarrhea (10–30 bowel movements/day or 10–15 liters/day) can be extremely difficult to overcome. Nutritional intervention often proves unsuccessful. In this event, proper hydration becomes essential. Nasogastric or nasointestinal feedings may be successful, but in cases where diarrhea cannot be controlled, total parenteral nutrition is the preferred route for repletion. *Lactobacillus acidophilus* can also assist in reestablishing the normal gut flora.[19]

Weight Status

Severe unrelenting weight loss appears to be a major component of the clinical picture for many AIDS patients. The catabolic stress of illness demands that additional calories be provided in an attempt to prevent such weight loss. Weight loss has been associated with a poor prognosis for AIDS patients with KS. Weight loss of the degree commonly occurring in AIDs patients places patients at risk of death because of resultant organ dysfunction. Moreover, severe weight loss may preclude recovery from infectious complications that otherwise would not represent a lethal challenge to the host.[20]

It is crucial to identify the mechanism of the weight loss associated with AIDS and to rapidly determine which agents are capable of altering or reversing this potentially lethal complication. Controversy exists over the best means of assessing ideal body weight in patients with AIDS. Pre-illness weight, or the patient's usual weight, is considered a meaningful standard of weight status for hospital patients.[21] Anthropometric measurements can be helpful in identifying patients with malnutrition and those at risk of developing malnutrition. One study determined that the average weight loss during hospitalization was 16% of admission weight.[22] It appears that most patients routinely receive oral diets without oral supplementation even when considered underweight at admission.[23]

More aggressive nutritional support could prove beneficial, preventing weight loss initially, or restoring a patient's weight closer to the ideal weight after weight loss has occurred.

Feeding Dilemmas

Oral diet supplementation should be the first method employed to prevent weight loss. Frequent snacks should be provided. High-calorie, high-protein liquid supplements containing adequate vitamins and minerals are easily accessible and can be used effectively between meals. These products contain 250–500 calories/8 ounces, and can provide a substantial amount of nutrition for a patient unable to consume a routine diet.

When nutritional needs cannot be met by this route, an alternative means of nutritional support must be considered. Naso-enteric feedings are appropriate when the patient has a functioning gastrointestinal tract but is unable to consume enough nutrition orally. A lactose-free, low-residue enteral formula is recommended. Intravenous hyperalimentation is the preferred mode of nutritional support for patients with infectious diarrhea and malabsorption. Peripheral parenteral nutrition may be considered if the intestinal tract is expected to resume normal function within 2 weeks. If intestinal function is not likely to return within 2 weeks, a central line catheter may be placed for total parenteral nutrition. A complete nutritional program can be provided by both enteral and parenteral methods.

Like most forms of treatment, nutritional therapy is expensive, especially when the parenteral route is employed. If third-party reimbursement is not available, patients may have to turn to their own resources, which may be depleted in a short time. In addition, many patients are unable to continue to work because of weakness and viral central nervous system involvement associated with the syndrome, so employment benefits may be quickly exhausted. As a result, there is often no other alternative to sending the patient home on oral nutritional support. Patients already experiencing nutritional problems may continue to lose weight, resulting in further deterioration of nutritional status. This in turn increases the patient's risk of further infections. Therefore, nutritional support should be regarded as a high priority during discharge planning.

Trace Metals

Selenium (a trace mineral) plays a role in immune response. A selenium deficiency may depress the ability of leukocytes to kill yeast cells. Selenium deficiency may affect the secondary antibody response to T-cell-dependent antigens. Vitamin E and selenium are interrelated. A suppressed antibody response that results from a selenium deficiency can be reversed by vitamin E.[24] Selenium deficiency is a common component of malnutrition in AIDS patients.[25] Consuming a wide variety of foods usually provides adequate selenium. In 1980, the National Research Council stated that a safe and adequate daily selenium intake for adults is 50–200 mcg. Seafood and organ and muscle meats are high in selenium, whereas fruits and vegetables are relatively low in selenium. Selenium content of grain varies depending on where it is grown.[26] If an AIDS patient is receiving enteral or parenteral nutrition, selenium should be provided.

Renal Function

Reversible acute renal failure due to toxicity, ischemic injury, or both has occurred in AIDS patients. Some patients lose massive amounts of protein through urine; in some a building of protein in the blood occurs; and occasionally irreversible uremia occurs. If kidney dysfunction is severe, dialysis may be required. In that case, nutritional recommendations would be similar to recommendations for a non-AIDS dialysis patient.[27] Adequate calories should be provided, and blood urea nitrogen, serum creatinine, and serum albumin levels monitored to determine the level and type of protein that should be provided. Serum potassium and sodium levels and water balance require monitoring, and nutritional support should be adjusted accordingly.

The Pediatric Patient With AIDS

Treating a child with AIDS is especially challenging because of the complications of the disease itself superimposed on the need of the child to continue growing. The complications of infection, fever, diarrhea, feeding problems, and decreased intake all lead to malnutrition. Once malnourished, the child is more likely to experience infection and malabsorption. Because rate of growth is faster in childhood, children require more kilocalories per kilogram than adults do. In order to maintain an adequate rate of growth in the child with AIDS, additional kilocalories must be provided. Because weight change is one of the best indications of the adequacy of nutritional support, it is recommended that weight be assessed at least weekly. Visceral protein, serum potassium level, blood urea nitrogen level, creatinine level, and liver function tests should be performed when indicated. To promote growth and stave off the effects of malnutrition associated with AIDS, high-calorie, high-protein feedings and vitamin supplements should be provided. If the child is unable to consume adequate amounts, gavage feedings or total parenteral nutrition is recommended.[28]

Support Through Home Care Agencies

A PWA who no longer requires acute care should still receive follow-up care at home from professionals trained to recognize nutritional deficiencies. Home health care agencies, family care agencies, and hospice programs employ nurses who are trained to make assessments and solve problems. Home visits can occur daily, weekly, or monthly depending on the patient's need. Dietitians can be consulted when a particular problem arises. Weekly weight changes should be reported and blood samples provided when necessary. Often, oral nutritional supplements are adequate and costs are reimbursed by the patient's insurance carrier. If enteral or parenteral nutrition is required, hospital-based home care agencies or independent home care companies can provide the home training and solutions necessary to meet the patient's nutritional needs. If a person is receiving enteral or parenteral feedings, a 24-hour on-call service is usually provided by the home care agency. Follow-up care involving routine physician visits provides an opportunity to make changes in the nutritional care plan.[29]

Aggressive Nutritional Monitoring and Counseling

Patients with AIDS often lose a significant amount of weight and their nutritional status often deteriorates. A study of the nutritional practices of HIV-positive patients in Atlanta, Georgia, revealed that most patients believed a well-balanced diet could help them remain healthier. Only 6% of patients in the sample, however, reported consuming a balanced diet. But of patients who stated that they had received dietary information, the majority reported that it had helped them change their diets.[30]

Will nutritional support and counseling improve the prognosis for HIV-infected persons? The answer lies in further investigation of malnutrition and its role in the deterioration of the immune system in AIDS patients. If such a role is reversible, perhaps development of opportunistic infections may be decreased. Until then, malnutrition should not be accepted as inevitable. Nutritional monitoring and counseling should be ongoing and aggressive, and nutritional intervention should be performed when appropriate.

DENTISTRY AND DENTAL HYGIENE

Obligation to Treat

Dentists and dental hygienists are faced with the distinct possibility that some of their patients are either HIV infected or have AIDS. While this possibility has led some HCWs in dentistry to refuse to treat PWAs,[31] the position of organized dentistry is stated clearly by the American Dental Association and the American Association of Dental Schools:[32,33] dental personnel may not ethically refuse to treat a patient whose condition is within their realm of competence solely because the patient has HIV infection or AIDS.

Precautions

The Centers for Disease Control (CDC) universal precautions do not apply to body fluids such as saliva, sputum, or vomitus unless they contain visible blood. Surveillance studies demonstrate a low occupational risk for AIDS among HCWs, including those in the dental field.[34] As of 1988, only 1 dentist, who identified himself as *not* belonging to a high-risk group, has been reported to have contracted the virus through dental treatment of a patient, and he apparently frequently treated his patients without wearing gloves.[35]

Guidelines for infection control with specific reference to HIV and hepatitis B have been established in dentistry.[36-38] These guidelines are designed to protect both dental workers and their patients. An effective infection control program must begin by dentists training their office staff in proper infection control and providing appropriate safeguards for staff to use.

During dental procedures, contamination of saliva with blood is predictable, trauma to HCWs' hands is common, and blood spattering may occur. Universal precautions call for wearing gloves while performing all dental procedures.[39] Gloves should cover the cuffs of long-sleeved gowns, and should be worn at all times during patient contact and when touching items or surfaces potentially contaminated with blood. After contact with each patient, the gloves should be removed and the hands washed and regloved with new gloves before treating the next patient. Washing or disinfecting the same gloves between uses is not acceptable; studies have shown that microorganisms adhere to gloves and are not easily washed off despite friction, use of a cleansing agent, and drying.[40] A second pair of gloves, such as examining gloves, may be placed over a first pair of gloves when it is necessary to briefly examine a second patient, or when handling patient charts or the telephone. The second pair of gloves should be removed before returning to the first patient.

Protection against splatter and splash of blood can be afforded by masks, goggles, and gowns.

Contaminated surfaces in the dental operatory should be thoroughly cleaned and disinfected after use. Areas such as light handles and x-ray heads may be wrapped with clear plastic during use; the wrap can be removed after treating each patient. Wear gowns and gloves when cleaning up.

Although no vaccine is yet available for the HIV, protection against hepatitis B is possible by vaccination. Dental personnel who have any contact with patients should receive the hepatitis B vaccine.

To provide protection for laboratory technicians, impressions, bite registrations, and appliances should be rinsed and disinfected before they are sent to the laboratory. Open intra-orally-used x-ray film packets in the darkroom with disposable gloves without touching the film.

Instituting universal barrier precautions in dental offices will increase the cost of rendering dental care. One study indicated an increase of $1.50/patient encounter for consumable supplies, with a yearly average of $7500/dental office.[41] Decreased productivity resulting from using these precautions raises the cost still higher.

Noting Evidence of Opportunistic Infections

Dental personnel may be the first health professionals to note evidence of opportunistic infections. A New York study of 150 HIV-infected patients reported that candidiasis involving the lateral borders and dorsum of the tongue, floor of the mouth, palate, buccal mucosa, and oropharynx was the most common manifestation (69%); treatment consisted of administering several antifungal drugs, depending on the severity and longevity of the infection.[42] Hairy leukoplakia (20%) was seen almost exclusively on the lateral borders of the tongue; treatment included antifungal and/or antiherpetic drugs, although lesions seemed to regress and recur independently. Gingival and periodontal problems (17%) included gingival pain resembling acute necrotizing ulcerative gingivitis and rapidly progressive periodontitis. Gentle debridement, careful scaling and root planing, and 0.12% chlorhexidine therapy eliminated most gingival problems. More aggressive treatment, including antibiotic therapy, was needed to resolve the rapidly progressive periodontitis. Oral Kaposi's sarcoma lesions (16%) were most commonly seen on the palate and gingiva. The researchers stated that lesions interfering with patient comfort and function may require chemotherapy, radiation, laser, or surgical treatment.[43]

Attitudes of dental personnel towards HIV-infected persons may interfere with providing an optimal level of care. Studies indicate, however, that misconceptions are clarified and attitudes improve as knowledge about HIV infection and AIDS increases.[44,45]

EMERGENCY MEDICAL SERVICES

Risk of Exposure

In view of the serious consequences of HIV infection, emergency medical service (EMS) personnel have reason to be concerned about their safety. After all, paramedics, emergency medical technicians (EMTs), fire and rescue personnel, and other "first responders" encounter frightening prospects: patients with unknown histories, trauma incidents involving spilled blood and other body fluids, resuscitation events characterized by transfer and spattering of vomitus and body secretions. In a recent study, 3% of trauma patients received in a major emergency department tested HIV positive, considerably above the rate expected in the general population.[46] EMS personnel thus appear to be at significant risk of exposure to the HIV.

The actual risk of infection, however, is very small. With HIV seroconversion estimated at 1:1000 by the CDC, EMS providers are at considerably greater risk of contracting other infections, such as the hepatitis B virus (HBV), meningitis, and tuberculosis.[47] Of the small number of medical care providers who have contracted HIV infection after exposure to infected patients, only 5 cases have been related to non–needle-stick exposure.[48] Most importantly, even this small risk is significantly reduced when EMS personnel adopt a few simple procedures.

The most likely means of exposure to the HIV is by accidental injury due to equipment and instruments used by first responders.[49] Needle punctures and scalpel wounds may carry the virus through the skin of a paramedic or EMT. Tools used by fire and rescue personnel may cause open wounds that, when exposed to HIV-contaminated body fluids, allow the virus to enter.

In trauma incidents, spillage of blood and other body fluids is common. Direct contact between an EMS provider's skin or mucous membranes and these body fluids may provide a mechanism for transmission. Unprotected abrasions, lacerations, or puncture injuries greatly increase the likelihood that the virus will penetrate.

Skin or mucous membrane contact with blood from samples drawn from HIV-infected patients could lead to infection in the EMS provider. Such contact might result from accidental needle-stick injuries, breakage of a sample container vial, or spattering of a blood sample that is being transferred.

During resuscitation procedures, mucous membrane contact with saliva and other secretions from the patient's oral and nasal passages may result in HIV exposure. The CDC[50] has stated, however, that universal precautions do not apply to saliva.

Preventive Measures

Although EMS personnel treat patients before they reach the hospital, maintaining an adequate level of protection is feasible. The CDC recommendations for prevention of HIV transmission in health care settings (see Chapter 4), if adapted and applied, should leave EMS providers facing no greater risk than in-hospital personnel face.

First, EMS agencies should establish administrative structures and procedures conducive to control of infection in general and prevention of HIV transmission in particular. The administrative structure should identify an infection control officer (ICO) with responsibility to recommend procedures, monitor conditions, and evaluate the effectiveness of programs in place. Standard operating procedures (SOPs) should provide consistent guidance. On-scene responsibility to see that appropriate protective measures are implemented should be assigned to the EMS crew leader or the fire or rescue company officer. Individual crew members should not have to decide what level of protection to employ.

The most important standard operating procedure (SOP) to emphasize is handwashing. Next, appropriate handling of sharp instruments at emergency scenes is essential. Preventing accidental punctures and lacerations helps prevent the most likely mechanism of HIV infection for paramedics and EMTs. Appropriate disposal of used items is also important. The CDC recommends that needles be disposed of in a standard container carried to all emergency scenes, and that needles not be recapped, bent, broken, disassembled, or mutilated. Because EMS personnel must often carry all their equipment to a scene, the additional disposal container can become a burden. It is possible, however, to use a small, red-coded plastic box that fits into a section of the paramedic's drug box tray. The plastic box can be dropped into the standard disposal container when the box becomes full.

Barrier precautions should be a part of the SOPs of any EMS organization. Gloves should be worn any time an incident provides a possibility of contact with body fluids. Becaue there is no way to determine on-scene whether a patient is HIV-infected, the same precautions should be used for all patients. Wearing double gloves may even provide a tamponade effect hindering contaminated fluids from entering any wounds in the EMS provider's skin. Masks and goggles or shatterproof glasses protect mucocutaneous membranes against possible exposure. Appropriate dressings should always be used to protect broken skin (*e.g.*, abrasions, lacerations, insect bites).

Protection of EMS personnel during resuscitation and respiratory support procedures requires using ventilatory equipment that prevents contact between the provider and the patient's mucous secretions. Treatment should be initiated using bag masks and integrated protective airways, rather than by beginning mouth-to-mouth resuscitation and then switching to use of the mask. EMS personnel should be encouraged to carry personal ventilating masks in case they must initiate respiratory support with no equipment available. Every EMS agency should provide the necessary ventilatory equipment, strategically positioned to be available immediately when needed, and should require that personnel use the proper equipment and technique.

Exposure Management

Even using the best precautions, EMS personnel may occasionally be exposed to a patient's body fluids. When exposure occurs, agency SOPs should provide guidance for the appropriate follow-up to ensure the best protection for the provider. An exposure report system should exist that provides for recording each exposure, the conditions under which it occurred, and the follow-up that was initiated.

Procedures to initiate immediately following exposure to a patient's body fluids are simple and based on common sense. In the case of percutaneous exposure, immediately wipe and cleanse the wound with an antiseptic wipe. For mucocutaneous exposure, irrigate or rinse the exposed areas with sterile water or saline solution. Hands should always be washed with water and bacteriostatic cleanser as soon as appropriate facilities are available. If facilities are not available at the scene, it may be necessary to wash immediately using antiseptic wipes, and then wash thoroughly as soon as the crew can reach an appropriate facility. All contaminated equipment should be cleaned immediately and wiped with a disinfectant solution[51] (*e.g.*, 1:10 solution of chlorine bleach, Lysol, and so forth). If the crew will not be returning directly to its station, the cleaning should be done before leaving the hospital and returning to service.

CDC recommendations[52] for follow-up care for exposed health care personnel are valid and should be implemented whenever an EMS provider has been exposed to body fluids of a patient who could be a carrier of the HIV.[53] When such an exposure has occurred, the source patient should be tested for the HIV. If the source patient turns out to be HIV-positive, then the exposed EMS provider should also be tested, and retested at 3-month intervals over the next year. During this time, the EMS provider should receive counseling about transmission of the HIV and about the precautions the provider should take in his or her personal life to prevent transmission, in case he or she is actually infected. If the source patient has tested positive for HIV antibodies, but presents no clinical evidence of infection, blood testing of the EMS provider may be discontinued after 1 year. If, however, the source patient presents signs of infection, then follow-up testing and counseling the EMS provider should be continued, according to the needs of the individual case.

Legal Considerations

Although it seems necessary for the protection of EMS personnel, identifying HIV-positive patients may not always be permissible. In some states, laws prevent divulging the health status of persons who have tested HIV-positive.[54]

> **STATES EXPAND AIDS-notification requirements for workers.**
>
> *From 1983 through 1988, 32 states—16 in '88—passed laws requiring emergency medical technicians, funeral personnel, police and others to be notified if exposed or possibly exposed to the human immunodeficiency virus and some other diseases. HIV, the AIDS cause, is the most common trigger, with at least 30 states making it a notifiable condition, the State AIDS Policy Center at George Washington University reported.*
>
> *Half the states say the patient must be already confirmed HIV-positive, or later diagnosed, before the worker is notified. By 1988, 16 state laws provided for patients to be tested after a worker's HIV exposure, but only Utah required testing of patients for the more-common, non-AIDS-related hepatitis B virus, the center said.*[128]

MEDICAL ASSISTING

The first encounter an HIV-infected person has with health professionals may be in the medical office. The undiagnosed HIV-infected patient may come to a physician's office with vague and varied symptoms. The physician may suggest testing for the HIV, based on the patient's history and physical examination. If the test result is positive, regular monitoring and treatment may continue through the medical office. Medical assistants should be knowledgeable about HIV infection and transmission and about treatment of infected persons. Assistants should also recognize their responsibility in educating HIV-infected patients about health protection, high-risk activities, and home care procedures.

Medical assistants should learn and know how to apply the CDC's universal precautions for handling body fluids. Blood is the single most important source of blood-borne pathogens. Universal precautions also apply to semen and vaginal secretions, cerebrospinal fluid, synovial fluid, pleural fluid, peritoneal fluid, pericardial fluid, and amniotic fluid.[55] They do not apply to feces, nasal secretions, sputum, sweat, tears, urine, and vomitus unless these substances contain visible blood. Adhering to the following procedures when treating *all* patients will protect both office staff and patients.

Protective Skin Care

1. Wash hands using aseptic technique before and after patient care; after removal of gloves; after accidental contact with blood or other potentially infectious body fluids; and after specimen collection, even if gloves are worn.
2. Avoid patient contact or contact with patient care equipment or materials when his or her skin is broken (around fingernails, on the face, or on other exposed body surfaces).
3. Wear gloves when expecting to be exposed to blood or potentially infectious body fluids (see listing in Chapter 4). Do not reuse gloves.
4. Wear mask, gown, and goggles when there is a risk of splash and splatter of blood.

Protective Use of Barriers

Gloves should be made of durable, resilient material. Nonsterile gloves may be used unless there is a risk of transmitting infection to the immunosuppressed patient. When purchasing gloves, consider the average size needed by office personnel and the number of pairs needed. Gloves should be worn when:

1. Exposure to blood, potentially infectious body fluids, or bleeding lesions is possible.
2. Handling or disposing of blood-soiled specimens, linens, materials, dressings, or instruments.
3. Cleaning areas contaminated with blood, semen, or vaginal fluids.

4. Drawing blood, especially from an uncooperative patient, and when performing finger and/or heel sticks.

Gloves should be changed after caring for each patient, or immediately when tearing or puncture occurs. They should be removed by pulling at the cuffs and rolling them off the hands inside out.

Gowns and/or aprons, usually made of plastic or disposable materials, should be worn when there is danger of soiling or splashing with blood when assisting with or performing invasive procedures and cleaning.

Masks, goggles, and/or glasses should be worn to shield the face and eyes from splashing and splattering of blood. Masks are usually made of disposable materials. Goggles can be reused after washing with disinfectant. Eye glasses are regarded as barriers; goggles, however, offer better protection around the corners of the eyes and are preferable when splash or splatter is expected. Risk situations include suctioning or aspirating fluids used for irrigation and performing medical laboratory procedures such as mixing or centrifuging (see next section, on Medical Technology).

Protective Handling and Disposal of Sharp Instruments

Do not break, bend, or recap needles after administering injections, or recover scalpel blades after use. Dispose of intact disposable needles and syringes in a special, closed, puncture-resistant disposal container. Use disposable needles, syringes, and scalpels whenever possible. If using a reusable scalpel handle, remove the blade using a hemostat.

Protective Handling of Laboratory Specimens

Regard all specimens as potentially infectious. Take care not to contaminate the outside of the container with the collected substance. If the outside does become contaminated, use an approved disinfectant to clean the container. Wear gloves when collecting and handling specimens. For further protection, place the specimen in a specially designated tear-and-lock-resistant bag for transport. (See next section on Medical Technology for additional information.)

Cleaning Work Surfaces and Equipment

Work surfaces and equipment may be cleaned using high-level disinfectants such as glutaraldehyde, ethyl alcohol, stabilized hydrogen peroxide, or chlorine. Standard household bleach (5.25% sodium hypochloride) prepared fresh daily in a 1:10 dilution (1 part bleach to 10 parts water) is effective in killing the HIV on environmental surfaces. Following potential contamination of the environment, wash all instruments and surfaces that were splashed or splattered with blood or other infectious body fluids.

All disposable materials, including cleaning materials, should be placed in a hazardous waste bag according to state regulations. Blood and other body fluids usually may be poured down the toilet if connection to a sanitary sewer is certain; check with the local Health Department about this method of disposal.

Helping the HIV-Infected Patient Cope

All chronically ill patients must cope with the emotional, physical, and psychological repercussions of their illnesses; however, an HIV infection usually elicits severe emotional reactions from family, friends, and HCWs as well. Such patients are usually aware of the rejection and fear they may face and often feel so uncomfortable they postpone seeking help from health care professionals. Medical assistants need to be aware of their own feelings before they can focus on patients' needs (see Chapter 5 for ways of meeting the patient's psychosocial needs).

Interactions with HIV-infected patients should be based on honesty and fairness. Focus on patient's needs and concerns. In cooperation with the physician, make referrals to support groups and other sources of information. Have pamphlets and brochures available for distribution (see the resource list in the Appendices).

Patient Teaching

HIV-positive individuals should be taught to:

- Have regular physical examinations
- Obtain mental health counseling
- Refrain from donating blood, plasma, sperm, organs, or other tissues
- Refrain from sharing intravenous drugs
- Refrain from exchanging body fluids during sexual activity; use a condom with spermicide
- Refrain from oral–genital contact
- Refrain from sharing toothbrushes, razors, or anything contamined with blood
- Postpone pregnancy and discuss the matter with physician
- Inform physicians, dentists, and other HCWs who will be associated with their care of their condition
- Inform sexual contacts of their HIV infection before becoming intimate
- Enter a drug treatment program, if abusing drugs
- If using needles and syringes to inject insulin or other substances, soak in 1:10 bleach solution and then discard in a tamper-proof container to avoid recovery and reuse by others

Provide patients with the latest information about HIV testing and treatment. Enlist their active cooperation in coping with the infection and protecting themselves from opportunistic infections.

Privacy and Informed Consent

Laws vary from state to state and are constantly changing. The safest approach for the medical assistant to take regarding release of information on HIV status is *never to disclose* patients' names to anyone. Refer all inquiries to the physician. Disclose names to public health agencies only with a physician's written order.

Medical assistants must keep abreast of state laws and local regulations. They must recognize their responsibilities to all patients regarding right to privacy and informed consent. The legal definition of informed consent includes the patrient's right to know what procedure will be performed, by whom, why, the risks, the predicted or desired outcomes, and the nature of the procedure itself. Office policy on informed consent should be clearly developed and closely followed.

Medical assistants must actively educate themselves and their patients about HIV infection. Only through education can people distinguish fact from fiction. Through their participation in patient teaching, administering care, and interacting with patients' families and friends, they can significantly contribute to the control of the AIDS epidemic—and its accompanying epidemic of fear.

MEDICAL TECHNOLOGY

General Precautions

For more than a century it has been recognized that infections and infectious body specimens pose an occupational hazard to laboratory workers. Safety guidelines have come a long way since the time of Koch and Pasteur, especially in the arena of containment and protection for biologic agents. Biologic safety hoods and cabinets have made the laboratory environment a safer place in which to work.

Biosafety level 3 practices are generally recommended for handling *concentrated* preparations of the HIV, whereas Biosafety level 2 practices are recommended for handling routine HIV specimens in the typical clinical laboratory setting.[56] Laboratories routinely working with HIV specimens should review their biosafety containment policies. Proficiency and strict adherence to laboratory procedures should be an ongoing and frequent educational emphasis.

The integrity of all equipment used to transport fluids containing the HIV should not be overlooked. Any spill or leakage should initiate a formal review to assess exposure potential for workers and to identify corrective actions to prevent recurrence.[57] Laboratories must be especially attentive when continuous flow zonal centrifuges are used in processing HIV material. Technicians must be trained in the proper use of centrifuges and in decontamination methods to control centrifuge biohazards.

The rarity of AIDS and HIV seroconversion among laboratory personnel should not lull technologists into complacency. Medical technologists have a professional responsibility to protect themselves and their coworkers from exposure to potentially contaminated specimens. *All specimens should be handled as if they were contaminated.* The notion that hepatitis and HIV are the only specimens to be singled out for extra precaution is dangerous. The risk of hepatitis B virus (HBV) transmission far exceeds the risk of HIV transmission. The likelihood of acquiring HBV infection after an accidental needle-stick is estimated to range from 6%–30%, compared with less than 1% for the HIV.[58]

The AIDS epidemic has changed the attitudes of laboratory workers. They are more aware of what they are doing and how they are doing it. Since 1982, the CDC has published recommended precautions for HCWs, doctors, dentists, nurses, medical technologist, and others.[59–62] The recommended precautions for laboratory workers are as follows:

1. Avoid contaminating the outside of containers when collecting specimens. All specimens of blood and body fluids should be placed in well-constructed containers with secure lids to prevent leakage during transport.
2. Gloves must be worn when processing patient specimens, including blood, body fluids containing visible blood, and other fluids (see Chapter 4). Masks and protective eyewear (goggles or face shields) should be worn if splashing or aerosolization is anticipated. Change gloves and wash hands after processing each specimen. Workers with active dermatitis or skin lesions on the hands or wrists should not perform procedures that involve the transfer of concentrated HIV materials, even if their skin is protected by gloves.[63]
3. Use biological safety cabinets (class I or II) for blending, sonicating, and vigorous mixing whenever there is a potential for generating droplets. For routine procedures, such as histologic and pathologic studies, a biological safety cabinet is not necessary.
4. Mouth pipetting is not permissible. Mechanical pipetting devices must be used for the manipulation of all liquids in the laboratory.
5. Use extreme precaution when handling needles. Bending, breaking, recapping, and removing needles from disposable syringes are prohibited. Disposable syringes with needles should be placed in a clearly marked puncture-resistant container.
6. Decontaminate work surfaces with a hospital-approved chemical germicide after spills and *daily* when work is completed.
7. Infectious waste from the laboratory should be processed in accordance with institutional policies for disposal of infectious waste.
8. Decontaminate equipment before repairing or shipping.
9. Tissue or serum specimens to be stored should be clearly and permanently labeled as potentially hazardous.
10. Eating, drinking, and smoking should be prohibited in the laboratory environment.
11. Remove protective clothing and wash hands *before* leaving the laboratory.
12. Direct handling of blood or other body fluids requires the use of gowns that should be changed immediately when contaminated. The traditional lab coat

is appropriate for technologists whose work does not directly involve patient specimens.

Precautions for Phlebotomists

In addition to following the recommended precautions for laboratory workers, phlebotomists should note that wearing gloves reduces the likelihood of contaminating the hands with blood when drawing blood samples from patients (phlebotomy). Gloves cannot prevent injuries caused by needles or other sharp instruments that may penetrate the intact skin, however. The likelihood of hand contamination with blood containing the HIV, the HBV, or other blood-borne pathogens depends on a number of factors:[64]

- The skill and technique of the phlebotomist
- The frequency with which the phlebotomist performs the procedure; obviously, the more procedures performed, the higher the risk
- Whether the procedure is a routine draw (removal of blood from the patient), or occurs in an emergency situation, in which case blood contact is more likely;
- The patient population; a greater risk occurs in areas where the incidence of HIV and HBV infection is high

Universal precautions are based on assuming that all blood carries infective pathogens. In settings where blood-borne pathogens are not found frequently, some institutions have relaxed the requirement that skilled phlebotomists wear gloves. However, gloves should be available to all HCWs who are responsible for obtaining blood from patients. Their use should be encouraged.

The CDC's[65] general guidelines for phlebotomists are as follows:

1. Use gloves for performing phlebotomy when the HCW has cuts, scratches, or other breaks in the skin
2. Use gloves in situations where the HCW judges that hand contamination with blood may occur, for example, when performing phlebotomy on an uncooperative patient
3. Use gloves for performing finger and/or heel sticks on infants and children
4. Use gloves when an HCW is receiving training in phlebotomy

MEDICAL RECORDS

Because of the potential for discrimination and social stigma associated with AIDS, information about persons screened for HIV antibodies, or diagnosed or treated for AIDS or its related manifestations must be scrupulously managed. Improper, unnecessary, or inaccurate disclosure must be avoided, but information must be disclosed if required by law or medical necessity. With all sensitive information, there is an inherent ethical and legal obligation to balance the patient's right to privacy with the rights of caregivers and other third parties to information needed for legitimate purposes (see Chapter 9 for further discussion). The medical record practitioner (MRP) must be aware that laws are changing rapidly because of the volume of AIDS legislation introduced at the state and national levels.

Consent for Screening and Diagnosis

Although the eventual direction of testing legislation is yet to be decided, it is clear that mandatory HIV screening is not presently permitted. Thus any testing policy being considered should be carefully evaluated to ascertain that the purpose is clinical management (gaining information on how to treat, not whether to treat), management of employee exposure (consistent with CDC and Occupational Safety and Health Administration [OSHA] guidelines), or screening of blood or organ donations. Testing for purposes of discrimination (refusal to treat) is illegal.[66]

It is particularly important where HIV testing involves minors or persons unable to give informed consent that consent be obtained as stipulated by law. For example, under some state laws, minors as young as age 12 may give their own consent for testing.[67] An attorney at fact (durable power of attorney) may be empowered to give consent for testing only when a patient is mentally incompetent as determined by a physician; if unclear, hospitals seek legal counsel or clarification by courts. The MRP should be aware of procedures for proper authorization for testing, because ordinarily under state law the person empowered to consent to testing also has the legal authority to receive and release the medical information regarding the test results.

The MRP also should know the situations under state law where no consent is required for HIV testing. In California, for example, consent is not required for unlinked testing, when persons treated in a health care facility are not identified. Anonymity of persons tested at HIV screening clinics may be preserved under state law. Consent is not required to test blood donors (consent forms for blood donation should state that blood will be tested for HIV antibodies; thus consent is merely implied).

State law may permit cadaver testing during autopsy, or testing of body parts donated for transplantation (under the Uniform Anatomical Gift Act).[68] Dilemmas exist when physician judgment indicates HIV testing is medically indicated but the patient refuses. This public health issue of containment of a deadly infectious disease has yet to be addressed legally.

Documentation and Storage

Policies that ensure careful handling of sensitive information should be implemented. Rules used to prevent inadvertent or inappropriate disclosure of information from substance abuse, psychiatric, and similar records may be adopted.[69] MRPs must be actively involved in the following issues.

Consent for HIV Testing. When individual identity is not revealed to the facility (for instance, if reporting to state health authorities is not mandated), an alternative identifying system must be used to link the patient, blood sample, and test results. Even when the individual's identity is revealed and written consent has been obtained for testing, it may be advisable or required under state law to protect the individual's identity as fully as possible by employing an identifying system other than attaching the person's name to the blood sample and test result that will circulate outside of the medical record.

The health care facility should adopt a policy specifying where consents will be permanently filed. State law may or may not require that the same policies for handling HIV test results apply to the consent forms. Given the possibility for discrimination, however, special handling is appropriate even if not legally mandated. Extraordinary security measures, such as the use of a locked safe for consent and/or test results, may be required by law. Legal opinions about the necessity of extraordinary measures have varied widely.

Consent forms for HIV testing, where allowed or required, must conform to specifications of state law.

Handling of HIV Antibody/Virus Test. State or federal law may stipulate circumstances under which HIV test results must be especially restricted to maintain confidentiality. For instance, the law may stipulate that test results may not be filed within the medical record, or that they must be kept in a special portion of the record or within a sealed envelope. Scrutinize the law for applicability. For example, in some states special confidentiality restrictions may apply to HIV antibody test results but not to the virus test results.[70] Some health care facilities, in an attempt to prevent inadvertent release of HIV test results, have chosen not to file the laboratory slip within the medical record, using special locked storage instead. Such a policy, however, violates the current standards of the Joint Commission of Accreditation of Health Care Organizations[71] and most likely state licensure law,[72] which generally stipulate that all medical record information be retained within 1 record. If state law requires separate filing of test results, the facility's legal counsel should be consulted. Whenever test results are not filed in the record, the record should contain a written reference to the fact that the test results are available in a designated place.

The American Medical Record Association (AMRA)[73] recommends handling records regarding HIV-seropositive status using the "usual" institutional policies. Presumably this recommendation also extends to HIV-seronegative status.

Order for Test. State law may or may not address whether documenting a physician's order for HIV testing in the medical record is permitted or required. Ordinarily it is legally more advisable to document any physician order, even a sensitive one, than to omit permanent reference to a medical decision.

Record That Testing Was Done. State law may or may not address whether documenting the fact that HIV testing was done (as distinct from test results) is permitted or required.

HIV Test Results. State law usually prohibits unauthorized disclosure of HIV antibody or virus testing, even if it does not prohibit disclosure of a diagnosis of AIDS. Protection of the laboratory slip containing HIV test results, however, does not ensure protection of the person's privacy; it is virtually impossible to ensure that the rest of the medical record does not contain references to the results of HIV testing. Until recently, for example, California law forbid unauthorized disclosure of HIV test results to a "third party." It was unclear whether the law allowed disclosure by the physician ordering the HIV test to (a) anyone other than the patient or (b) anyone outside the health care facility (implying free access to anyone *within* the facility connected with giving care or providing support services, such as abstracting statistics.)[74] However, in California health care facilities treating significant numbers of HIV-infected and AIDS patients, it was found that unauthorized documentation of HIV status within medical records was pervasive and difficult to control, because health care professionals believed they had a legitimate right to know a patient's HIV status, either for personal reasons or patient management. Recent legislation clarified this dilemma by explicitly stating that inclusion of HIV test results in the medical record is not a disclosure, and that the test results may be provided to agents or employees of health care providers involved in direct patient care and treatment.[75]

Additional questions that must be addressed by institutional policy, and ones in which MRPs should be involved, include the following.

Should HCWs document a patient's HIV status if he or she offers this information? Should there be written consent from the patient to document HIV information in the medical record? Should there be corroborative evidence from the testing facility?

How should inappropriate documentation of HIV testing be handled? The MRP must ensure that capable persons within the facility are screening records for inappropriate HIV documentation and initiating follow-up and corrective action when it occurs. The burden of protecting confidentiality falls to persons or departments who monitor release of information within the facility (e.g., hospital copy services).

Whether HIV test information is inadvertently or inappropriately recorded, or recorded properly in accordance with state law, should medical records be marked in a special way to alert employees releasing information that special laws and precautions apply? A common medical record practice is flagging records containing sensitive documentation as a precautionary measure. A 1987 survey of medical record practitioners[76] indicated that a majority of respondents did use some special marking to indicate HIV testing. The most commonly employed marker was a colored sticker attached to the record folder.

The ease with which most HCWs identify the significance of colored stickers should create serious reservations about their use, given the potential for misuse of such a system. The AMRA[77] suggests that "health records of infected patients should not be marked in any special way, for such designations are more likely to cause the privacy of the patient to be violated than routine handling of health records," but acknowledges that it may be necessary to mark such records in an obscure manner to prevent inadvertent release.

How ethical and/or legal is the practice of innuendo documentation to bypass any prohibition on reporting test results? An example of such documentation is, "Patient with signs and symptoms suggestive of an immune deficiency syndrome," with no direct reference to HIV-positive status.

What is the likelihood of being sued for documenting a patient's HIV-positive status when such documentation is not permitted by law? This problem is especially important when documenting HIV status is essential to managing patient care. For example, organ transplantation is not performed unless it is certain that both donor and recipient do not have HIV infection. One may find that legally prohibited documentation is medically mandated.

Release of Information

Laws governing the release of information about HIV testing or AIDS should dictate the circumstances for *mandatory/compulsory* disclosure (e.g., notification of a central blood donor registry), *permission/discretionary* disclosure (facility creates its own policy about information release), or *prohibited* disclosure (e.g., no disclosure of information to specified parties without express written authorization of the patient).

Mandatory Disclosure. When disclosure is mandatory, the MRP must ensure that the appropriate persons are complying with the law in the manner prescribed and within the required time frame. Generally, where state laws mandate disclosure, there is a civil or criminal penalty for failure to comply, and statutory immunity from liability for the disclosure. In some states, a diagnosis of AIDs must be reported to state health authorities; in others, HIV-positive status must also be reported, or indirectly reported (for instance, to a nonspecific blood-donor-deferral register).

Prohibited Disclosure. Where the law clearly stipulates that disclosure to a third party is prohibited without the patient's express authorization, or requires concurrent consent by a health care professional, the MRP must ensure use of authorized forms (which sometimes require special wording, format, or type size) and must guard against inadvertent disclosure or disclosure without proper authorization. The AMRA recommends stamping all released material with a statement prohibiting redisclosure and also requesting that the information be destroyed when no longer needed.[78]

State law should be carefully reviewed to determine if restrictions on release of HIV information supersede duty to comply with subpoenas or court orders for civil, criminal, legislative, or administrative legal actions.

Permissive/Discretionary Disclosure. Management of discretionary disclosures is the most problematic. For example, in some states, a physician is permitted, though not required, to inform the presumed spouse of the patient's

HIV-positive status. It is unclear if this permission extends to common law spouses or live-in partners. Could there be liability for failure to warn these persons? Could the MRP be liable for failure to release this information upon request? Should one trust the word of the patient that the spouse has been told of the HIV-positive status, or attempt independent notification or verification? Should there be written verification in the medical record that the spouse was told, or that attempts were made to contact the spouse? Although the decision to notify is made by the attending physician, the MRP must be able to provide current information on legislative trends related to the duty to notify, and must be able to help implement facility policy on discretionary disclosure.

Release of HIV Information to the Patient. It is suggested that when a patient requests copies of his or her medical record regarding HIV infection, this request be handled according to the policy governing any release directly to the patient. Ideally, a written authorization should be filed in the patient's record along with verification of the physician's approval of the release.

Reverse Disclosures. Health care facility policy should stipulate that HIV-positive health care professionals must inform patients of the risk they incur by accepting treatment from them. Such disclosure should be documented, preferably in the patient's medical record.[79]

Employee Health Records. Medical records are generally maintained separately from personnel records to ensure medical confidentiality. A difficult issue is appropriate handling of documentation for employees potentially exposed to the HIV or diagnosed as having AIDS.[80] Exposed employees may want to take advantage of free testing but not wish the employer to gain access to the test results. Under current OSHA regulations, hospitals must document employee exposure and make this information available to OSHA inspectors.[81] Legal experts have recommended, however, that employee records not be released without consulting hospital counsel.[82]

Billing Information. Where state law mandates that HIV test results or information about an AIDS diagnosis may not be released to a third party without the patient's authorization, the MRP must ensure that this information is not released to third-party payers in either diagnostic narrative or coded form unless (a) valid authorization is received, or (b) an alternate system of billing is used. Ordinarily it is acceptable to release without patient consent the information that the test was done; information may also be released for Medicare claims, because this is required under federal law.[83] Some hospitals have chosen to use a nonspecific procedure code for HIV testing, for instance, a standard blood work or antibody test code and a nonspecific diagnostic code, for instance, a code for unspecified communicable disease exposure. In any case, billing personnel must adhere to the same standards of confidentiality that are expected of other professionals handling sensitive data. Because access to disease or operation codes is readily achieved, the use of International Classification of Diseases (ICD) codes is inadequate to protect diagnostic confidentiality. The AMRA suggests that institutional policy should stipulate that no billing claim relative to HIV infection may be submitted without ensuring that the patient has been informed of this diagnosis and knows that a claim listing this diagnosis will be submitted for billing.[84]

AIDS Research. MRPs should ascertain state law regulating the use of research-generated information. Generally, there should be no disclosure of information in which research subjects are personally identifiable without the subjects' written consent.[85]

Protection of Secondary Records. Diagnostic and demographic information about patients is transferred to many secondary records, such as indexes of disease and surgery, physician profiles, and billing records. Relevant policy issues include the following:

Indices and Logs. Consult state law about which information regarding the HIV must or must not be maintained in secondary records. In general a diagnosis of AIDS has no special legal protection and so should be included in disease or other indexes. Review the institutional ability to control access to the disease index and decide if special protection, such as deletion of the name of the AIDS patient, is warranted. In facilities where a large volume of research is conducted (quality assurance studies, and so forth), providing access to selected portions of the patient data base is indicated, but access is difficult to control.

HIV test results are more frequently protected by law than are AIDS diagnoses. If state law makes no stipulation about secondary records, the facility must determine its own policy. If the facility chooses not to file HIV test results in patients' medical records, then this information should not be collected from the laboratory to be used in secondary records. Where HIV test results are readily available for inclusion in secondary records, the facility must determine its ability to limit access to this data, ensuring user and terminal security, before deciding to include this data in secondary records. Separate logs of HIV infection should be maintained with discretion or not at all because of the potential for their misuse.

Disease Classification and Statistics

A number of published guidelines exist for coding HIV infection within the ICD for mortality classification and its *Clinical Modification* for morbidity classification. The MRP must be aware of current official guidelines and interpretation of any federal guidelines and ensure their consistent application within the health care facility. As the official codes for HIV viral disease are revised, the MRP must ensure that coding changes are implemented as mandated by federal (and possibly state) regulation and that these changes are precisely referenced by time and type of change, so that correct data can be retrieved from the disease index and other pertinent secondary records.

Correct classification of HIV disease is challenging because it requires that a rapidly changing disease nomenclature be placed within a slowly changing classification.[86] The ICD differentiates among AIDS (ICD code 042.X), AIDS-related complex (ICD code 043.X), and acute infection with the HIV (ICD code 044.X);

the correct code is determined by the type of infection, neoplasm, or other manifestation. The CDC has constructed a useful though artificial system with strict criteria for code selection.[87] For example, HIV infection with oral candidiasis is coded within the AIDS-related complex (043) rubric, whereas HIV infection with progression to lung or esophageal candidiasis is coded within the AIDS (042) rubric. Because HIV terminology is continually changing (for example, the category AIDS-related complex [ARC] has been eliminated), the MRP must be knowledgeable of CDC coding guidelines and work closely with medical staff to promote uniformity and accuracy in diagnostic wording and code assignment.

Other codes to identify HIV-related problems include the following: 795.8 identifies HIV-seropositive status; V02.9 (carrier or suspected carrier of other specified infectious organism—definition of "carrier" unclear) may be used to identify the HIV carrier; V01.8 (contact with or exposure to other communicable diseases) may be used to identify exposure to the HIV virus.

Confidentiality Implications. Because both V02.9 and V01.8 represent broad residual categories not specifically identifying AIDS, there are no special confidentiality problems associated with their use. Where a diagnosis of AIDS or pre-AIDS (ARC) carries no special confidentiality protection, using the codes 042.X or 043.X is acceptable; however, it is suggested that these codes be given the special protection psychiatric or other sensitive codes are given.

Where state law mandates special protection of HIV test results, however, the use of either 795.8 or 044.X becomes problematic, because use of either code virtually identifies the person as HIV-positive.[88] Where relevant, legal counsel should be consulted about whether the codes should be used. It is unlikely that either of these codes would represent a patient's reason for admission (principal diagnosis), but they would represent important secondary information.

Morbidity and Mortality Statistics. From a statistical perspective, it should be noted that current reporting systems generally allow for only 1 ICD code to indicate a patient's reason for admission. With AIDS illnesses, however, 2 codes are frequently required, one to identify AIDS and another to identify the manifestation for which the patient is being treated. The code for the manifesting, or secondary, disease is usually recorded first. Thus AIDS could be underreported as a reason for admission if only the principal (first) diagnosis code is considered when compiling statistics.

MRPs have noticed that because they fear lawsuits, some physicians hesitate to list AIDS as a diagnosis. MRPs must ensure that all relevant diagnoses are recorded to avoid skew in statistical reporting, and must follow facility procedure in correcting problems of documentation.

Another concern is under-reporting of AIDS on death certificates. Under-reporting occurs in part because death certificates are constructed to report only 3 causes of death, and AIDS may be fourth or fifth in the chain of events of underlying cause.[89] MRPs must ensure adequate documentation of cause of death on hospital medical and secondary records and recognize that under-reporting of AIDS in mortality statistics exists.

NURSING

M. Patricia Donahue[90] writes:

> *From the dawn of civilization evidence prevails to support the premise that nurturing has been essential to the preservation of life. Survival of the human race, therefore, is inextricably intertwined with the development of nursing. . . .*

The AIDS epidemic presents what may be one of the greatest challenges to nursing in modern times. The role of nurses in the AIDS epidemic is central. Nurses nurture, comfort, and support persons with HIV infection along the entire continuum of illness, and often provide the last human touch for a PWA at the time of death.

Yet the focus of much that has been written about nurses in the era of AIDS is about nurses' fear, anxiety, and personal safety concerns. In many ways, this focus is inconsistent with how nurses have behaved in other eras when personal risk for diseases such as tuberculosis, influenza, rubella, or viral hepatitis was considered just "part of the job." Occupationally acquired cases of all of these diseases may also result in serious illness or death, albeit not with the same degree of certainty that infection with the HIV seems to present. On the other hand, we now have vaccines to prevent rubella and hepatitis B. Unfortunately, many health care personnel have not yet been vaccinated against hepatitis B, a well-recognized risk reduction strategy for any HCW who has contact with blood.

Nurses should learn more about ways to enhance their nurturing, caring role while becoming more technically competent in meeting the multifaceted and complex needs of persons with HIV infections and AIDS. Learning the ways the HIV is transmitted, as well as the ways it is not, should alleviate much of the fear that many nurses—and prospective students of nursing—feel.

Nurses must learn the facts about the disease, whom it affects, and the risks to themselves. Then they must use that information to modify behavior. This means becoming skilled at recognizing clinical signs and symptoms that signal difficulties in the patient, and becoming adept at dealing with the many psychological and social problems associated with this complex illness.

Nurses need to evaluate their own standards of practice to ensure that they are appropriately using interventions known to reduce personal risk, while avoiding using excessive protective garments and distancing maneuvers that patients further isolate. Nurses often serve as health care team leaders, especially in home and hospice care. Their example is likely to be followed by other team members. Theirs is a signal responsibility to set the stage for compassionate care.

The AIDS epidemic offers nurses the opportunity to participate in the excitement of learning about a new disease, while at the same time questioning their own values and prejudices. The epidemic also offers the opportunity for nurses to set standards of quality patient care and infection control for both patients and personnel.

OCCUPATIONAL THERAPY

Occupational therapists accept responsibility for treating persons who exhibit neurological and/or psychosocial–cultural dysfunction in life roles and tasks resulting from HIV infection and AIDS. Therapists confront the same fears and challenges other team members do, such as fear of the unknown, dealing with the dying patient, homophobia, the drug culture, helplessness, and uncertainty.

Occupational Behavior

The concept of occupational behavior is the frame of reference occupational therapists have developed to treat patients who have difficulty controlling and mastering life situations. Kielhofner[91] defines occupational behavior as "the purposeful use of time by humans to fulfill their own internal urges toward exploring and mastering their environment that at the same times fulfills the requirements of the social group to which they belong and personal needs for self maintenance."

Many terminally ill persons are not able to follow the process of normal development by exploring their environments, and cannot make appropriate choices in dealing with life tasks. Physical, cognitive, and psychosocial dysfunctions disrupt mastery of life skills. The occupational behavior frame of reference, also called the *model of human occupation,* is the basis of occupational therapy for terminally ill persons. This approach effectively integrates the psychosocial, physical, and environmental aspects of health care of the person with AIDS.[92]

According to the theory of occupational behavior, the individual is an "open system" who dynamically interacts with his or her environment. Occupational behaviors can be categorized into 3 subsystems, or groups, of behaviors within the person's environment. PWAs may experience dysfunction in any or all of these subsystems.

The first category (subsystem) of occupational behavior involves volition, or the act of willing and choosing behaviors. Regardless of how a person acquired HIV infection, having AIDS diminishes his or her belief in self and abilities, expectations of success, and control of his or her environment. A PWA may suffer a serious change in value system, partly because he or she cannot maintain the usual pace of daily activities. Formerly valued activities become meaningless; work and lifestyle goals change. Interest patterns and the values attributed to skills and feelings change.

The second category is habituation, or the ability to maintain activities through routine behaviors. Habituation involves role delineation, the ability to internalize expectations and to balance those expectations. PWAs cannot organize the habits necessary for social interaction. They are threatened with loss of habitual living skills and fear their inability to continue functioning.

The third category of occupational behavior is performance, involving the skills producing action. Skills include interpersonal, communicational, perceptual, and motor skills, and neurological and musculoskeletal functions.[93]

The role of the occupational therapist is to assist the patient in identifying changes, deficiencies, strengths, potential skills, and habits in order to organize and develop life roles and skills that will provide identifiable values and choices. Therapy includes occupations and activities that help the patient integrate psychosocial, physical, and environmental functions. Through the use of their hands, many patients are able to develop a meaningful lifestyle.

Threats to Independence in Daily Life Roles and Tasks

The developmental tasks of the young adult (23–45 years of age) include assuming new roles at home, at work, and in the social world, after leaving home and and school. Values, attitudes, and interest develop with these changing roles and affect the types of daily tasks and the manner in which they are accomplished.[94]

In young adulthood, a person becomes independent of parental care and focuses on an occupational role which becomes his or her new way of life, in order to meet survival needs and achieve satisfaction. The person chooses leisure activities, including exercise, sports, and hobbies. Although work roles and goals occupy most of the young adult's time, a struggle to balance self-care, work, and leisure roles usually takes place. The young adult must often balance roles chosen to meet his or her own needs with the responsibility for a family or "significant other" persons or animals.

During this period, the young adult functions at his or her highest level. The young adult experiences an emotional developmental crisis when making a commitment to an intimate relationship, to a cause, or to an institution.

A PWA in this age range is likely to become withdrawn, lonely, or self-centered. Finding adequate and satisfying sexual experiences, which are very important to young adults, is thwarted by the disease.

From their experiences with developmental problems in severely disabled and terminally ill young adult patients, occupational therapists are thus able to adapt evaluation and treatment skills to assist PWAs in confronting and adapting to a different level of function in life tasks. PWAs must face the developmental challenge of persons 20–40 years old (98% are workers) without the opportunity to master the life tasks of their own age group.

Rather than becoming independent in self-care and work roles, PWAs suddenly become dependent again on family and society. Unlike other young adults, who have a high level of energy in both physical and mental activities, PWAs are unable to perform adequately in work and leisure activities. Being out of work, perhaps for the first time, losing intimate relationships because of physical weakness, and experiencing guilt or fear of transmitting the disease all disturb social interactions. Self-concept is shattered. Habits change drastically.

AIDS patients find it nearly impossible to make temporal adjustments to the here-and-now, to a shortened life span, to a meaningful and purposeful lifestyle. Sometimes they must abandon life goals, change, work choices, and enduring intimate relationships. These problems cut short the ability to solidify identity, and may force the person to accept a warped or rejected role in his or her social group. Not feeling accepted by one's social group is the most hurtful and difficult change to accept, because it deprives the person of ways to meet needs for intimacy, sexuality, and belonging.

The goal of occupational therapy is to help PWAs face a shortened lifespan through meaningful activities within the patient's ability to understand and function. Ways of meeting this goal range from self-care sessions involving learning to use make-up, hair style, clothes, and body movements to increase self-worth, to work evaluation programs that identify remaining work skills that can be performed with limited physical energy. Each patient's needs should be addressed individually to enable him or her to master the changed environment as much as possible.

Evaluation and Treatment

Within the occupational behavior model, the occupational therapist first assesses how the patient performs each of his or her life roles and assists the patient in developing goals within reach.

Although each patient has different problems, common problems include:

- Decline in function caused by the disease and resulting in diminished self-esteem and confidence about skills
- Fluctuating ability to function and fluctuating health status, with lower expectations and success in performing usual activities
- For adults, loss of meaningful work and income, loss of identity, and loss of relationships (support system), daily habit change, and dependency on others, which affects ability to live productively; for children, dysfunctional play and altered concepts of self (the sociopolitical nature of AIDS involves discrimination against both old and young in their daily occupational roles)
- Roles are affected by an uncertain future; daily activities change meaning, new hobbies and interests take precedence, value systems shift
- Quality of life takes on a different meaning; new occupational goals are adopted; frequently, more time is spent with family and significant others
- Changing standards for productive and meaningful living affects occupational behaviors
- Interests in meaningful daily tasks change in intensity; work investment may shift to leisure and family skills

To reduce the impact of terminal illness on AIDs patients, occupation is used as a tool to enhance the quality of life. Through evaluating existing skills and establishing goals and priorities for desirable activities, therapists help patients maximize attainable occupational roles. The patient can gain a feeling of mastery and competence of the immediate environment, self, and the disease.[95]

Using the concepts of occupational behavior,[96,97] the therapist helps the patient explore and achieve physical, cognitive, and psychosocial tasks. Trial and error are allowed but levels of competency are identified in the process of developing problem-solving and decision-making skills.

It is also important to help the patient achieve a sense of productive living in the midst of fluctuating habits. The impact of performance, volition, and the environment on the ability to maintain routine activities (habituation subsystem) affects the quality of evaluation and treatment.[98]

The patient who exhibits muscle weakness, incoordination, and poor endurance in accomplishing life tasks frequently lacks self-confidence and is depressed. The occupational therapist helps the patient select activities at which he or she can succeed and that will provide an opportunity to make choices in a supportive environment (for example, grooming activities such as shaving, putting on make-up, or dressing). Energies necessary for making desirable neurophysiological movements are identified, giving patients choices in working towards self-care skills within the parameters of their physical and psychosocial abilities. Activities are graded by levels of difficulty within patients' present and projected abilities. Pursuing one goal at a time results in feelings of accomplishment, success, and self-control and promotes quality living.

Caring for the Child with AIDS

Even though the number of children estimated to have AIDS by 1991 is only 2000, many occupational therapists, especially those working in areas where the rate of intravenous drug use is high, will be treating children with AIDS.

Evaluation of dysfunctions in children is similar to evaluation of dysfunction in adults, but is adapted to childrens' world of play and school. Building self-concept, encouraging enjoyment of here-and-now activities, and helping the child achieve temporal goals can add meaning and quality to the life of a child with AIDS.

Caring for the Home-Bound AIDS Patient

Because of the nature and cost of AIDS medical care, home care programs are often the most cost-effective way of treating AIDS patients. Because life activities are home or family centered, the home is the logical treatment environment. Community-centered clinics can be effective in supporting interaction between choosing behaviors, maintaining activities, and producing action (the subsystems of human occupation).

Occupational therapists have traditionally been responsible for assessing the physical environment and suggesting modifications such as removal of barriers to independent living. Adaptive and assistive devices, energy conservation techniques, and work efficiency strategies contribute to modification of daily living skills.

An AIDS patient may need assistance in the following:

- Working out a daily activity program within energy levels
- Rearranging cooking tools, dishes, and supplies within limited reach
- Removing loose carpets easily tripped over
- Installing grab bars by toilets for easier sitting and rising
- Removing door closures and installing lever openers to make doors easier to open
- Installing simple ramps and hand rails in place of hazardous steps
- Adapting to public transportation
- Learning to use "dial-a-ride" services to reach appointments
- Selecting and accomplishing recreational and avocational activities
- Adapting and using environmental controls for home appliances, lights, phones, and communication

The patient's support system should be recognized and included in an educational program for the family and significant others. Therapy will identify environmental barriers and daily activity patterns and design a program specific to the person's needs.

Barrier-free Living in the Community

Many AIDS patients will experience muscle weakness, incoordination, and lack of endurance, all of which limit mobility and independence in daily living. Although communities are becoming more accessible to physically handicapped people and homes are being designed to accommodate people with permanent disabilities, AIDS patients present a new demand for an accessible environment. AIDS patients may need guidelines and assistance as they confront barriers and strive to maintain their independence. New barriers may confront them as their illness progresses.

Although preparing a barrier-free environment is the responsibility of the family and the community, AIDS projects and other interested groups may need to become politically active to encourage communities to respond. Universal accessibility includes wide, level parking; maneuvering space in parking and restroom facilities; ramps; grab bars; wide and easily opened doors; amenities such as phones, service counters, and mail drop boxes placed at lower levels; in supermarkets with lighter packages, carry-out assistance, and assistance reaching higher shelves; space to move at work and home; furniture placed at strategic spots for walking, transferring, and moving; and adaptive shower heads and storage units.

Loan Centers. Occupational therapists can assist AIDS patients by setting up a community evaluation clinic with a network of resources that provides adaptive and assistive devices on loan when needed. The value of such a resource center will be demonstrated psychosocially as patients and families share and care, and economically as equipment is used more efficiently.

Adaptive and assistive devices that such resource centers could make available include:

- Reachers
- Built-up handles for utensils, grooming aids, and home tools
- Grippers for dishes, appliances, and tools
- Tub/shower benches and grab bars
- Lever handles/knobs
- Food- and pot-holding boards/clasps
- Lap boards
- Storage units
- Computers and computer-assisted controls

To protect against possible transmission of HIV infection, all loan equipment should be cleansed using a tuberculocidal chemical germicide (see Chapter 4) and allowed to air dry.

Although much of the new assistive technology is expensive, occupational therapists can assist AIDS patients by finding creative ways to help them achieve independent living.

PHYSICAL THERAPY

Goals

Physical therapy goals for patients with HIV infection or AIDS are different than goals for patients whose full recovery is expected. Patient goals may become less rather than more ambitious as the disease progresses. Goal setting has psychosocial overtones. A therapist should not take away a patient's hope. If returning to employment on a part- or full-time basis is realistic, then both the physical and occupational therapist can assist the patient in learning ways to save energy. While working with the patient to set goals, the therapist should be a good listener. Help the patient decide which goals are most important. Evaluate whether these goals are realistic. Remember that the patient's emotional support system may make or break his or her desire and will to live.

Barbara Bezalel[99] reports from her work with AIDS patients at San Francisco General Hospital that physical therapists must be "in tune" to the needs of patients with AIDS. Therapists must accept the patient's support system and all manifestations of the disease. Also, they should listen when patients report how they are feeling, because their health status can change very rapidly. When giving AIDS patients assistive devices for ambulation and wheelchair mobility, be open to options. One day the patient may require a cane and the next day a walker. Flexibility of treatment approach is important. The patient's health should be constantly re-evaluated.

The goal of physical therapy is to evaluate and appropriately treat patients based on their physical therapy needs. The physical therapist should focus on functional mobility and prevention of disability. For each AIDS patient, the therapist should evaluate the following, if applicable:

Muscle strength and coordination
Joint mobility
General level of physical fitness, including cardiopulmonary function
Ambulation and balance deficits
Neurological deficits due to involvement of the central and peripheral nervous system
Pain
Skin integrity

The patient and therapist then work together to maintain or enhance quality of life using the therapist's knowledge and treatment tools. Goals may be reached by use of endurance and strengthening exercises; coughing and deep breathing exercises (except when the diagnosis is *Pneumocystis carinii* pneumonia); manual neurological techniques such as neurodevelopmental treatment, proprioceptive neuromuscular facilitation (PNF), Rood, Brunnstrom; Transcutaneous electrical nerve stimulation (TENS); patient education for energy conservation, joint protection, and safety; and discharge plans for the patient.

Physical Therapy Department Practices

A telephone survey of physical therapy departments was conducted by Rogers* in May 1986. Rogers found that 2 of the 12 large institutions where AIDS patients were treated did not refer them to physical therapy. The directors of physical therapy indicated this was because the purpose of treatment for AIDs patients was considered maintenance only. With no reimbursement for service, the physical therapy departments in these institutions were not involved in evaluation and treatment of AIDS patients.

Figure 10–1 shows that in the 10 institutions Rogers contacted where the physical therapy department was involved in treatment of AIDS patients, endurance and strengthening exercises were the most frequently reported activity (9 out of 10 hospitals). Improving mobility by gait analysis and use of assistive devices was the second most frequently mentioned goal of physical therapy (7 out of 10). Maintaining or restoring the ability to perform activities of daily living (ADL) was next (6 out of 10). Three of the 10 departments reported splinting patients with central nervous system involvement. TENS units were used for pain control. Home exercise programs with appropriate equipment were re-

*Rogers, EA: Unpublished survey, 1986.

SERVICES

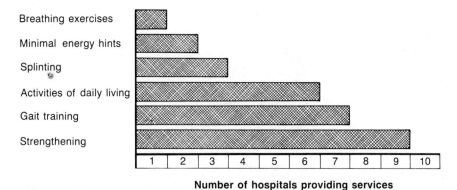

Number of hospitals providing services

FIGURE 10-1. May 1986 telephone survey of 12 health care institutions regularly treating AIDS patients.

ported. Two of the 10 departments taught patients methods of minimizing energy expenditure. One of the 10 departments taught breathing exercises.

In July 1987, the survey was repeated* (Fig. 10–2). Rogers attempted to talk with the same therapists she had interviewed the previous year. Of the 12 hospitals, 1 had instituted a new policy indicating that therapists could not talk to anyone about treatment guidelines for AIDS patients; therefore, the following results are based on data from 11 hospitals.

Help with ADL and exercises for strengthening were part of treatment in 8 of the 11 hospitals. Gait analysis and gait training occurred in 7. Physical therapy evaluation of AIDS patients was common in 5. Home health care was provided by 5. Equipment evaluation occurred in 4. Hydrotherapy was a part of treatment in 2. Safety education for the patient and instruction of family members was taught in 1 institution.

When comparing the results of the 2 surveys, there appears to be a slight increase in awareness of physical therapists' role in evaluating and instructing patients and family members about safety and functional activities. Use of the services of a home care physical therapist became an option for patients at 2 hospitals. Three of the 11 institutions indicated that referring physicians were being more selective about which AIDS patients should be referred for physical

---

*Rogers, EA: Unpublished survey, 1987.

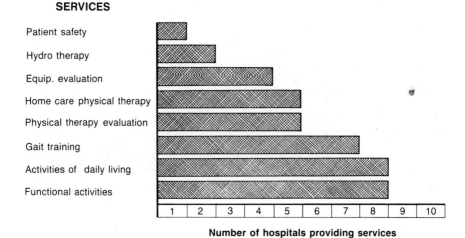

FIGURE 10-2. July 1987 repeat of telephone survey to 12 health care institutions regularly treating AIDS patients.

therapy. Additionally, 2 of the institutions now reported seeing AIDS patients on an outpatient basis in the physical therapy department.

In the 1986 survey, physical therapy staff at 4 of the 11 institutions learned that patients had HIV infections *after* evaluation and treatment had been given. This was very upsetting to the staff. These occurrences re-emphasize the importance of using universal precautions in treatment of all patients.

Galantino,[100,101] director of physical therapy at the Institute for Immunological Disorders in Houston, Texas, describes the role of the physical therapist in working with HIV-infected patients. She advises that therapists can and should play a major role in the AIDS epidemic just as they did in the past during the polio epidemic. She stresses that opportunities for therapists in evaluation, treatment, and research are excellent.

The treatment approach must be patient centered; that is, the therapist must be attuned to patient needs. As the disease progresses, the therapist must revise treatment goals. Galantino and Levy[102] believe that HIV infection should be considered an actual or potential neuromuscular degenerative disorder. As a result, they urge early physical therapy intervention with HIV-infected persons to prolong their lives and improve the quality of their lives.

Muscle Fatigue

Fatigue is a major musculoskeletal problem affecting patients with HIV infection or AIDS. Muscle strength may appear good but endurance is often poor. Therefore, it is important when setting up a treatment program to monitor vital signs and blood gases.

Neurological symptoms may occur in HIV-infected persons as the central nervous system and peripheral nerves are attacked by the HIV directly. These patients suffer spasticity, gait disorders, paraparesis, hemiplegia, and dystonias. Physical therapists can work with the patient to improve balance, coordination, and mobility.

Central Nervous System Involvement

As research reveals more about central nervous system involvement in HIV-infected patients, physical therapists will see more patients who have neurological problems but in whom HIV infection or AIDS has not yet been diagnosed. This may prove helpful to patients because therapists' approach to these patients will probably be more oriented towards function and life. This fact should also remind therapists of the importance of treating all patients as though they were potentially HIV-infected. The patient with hemiplegic-like symptoms or other neurological deficits may have incipient AIDS.

Precautions

Protection from potential transmission of HIV infection during physical therapy procedures should follow the universal precautions for all HCWs outlined in Chapter 4. The use of a standard tuberculocidal chemical germicide to disinfect equipment between uses where there is a potential for transfer of body fluids such as blood, semen, or vaginal secretions is sufficient. The chemical disinfectants ordinarily used in such devices as whirlpool baths are sufficient to prevent the transfer of HIV.

Physical therapists need to respond positively to HIV-infected patients by providing quality care. These patients deserve all the benefits the profession can offer. Physical therapy is part of the comprehensive multidisciplinary team approach that can enhance the quality of life for HIV-infected persons.

RADIOGRAPHY AND RADIOLOGIC TECHNOLOGY

HCWs in the fields of radiography and radiologic technology should follow the same universal precautions other health professionals follow when dealing with blood, semen, vaginal secretions, cerebrospinal fluid, synovial fluid, pelural fluid, peritoneal fluid, pericardial fluid, and amniotic fluid.[103]

For a student entering the field of radiology, the main problem regarding HIV transmission is often one of application rather than of knowledge. When students begin practicing in the various imaging and therapeutic modalities of radiology, they may not see universal precautions uniformly applied. Many current practitioners began professional practice before the advent of AIDS. Students must know and apply what they have been taught about universal precautions, regardless of what they see practiced. Of course, student learners should always respect and be ready to learn from employees with whom they train.

Universal Precautions

Many radiographic examinations do not involve routine exposure to a patient's blood, body fluids, or tissues. The possibility of such exposure, however, can exist when examining almost any patient and cannot be determined simply by reading the type of examination to be performed from the x-ray order form. The age and condition of the patient or the presence of pathological conditions such as lesions or trauma may turn a simple examination into one that poses a risk for HIV transmission.[104] Table 10–1 outlines the various categories of risk in radiography. The following radiographic examinations present little chance of body fluid contact: x-rays of the chest, extremities or joints, pelvis, or abdomen; mammography; spine and skull examinations; and most ultrasound examinations. A technologist might choose to wear nonsterile gloves as a precautionary factor when performing any of these examinations, or might choose to wear gloves for such examinations only when individual patient circumstances dictate. If technologists choose not to wear gloves for such low-risk examinations, they should at least wash their hands thoroughly after examining each patient, and should consider wearing gloves if they have cuts or abrasions on their hands that may come in contact with the patient, because immune-suppressed patients are more susceptible to nosocomial infections.[105]

Many radiographic examinations fall within an intermediate risk category where exposure to blood, body fluids, or tissues is possible but the risk is minimal if proper precautions are followed. In these types of examinations, the risk of exposure is normally much greater for the radiologist or physician performing the examination than for the student or technologist. Gloves should normally be worn for all types of examinations in this category. Gowns may be appropriate for certain examinations in these areas, but masks or protective eye wear would be needed in only a limited number of cases.

On the lower risk end of this category are contrast examinations that present potential exposure to saliva or urine. These fluids have low levels of the HIV with little possibility of infectious transmission. Examinations such as upper gastrointestinal examinations (UGIs), esophagrams, cystograms, voiding cystourethrograms, and endoscopic retrograde cholangiopancreatography (ERCPs), should be performed using proper precautions for body fluid contact. Soiled linens or disposable items used in these examinations should be properly discarded.

Of intermediate risk are a wide variety of contrast examinations in which needles are used to inject contrast into veins, joints, cavities, lymphatics, and so forth, and/or in which fluids are withdrawn for laboratory analysis. Although

TABLE 10-1. Potential Risk Factors for Exposure to Patients' Body Fluids by Radiographic Examinations and Areas

Lower Risk Examination/Areas			
Chest	Mammography	Skull	Ultrasound
Spine	Extremities	Abdomen	Pelvis

Intermediate Risk Examination/Areas			
Gastrointestinal tract (esophagus, stomach, small bowel)			
Myelography	Venography	Cystography	Urograms
Arthrography	Amniocentesis	MRI w/contrast	Most contrast
Endoscopic examination	CT w/contrast	Trauma examinations (stabilized patient)	examinations

Higher Risk Examinations/Areas		
Barium enemas (colon)	Angiography/arteriography	Hysterosalpingography
Biopsies	Interventional radiographic procedures	Trauma examinations (ER)
Surgical examinations	Nuclear medicine injections w/needle recapping	

CT = computed tomography; MRI = magnetic resonance imaging; ER = emergency room.

needle-stick may be considered a serious consequence of any of these examinations, widespread splashing or spreading of blood or fluids is usually not involved. Risk is usually limited to the physician responsible for injecting contrast and to the technologist responsible for needle disposal. Gloves should be mandatory for these examinations; gowns are often appropriate; masks and protective eyewear may sometimes be needed. Needles should never be recapped, and manual manipulation of needles should be limited to placing them in puncture-proof containers for disposal or transport, if reusable. Safe collection, storage, and labeling of fluids for laboratory analysis should be practiced. Follow the procedures outlined in Chapter 4 for care of soiled linens and cleansing of soiled surface areas. Radiographic examinations in this risk category include myelography, arthrography, all intravenous examinations such as urography and cholecystography, intravenous injection for computed tomography (CT) and magnetic resonance imaging (MRI), biopsies, and amniocentesis.

The last category of radiographic examinations includes those that present a high risk of exposure to blood, body fluids, or tissues if proper precautions are not taken. Fortunately, this category contains fewer routine radiographic examinations than the other categories. Many of the high-risk radiographic procedures are performed only in specialized areas. A full complement of protective coverings should be worn during these examinations, including eyewear if splashing of blood or fluids commonly occurs. This category includes administering barium enemas, colostomy examinations, and hysterosalpingography. Radiographic examinations that take place in surgery or in the emergency room and involve trauma patients are also high-risk. For these type of examinations, radiographic cassettes may be placed in sterile/nonsterile plastic bags to avoid contamination from body fluids. Also, gloves must be removed/changed between touching the patient and touching any other radiographic equipment or personnel. If enough technologists or students are available for an examination, one technologist can remain gloved and handle all patient contact, while another handles all non-patient contact situations. Any radiographic equipment or positioning aids that become contaminated during such procedures should be cleaned or sterilized after the examination.

Other high-risk areas in radiology include nuclear medicine and angiography/intraventional procedures. In nuclear medicine, most patients must be injected with radiopharmaceuticals before scanning is performed. Because radioisotopes may remain in the needles used for injection, these needles must be recapped and stored separately as low-level radiation waste products.

Angiographic/interventional studies probably pose one of the highest levels of risk for exposure to blood and body fluids in all of radiology. The insertion of guide wires and catheters into the arterial system provides opportunities for blood to spray under pressure at the beginning of a procedure, and contact with blood is possible throughout the procedure until the patient has left the radiographic suite. Use of new mechanical apparatuses designed to reduce blood spray on arterial puncture should be considered for these exams.[106,107] Because this is a sterile procedure, physicians, nurses, and technologists have always worn protective clothing and gloves, but must now include mask and goggles. These precautions apply to anyone who will be in close contact with the patient. Catheters, guide wires, and other items used during the procedure must be disposed of according to the steps in Chapter 4.

Radiology presents students and technologists with a full range of possibilities for exposure to the HIV and other infectious agents. HCWs in radiology should know and follow protective measures. But they must also remember that patients are people who need care and concern. AIDS patients must not be made to feel that HCWs view them only as potential sources of infection. Concerned technologists will avoid giving that impression.

RESPIRATORY CARE

Respiratory care practitioners (RCPs) often play a key role in the treatment of HIV-infected persons and PWAs because the most common complications of AIDS involve the respiratory tract. Since the lung provides a portal of entry for many possible opportunistic infections, the immunosuppressed patient frequently develops lung infections that are a major cause of morbidity and mortality. In fact, respiratory failure due to PCP is a common cause of hospitalization and death in HIV-infected patients.[108,109] This section reviews the specific precautions RCPs should take in order to provide appropriate respiratory care for these patients while protecting themselves from infection.

The goals of infection control are to protect the AIDS patient from opportunistic infections and to prevent spread of the HIV and any AIDS-related pulmonary infection, such as tuberculosis or cytomegalovirus, to clinicians and other patients. Specific considerations for different types of respiratory care are outlined below; however, a few general guidelines are presented first. Universal precautions call for all RCPs to use a mask, gown, gloves, and eye protection when performing any procedure that may result in splashes or spraying of the patient's blood.[110] These precautions should be taken when caring for *all* patients regardless of the diagnosis.

Standards of Care

The standards of care that call for proper hand washing before and after caring for each patient, and for cleaning and sterilizing all respiratory therapy equipment before use are adequate for the HIV-infected patient. The standard for processing nondisposable equipment that touches or indirectly contacts mucous membranes (i.e., mouth pieces, circuits, and nebulizers) requires that it be disassembled, cleaned with detergent and water, and then disinfected with a high-level disinfectant such as glutaraldehyde, ethyl alcohol, stabilized hydrogen peroxide, or chlorine.[111] If possible, the equipment should be autoclaved or gas-sterilized with ethylene oxide. Use of disposable mouthpieces, nebulizers, and tubing whenever possible is helpful for respiratory care departments that do not have the resources to effectively process nondisposable equipment. Special precautions are advisable when performing the following procedures for an HIV-infected patient.

Suctioning

Pneumocystis carinii pneumonia and other lung infections may result in respiratory failure and the retention of excessive pulmonary secretions. The patient may need assistance in the removal of these secretions with suctioning. If not performed properly, aspiration of the patient's airway can result in contamination of the patient's respiratory tract. To avoid this problem, strict adherence to sterile technique is necessary. If the patient has a strong cough, which is often stimulated when the catheter is inserted, spraying of droplets into the air may result.

Spraying of droplets into the room can also occur when a patient receiving mechanical ventilation is disconnected from the circuit. In such cases, the RCP should wear a mask, gown, and goggles in addition to gloves. This type of garb is also recommended when the RCP must intubate a patient or assist the physician during a bronchoscopy. Bronchoscopy is often needed in the care of HIV-infected patients because it is an effective tool for diagnosing *Pneumocystis* infections.[112]

When sputum specimens are collected for analysis, the outside of the container should not be contaminated and the lid must be securely attached. Gloves should be worn by anyone handling the container. The specimen should be labeled "body fluid precautions." Labeling the specimen "HIV-infected" does not serve any purpose.

Aerosol Treatments

Because sputum from the patient's mouth could fall into the nebulizer cup, RCPs should wear gloves when handling the nebulizer. Placing a bacterial filter on the exhalation port is probably not necessary but is a reasonable precaution.

Aerosolization of pentamidine for the prevention and treatment of *Pneumocystis carinii* pneumonia has been done and appears to have promising results thus far.[113] This technique allows more direct application of the drug to the lung with fewer and less severe systemic side-effects compared with intravenous administration. Experience with the drug is limited and the Food and Drug Administration considers it investigational therapy at this point.

Two types of nebulizers, ultrasonic and jet, have been used to deliver aerosolized pentamidine. It is not yet clear which method is optimal. Particle size is important because alveolar deposition of the drug is ideal. A jet nebulizer such as the Respirgard II* is helpful because it has appropriate particle size output, a reservoir to collect aerosol during exhalation, and an expiratory filter to prevent contamination of the environment. Because the nebulizer output per unit of time decreases at pressures less than 20 psi, small home compressors are not recommended for aerosolization of pentamidine.[114]

Arterial Puncture

The use of needles and any sharp instruments requires special consideration to avoid accidental cuts or stick injuries. Recapping needles with the standard 2-handed technique is the act most often resulting in accidental puncture wounds and therefore should not be standard practice.[115] Commercial products are avail-

---

*Produced by Marquest Medical Products, Englewood, Colorado.

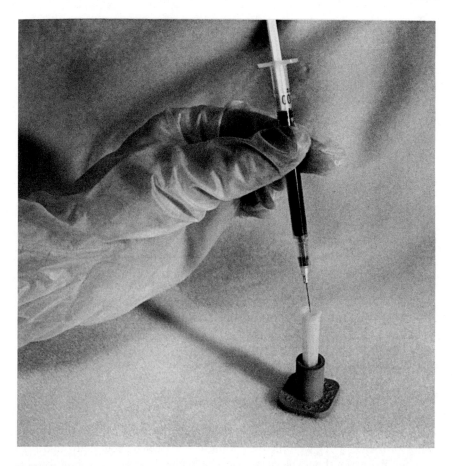

FIGURE 10-3. Demonstration of a safe technique for recapping a contaminated needle with one hand. (Photograph by Mark A. Valley, R.R.T.)

able that allow the contaminated needle to be recapped or secured with only 1 hand holding the barrel of the syringe (Fig. 10–3). Under no circumstances should the needle be reinserted into the sheath using the 2-handed technique. Also, an uncapped needle should never be removed from a syringe. Disposable syringes and needles should be placed in puncture-resistant containers located as close as possible to where needles are used.[116] To avoid direct contact with the blood sample, glvoes should be worn during the puncture procedure and when handling the sample for any reason. Spilled blood samples should be cleaned up with a 1:10 solution of sodium hypochlorite (household bleach).

Cardiopulmonary Resuscitation (CPR)

In the hospital setting, mouth-to-mouth resuscitation should not be performed. Strategic placement of resuscitator bags with appropriate size adapters and masks is essential. These bags provide artificial ventilation with an increased oxygen concentration and obviate the need for mouth-to-mouth resuscitation. Gloves should be worn during maneuvers to clear the airway with finger sweeps.

Ventilator Care

When caring for AIDS patients receiving mechanical ventilation, many of the precautions already mentioned will be helpful. In addition, the ventilator tubing can collect a combination of water from the humidifier and sputum from the patient. The fluids within the circuit should never be drained back into the humidifier reservoir because this can result in contamination of the humidifier. Gloves should be worn when draining water from the tubing. If droplets from the tubing might be sprayed into the room, a mask, gown, and goggles are needed. Spraying is more common when high peak pressures or continuous positive airway pressure is used.

The surface of the ventilator is frequently soiled with the patient's blood or sputum and should be wiped clean with an appropriate solution. Regular changing of the circuit (every 24–48 hours) helps reduce the incidence of nosocomial infections. The internal parts of the ventilator do not need to be treated any differently following use by an HIV-infected patient.

Home Care

Special considerations should be observed when HIV-infected patients receive home care for the treatment of any chronic pulmonary disease. In such cases, family or friends living with the patient must be educated about body fluid precautions. Extra care should be taken to teach all household members how to keep the home equipment as clean as possible, because the patient's immune system is compromised. A 1:10 chlorine bleach solution, freshly prepared, is inexpensive and effective. Whenever possible, disposable circuits and nebulizers should be used. After use, all equipment should be brought to the hospital for appropriate disposal. Dumping contaminated equipment into home trash containers is not acceptable because it could result in exposure of sanitation workers to potential infection.

RCPs can also provide both support and education to HIV-infected persons. RCPs can establish team relationships with their patients to help them to understand the disease and the potential offered by various treatments.

SPEECH–LANGUAGE PATHOLOGY

Speech–language pathologists (SLPs) will assume a greater role in treating HIV-infected persons as research provides methods to enable such persons to live longer. Patients who live longer will need to communicate with others at their jobs and in the community before reaching the terminal phase. Currently, however, few SLPs are involved in diagnosis or in treatment during the early stages of the disease. Most often, if involved at all, the SLP may be called upon to provide some augmentative or alternative means of communication when an AIDS patient is critically ill.[117] This section outlines what is currently known about the manifestations of HIV infection most likely to underlie communication disorders and discusses clinical implications for SLPs.

At present HIV infections are implicated in communication disorders in 4 broad areas. First, neurological manifestations of HIV infection due to central nervous system (CNS) damage may be implicated in motor speech disorders (dysarthria, apraxia), language disorders (aphasia), and deterioration of cognitive functions (AIDS dementia complex, or ADC). Second, primary and secondary infections and secondary cancers, especially Kaposi's sarcoma (KS), may be found throughout the ear, nose, and throat areas. Third, both conductive and sensori-neural hearing losses have been found in many AIDS patients. Fourth, the logistics of caring for the critically ill AIDS patient in the hospital (e.g., intubation, respirator dependence, and so forth) may exacerbate communication disorders. These disorders have implications for the delivery of speech pathology services throughout the course of the disease in both chronic and acute care settings.

Neurologic Manifestions

Autopsy findings suggest that as many as 70% of AIDS patients develop CNS lesions.[118] Symptoms of ADC include difficulty concentrating, slowed thought processes, word-finding difficulties, slowing or slurring of speech, and personality changes. These symptoms were previously thought to be byproducts of depression brought on by facing terminal illness. More recently, however, experts have realized that these symptoms may be organic manifestations of CNS lesions.[119]

AIDS-Related Infections and Secondary Cancers in the Ear, Nose, and Throat

KS and a variety of infections (herpes zosteroticus, fungal infections, and others) have been known to affect the external ear and eardrum.[120] In addition, some AIDS patients manifest external and serous otitis media. These infections may cause middle ear dysfunction in the form of a conductive hearing loss. Nasal obstruction and drainage may be caused by KS or sinusitis. Although nasal obstruction may not directly result in a communication disorder, it may exacerbate it. Infections such as herpes, thrush (*Candida*), and hairy leukoplakia can occur in the oral structures. KS ococurs typically on the hard palate but can occur in any intraoral site. KS and other tumors in the oral and pharyngeal cavity are not likely to interfere with articulation but can cause hoarseness and even dysphonia. In some cases they have been implicated in recurrent nerve paralysis and airway obstruction.[121]

Hearing Loss

About half of AIDS patients suffer some hearing loss.[122] As mentioned above, infections in the outer and middle ear may result in a conductive loss. AIDS patients have also been known to suffer high-frequency sensorineural hearing losses as well as abnormal auditory brainstem responses. The exact cause of sensorineural losses is often unclear but may be infection along the auditory pathway.[123]

Communication Disorders Associated With Health Care

Some AIDs patients are too weak to raise their voices above the sounds of life-support equipment. The SLP can provide an amplifier or electrolarynx to assist communication. In addition, some AIDS patients may not be able to speak due to intubation and respirator dependence. In such cases, the SLP may provide augmentative and/or alternative communication techniques and equipment.

Clinical Implications

At present it is not known whether traditional speech and language therapy for aphasia, motor speech disorders, and ADC can improve AIDS patients' functioning. Until further research can delineate techniques specific to AIDS patients, it is suggested that speech and language therapy goals be the same as those for any patient with a degenerative disease.

Speech Therapy

Speech therapy should facilitate the patient's use of speech for as long as it can serve any communication need. The SLP should begin with traditional speech therapy designed to maximize intelligible communication. As speech degenerates, devices such as a palatial lift or amplifier may be used to help maintain speech intelligibility. Still further degeneration may indicate need for an alphabet board whereby the patient points to the first letter of each word he or she tries to say. This technique often acts as a pacing system for the speaker and gives a visual clue to the listener, thereby facilitating communication.[124] Handwriting, a word or picture board, an electronic communication device, and/or a computer are all possible alternative communication sytems that can be used when oral speech can no longer serve communication functions.

Language Therapy

Language therapy should begin with traditional techniques designed to maintain language processing and use and introduce compensatory techniques as they become appropriate. This approach traditionally involves educating the patient's communication partners. For example, partners may be advised to speak slower and with more simple sentences to the AIDS patient in order to help him or her understand. Partners may also be advised to introduce topic changes in a more salient way by explaining, "Let's talk about X . . . ." This can facilitate language processing by the patient.

For patients with a hearing loss, traditional aural rehabilitation techniques and amplification are appropriate. Communication partners should be instructed to make sure their face is in full view of the patient so that the mouth can be seen while speaking. It may be more difficult for the AIDS patient to hear speech in a noisy environment. The SLP may need to help the patient with lip-reading skills. A hearing aid may be beneficial.[125] Both the patient and his or her communication partners should be instructed in the benefits and limitations of amplification.

When working with AIDS patients in acute care settings, the SLP must be aware that patients are not always medically stable; cognitive, linguistic, and motor skills vary with their medical condition. The AIDS patient may only be able to tolerate short intervention sessions (5–15 minutes at a time), and schedules must be flexible.

When a hospitalized AIDS patient needs speech pathology services, more often than not he or she needs immediate, effective communication. To this end, Dowden and colleagues[126] recommend a hierarchy of intervention approaches. First, a preliminary screening determines whether the patient is responsive enough to have a reliable yes/no response. If so, a few questions are asked that tap attending responses (e.g., response to name), orientation (e.g., "Is this 1990?"), and direction-following abilities (e.g., "Close your eyes."). If the patient passes this screening, a communication needs assessment is conducted by interviewing nursing staff and family and reviewing the medical chart. This assessment will provide information about the types of things the patient needs to communicate and the ways he or she must do it (e.g., supine, intubated, and so forth). Based on these results, the SLP attempts to match communicative needs with optimum communication skills, keeping in mind that skills may deteriorate over time.

Facilitating oral communication should be considered first. If normal speech is not an option, the patient may be a candidate for a whisper technique or an electrolarynx. If oral approaches are not functional, consider a modification of oral approaches. At this stage the SLP must consult the physician and respiratory therapist. Temporary closure of the tracheostomy or use of equipment such as the PITT tube, communitrach, or ventivoice constitute ways to modify the patient and care plan to facilitate continued use of his or her own speech. If the above approaches are not feasible, then the SLP must resort to nonoral alternative approaches.

Handwriting is first assessed because communicating in writing will be the most normalizing for the patient and his or her partners. If handwriting is not feasible, consider devices that allow the patient to type messages, such as the Canon Communicator or the Sharp Memowriter. If the patient has inadequate motor control for the above devices, the SLP provides a scanning message selection technique as a means for communication. In scanning, the patient is presented with choices (words, letters, or phrases) by a partner, a word board, or an electronic device. The patient indicates when the partner or device has come to the word, letter, or phrase he or she wants. Scanning is slow but requires only limited motor abilities on the patient's part.

SLPs have the expertise to help AIDS patients with motor speech, language, and cognitive and hearing deficits during the course of the disease. Murphy and Cook[127] document that the communication systems for persons who have previously had intact speech must be provided in a timely fashion to prevent the patient from becoming a victim of learned helplessness, losing interest in taking an active part in social interactions. Health team leaders should recognize the ways SLPs can help AIDS patients in the early stages of the disease.

DISCUSSION QUESTIONS

1. Suggest research topics for each of the health professional areas discussed that could improve clinical practice and therapeutic modalities for HIV-infected persons or persons with symptomatic AIDS.
2. What steps should your profession take to develop and/or implement policy on the care and education of HIV-infected persons?
3. Explain the role your profession plays in educating for the prevention of HIV infection among various target populations.
4. Upon which of the health professions will the responsibility fall for care of HIV-infected persons who are adults? Children? Pregnant women?
5. What role can your profession play in confronting the international AIDS epidemic?
6. What role can your profession play in counseling people about HIV infection?
7. What are the current regulations or legislation in your state on disclosing the identity of HIV-infected persons?

REFERENCES

1. Institute of Medicine Committee Report: Allied health services: Avoiding the crisis. Quoted in American Society of Health Professions' Newsletter, July 12, 1988, p 2.
2. Kuhls, TL, et al: Occupational risk of HIV, HBV, and HSV-2 infections in health care personnel caring for AIDS patients. Am J Public Health 77:1306, 1987.
3. Weiss, SH, et al: Risk of human immunodeficiency virus (HIV-1) infection among laboratory workers. Science 239:68, 1988.
4. Beach, RR: Nutrition and the acquired immune deficiency syndrome. Ann Intern Med 99:565, 1983.
5. Kolter, DP, Wang, J, and Pierson, RN: Body composition studies in patients with the acquired immunodeficiency syndrome. Am J Clin Nutr 42:1255, 1985.
6. Gray, RH: Similarities between AIDS and PCM. Am J Public Health 73:1332, 1983.
7. O'Sullivan, P, Linke, RA, and Dalton, S: Evaluation of body weight and nutritional status among AIDS patients. J Am Diet Assoc 11:1483, 1985.

8. Coleman, N and Grossman, F: Nutritional factors in epidemic Kaposi's sarcoma. Semin Oncol 14(2) (Suppl3):54, 1987.

9. Nutrition and the M.D. 13(1):5, 1987.

10. Hathcock, JN and Coon, J: Nutrition and Drug Interrelations. Academic Press, New York; 1978, p 21.

11. Garcia, ME, Collins, CL, and Mansell, PW: The acquired immunodeficiency syndrome. Nutr Clin Pract June:108, 1987.

12. Patow, CA and Stark, TW: Pharyngeal obstruction by Kaposi's sarcoma in a homosexual male with acquired immune deficiency syndrome. N Engl J Med 311:20, 1286, 1984.

13. Nutrition and the MD. 13(1):5, 1987.

14. Patow, CA and Stark, TW: Ibid.

15. Garcia, ME, Collins, CL, and Mansell, PW: Ibid.

16. Garcia, ME, Collins, CL, and Mansell, PW: Ibid.

17. Garcia, ME, Collins, CL, and Mansell, PW: Ibid.

18. Modigliani, R and Bories, C: Diarrhoea and malabsorption in acquired immune deficiency syndrome. Gut 26:179, 1985.

19. Garcia, ME, Collins CL, and Mansell PW: Ibid.

20. Chelbowski, RT: Significance of altered nutritional status in acquired immune deficiency syndrome (AIDS). Nutr Cancer 7:85, 1985.

21. O'Sullivan, P, Linke RA, and Dalton, S: Ibid.

22. Rohde, CL and Braun, RN: Home Enteral/Parenteral Nutrition Therapy: A Practitioner's Guide. The American Dietetic Association, Chicago, 1986.

23. Gray, RH: Ibid.

24. Dworkin, BM and Rosenthal, WA: Selenium deficiency in the acquired immunodeficiency syndrome. Journal of Parenteral and Enteral Nutrition 10:405, 1986.

25. Dowrkin, BM and Rosenthal, WA: Ibid.

26. Shils, MR and Young, VR: Modern Nutrition in Health and Disease, ed 7. Lea & Febiger, Philadelphia; 1988, 265.

27. Rao, TK, Friedman, EA, and Nicastri, AD: The types of renal disease in the acquired immunodeficiency syndrome. N Engl J Med 316:1062, 1987.

28. Bentler, M and Stanish, M: Nutrition support of the pediatric patient with AIDS. J Am Diet Assoc 87:488, 1987.

29. Rohde, CL and Braun, RN: Ibid.

30. Hunt, NM, Miner, KR, and Thompson, S: Nutrition practices: An intervention survey of HIV-positive patients at a hospital clinic. Paper presented at American Public Health Association Convention, Boston, MA, November 1988.

31. The Los Angeles Times, August 11, 1985, View section, Part 6, p 1, "Few dentists willing to treat AIDS patients; West Hollywood clinic set up to handle cases rejected by private practice," Beth Ann Krier.

32. Logan, MK: Legal implications of infectious disease in the dental office. J Am Dent Assoc 115:850, 1987.

33. News item. Bulletin of Dental Education, American Association of Dental Schools 21:4, 1988.

34. Frieldnad, GH and Klein, RS: Transmission of the human immunodeficiency virus. N Engl J Med 317:1125, 1987.

35. Update: Universal precautions for prevention of transmission of human immunode-

ficiency virus, hepatitis B virus and other blood borne pathogens in health care settings. MMWR 37:377, June 24, 1988.

36. Centers for Disease Control: Ibid.
37. Update: Universal precautions. Ibid.
38. American Dental Association: Infection control recommendations for dental office and the dental laboratory. J Amer Dent Assoc 116:241, 1988.
39. Centers for Disease Control: Update: Universal precautions for prevention of transmission of human immunodeficiency virus, hepatitis B virus, and other bloodborne pathogens in health-care settings. MMWR 87:378, 1988.
40. Doebbeling, BD, et al: Removal of nosocomial pathogens from the contaminated glove. Ann Intern Med 109:394, 1988.
41. Demby, NA: The cost of compliance with CDC infection control guidelines in dental practice: Who pays? Paper presented at American Public Health Association, Boston, MA, November 1988.
42. Andriolo, M and Zakarian, AJ: Oral manifestations and dental management of HIV infection. Paper presented at American Public Health Association, Boston, MA, November 1988.
43. Andriolo, M and Zakarian, AJ: Ibid.
44. Coehn, L and Grace, E: Attitudes of dental faculty toward individuals with AIDS. Paper presented at American Public Health Association, Boston, MA, November 1988.
45. McCormack, KR: Dental hygienists' attitudes towarad AIDS: A descriptive study. Paper presented at American Public Health Association, Boston, MA, November 1988.
46. Rhodes, LV, Beideman, ME, and Samies, JH: Infection in traumatic extremity wounds. Emergency Care Quarterly 4:22, 1988.
47. Centers for Disease Control: Recommendations for prevention of HIV transmission in health care settings. MMWR 36(Suppl):2, 1988.
48. Baker, JL, et al: Unsuspected HIV in critically ill emergency patients. JAMA 257:2609, 1987.
49. AIDS: A guide for EMS. Maryland EMS News 14:1, 1987.
50. Centers for Disease Control: Update: Universal precautions for prevention of transmission of human immunodeficiency virus, hepatitis B virus, and other bloodborne pathogens in health-care settings. MMWR 87:377, 1988.
51. Stewart, C: AIDS and the emergency provider. Emergency Medical Service 17:24, 1988.
52. George, JE and Quattrone, MS (eds): AIDS: A challenge to EMS. Emergency Medical Technician Legal Bulletin 12:2, 1988.
53. Centers for Disease Control: Eight health care workers outside prospective studies test HIV-positive. MMWR 36:5S, 1988.
54. Gordon, D: Aeromedical personnel and AIDS. Emergency Medical Service 17:109, 1988.
55. Centers for Disease Control: Update: Universal precautions for prevention of transmission of human immunodeficiency virus, hepatitis B virus, and other bloodborne pathogens in health-care settings. MMWR 87:377, 1988.
56. Weiss, SH, et al: Risk of human immunodeficiency virus (HIV-1) infection among laboratory workers. Science 239:68, 1988.
57. Weiss, SH, et al: Ibid.

58. McCray, E, et al: Occupational risk of the acquired immunodeficiency syndrome among health care workers. N Engl J Med 314:1127, 1986.
59. Centers for Disease Control: Acquired immunodeficiency syndrome (AIDS): Precautions for clinical and laboratory staffs. MMWR 31:577, 1982.
60. Centers for Disease Control: Acquired immunodeficiency syndrome (AIDS): Precautions for health care workers and allied health professionals. MMWR 32:450, 1983.
61. Centers for Disease Control: Recommendations for prevention of HIV transmission in health care settings. MMWR 36:33, 1987.
62. Centers for Disease Control: Update: Universal precautions for prevention of transmission of human immunodeficiency virus, hepatitis B virus, and other bloodborne pathogens in health-care settings. MMWR 37:377, 1988.
63. Weiss, SH, et al: Ibid.
64. Centers for Disease Control: Update: Universal precautions for prevention of transmission of human immunodeficiency virus, hepatitis B virus, and other bloodborne pathogens in health-care settings. MMWR 37:377, 1988.
65. Centers for Disease Control: Update: Universal precautions for prevention of transmission of human immunodeficiency virus, hepatitis B virus, and other bloodborne pathogens in health-care settings. MMWR 37:377, 1988.
66. Scott, C (Hackman, Hoefflin, Shapiro & Marshal Law Corporation): AIDS: Legal issues. Presentation at California Medical Record Association convention, Anaheim, CA, May 5, 1988, pp 8 and 9.
67. California Health and Safety Code, Section 199.27 (a) (1).
68. California Health and Safety Code, Section 199.22.
69. O'Neill, J: Confidentiality concerns: The AIDS patient: Part II. Topics in Health Record Management. 7:77, 1987.
70. Jergeson, AD: AIDS codes create confidentiality problems. Newsletter of the California Medical Record Association, June 1987, p 6.
71. Joint Commission on Accreditation of Hospitals: Accreditation Manual for Hospitals. The Commission, Chicago, 1988, p 95.
72. 22 California Administrative Code Section 70749(a)(8).
73. American Medical Record Association: Guidelines for handling health data on individuals tested or treated for the HIV virus. Journal of the American Medical Record Association, October 1987, p 27.
74. Jergeson, AD: Ibid.
75. California Health and Safety code Sections 199.21(1), 199.22, and 199.24.
76. Jergeson, AD: Ibid, p 2.
77. American Medical Record Association: Ibid, p 27.
78. American Medical Record Association: Ibid, p 28.
79. Leonard, A: AIDS in the workplace. In Dalton, HL and Burris, S: AIDS and the Law. Yale University Press, New Haven, 1987, p 117.
80. Leonard, A: Ibid.
81. 29 CFR Part 19047.
82. Scott, C: Ibid, p 15.
83. Jergeson, AD: Ibid.
84. American Medical Record Association: Ibid, p 28.
85. California Association of Hospital and Health Systems: Consent Manual, ed 15. The Association, 1988, p 487.

86. Butler, K: Personal interview, September 1988.
87. Centers for Disease Control: Human immunodeficiency virus (HIV) infection classification. MMWR 36:5, 1987.
88. Jergeson, AD: Ibid, pp 1 and 6.
89. Kircher, T and Anderson, RE: Cause of death: Proper completion of the death certificate. JAMA 258:3, 1987.
90. Donahue, MP: Nursing: The Finest Art. CV Mosby, St. Louis, 1985, p 2.
91. Kielhofner, G: A model of human occupation: Part 2: Ontogenesis from the perspective of temporal adaptation. Am J Occup Ther 34:657, 1980.
92. Pizzi, M: Challenge of treating AIDs patients includes helping them lead functional lives. O.T. Week, Amer Occup ther Assn 2:32, 1988.
93. Pizzi, M: Ibid.
94. Christ, GH and Weiner, L: Psychosocial issues in AIDS. In Devita, V Jr, Hellman, S, and Rosenberg, S: (eds): AIDS: Etiology, diagnosis, treatment and prevention. JB Lippincott, Philadelphia, 1985, p 277–297.
95. Pizzi, M: Occupational therapy in hospice care. Am J Occup Ther 37:235, 1984.
96. Kielhofner, G: Ibid.
97. Kielhofner, G and Burke, J: A model of human occupation: Part 1: Conceptual framework and content. Am J Occup Ther 34:572, 1980.
98. Pizzi, M (1984): Ibid.
99. Bezalel, B: AIDS: The new challenge. Quoted by McDonnell, JM: Progress report. American Physical Therapy Association 15:6, 1986.
100. Galantino, ML: An overview of the AIDS patient. Clinical Management 7:23, 1987.
101. Galantino, ML: HIV infection: Neurological implications for rehabilitation. Clinical Management 8:6, 1988.
102. Galantino, ML and Levy, JK: HIV infection: Ibid.
103. Centers for Disease Control: Update: Universal precautions for prevention of transmission of human immunodeficiency virus, hepatitis B virus, and other bloodborne pathogens in health-care settings. MMWR 37:377, 1988.
104. Heller, RM, et al: AIDS awareness in the conduct of radiologic procedures: Guidelines to safe practice. Radiology 166:563, 1988.
105. Centers for Disease Control: Recommendations for prevention of HIV transmission in health care settings. MMWR 36(Suppl 25), 1987.
106. Olsen, WL, Jeffrey, RB, Tolentino, CS: Closed system for arterial puncture in patients at risk for AIDS. Radiology 166:551, 1988.
107. Van Sonnenberg, E, Casola, G, and Maysey, M: Simple apparatus to avoid inadvertent needle puncture. Radiology 166:550, 1988.
108. Douglas, S: Respiratory care and AIDS: Opportunistic infections of the AIDS patient. American Association of Respiratory Care Times 12:20, 1988.
109. Durak, DT: The acquired immune deficiency syndrome. Adv Intern Med 30:29, 1985.
110. Centers for Disease Control: Update: Universal precautions for prevention of transmission of human immunodeficiency virus, hepatitis B virus, and other bloodborne pathogens in health-care settings. MMWR 37:377, 1988.
111. Garay, SM and Plottel, CD: Nosocomial transmission. Clinics in Chest Medicine: Pulmonary Effects of AIDS 9:519, 1988.
112. Boroch, M and Boudin, K. Respiratory care and AIDS: Considerations for patient and clinician Safety. American Association for Respiratory Care Times 12:14, 1988.

113. Corkery, KJ, Luce, JM, and Montgomery, AB: Aerosolized pentamidine for treatment and prophylaxis of pneumocystis carinii pneumonia: An update. Respiratory Care 33:676, 1988.
114. Corkery, KJ: Ibid.
115. Boroch, M: Ibid.
116. Hmelo, CE: AIDS: Issues for the respiratory care practitioner. Respiratory Management 17:21, 1987.
117. Flower, W and Sooy, CD: AIDS: An introduction for speech-language pathologists and audiologists. American Speech and Hearing Association 29:25, November 1987.
118. Flower, W and Sooy, CD: Ibid.
119. Flower, W and Sooy, CD: Ibid.
120. Flowers, W and Sooy, CD: Ibid.
121. Flowers, W and Sooy, CD: Ibid.
122. Flowers, W and Sooy, CD: Ibid.
123. Flowers, W and Sooy, CD: Ibid.
124. Beukelman, D, Yorkston, K, and Dowden, O: Communication Augmentation: A Casebook of Clinical Management. College Hill Press, San Diego, CA; 1982.
125. Radcliffe, D: AIDS and the hearing professional: Low risk but no margin for error. The Hearing Journal 41:9, 1988.
126. Dowden, P, Honsinger, M, and Beukelman, D: Serving nonspeaking patients in acute care settings: An intervention approach. Augmentative and Alternative Communication 2:25, 1986.
127. Murphy, JW and Cook, AM: Limitations of augmentative communication systems in progressive neurological diseases. Quoted by Brubaker, C (ed): Proceedings of the 8th Annual Conference on Rehabilitative Technology, Washington, DC, Rehabilitation Engineering Society of North America, p 120–122, 1985.
128. Wall Street Journal. Tuesday, May 16, 1989, p A1.

ELEVEN

AIDS AND HEALTH CARE WORKERS: CASE STUDIES

David Pauley, Roland T. Sedillos

OUTLINE

WORKING WITH AIDS PATIENTS:
STAGES OF ACCEPTANCE
*Health Care Workers' Feelings
and Attitudes*

CASE STUDY NUMBER 1: A
VOLUNTEER WORKER WITH AIDS
CASE STUDY NUMBER 2: A HEALTH
PROFESSIONAL WITH AIDS

OBJECTIVES

By the close of this chapter, the reader will be able to:
1. State the stages through which health care workers may pass in relating to persons with AIDS.
2. Explore his or her own attitudes towards caring for persons with AIDS.

WORKING WITH AIDS PATIENTS: STAGES OF ACCEPTANCE

When health care workers (HCWs) treat AIDS patients, they are faced with caring for patients suffering a disease they frequently do not understand and often fear.

HCWs often pass through stages in their relationships with HIV-infected patients. Recognizing that such stages exist, and that exhibiting such behaviors or having such feelings is not abnormal, will help HCWs and students of the health professions to reach a level of acceptance with greater ease.

Stage 1: Avoidance. HCWs may find themselves avoiding the topic—and persons known to be HIV-infected or persons with symptomatic AIDS. "It won't happen here; only the big cities have cases of AIDS." "The doctor I work for never sees those kinds of patients." "If I had to take care of someone with AIDS, I'd ask for a transfer to another unit."

Stage 2: Demanding a Risk-Free Environment. In this stage, HCWs want proof that there is no danger in caring for an HIV-infected person. "Prove to me I won't get AIDS." "They don't know all the ways the virus is spread yet." "How can I be *sure* it isn't spread . . . through the air? By a patient coughing? By handling food?" This stage is characterized by lingering doubts in the face of mounting scientific evidence.

Stage 3: Resignation. HCWs see the number of patients in their facility or agency mounting, they realize that the AIDS epidemic is here to stay. It will not be made to disappear by not thinking about it.

Stage 4: Seeking Information. Once HCWs have accepted the fact that AIDS is here to stay, they seek information. They read articles and follow information presented on television and in news magazines alertly. They attend workshops and continuing education programs. Often their first concern is still personal protection in the work environment. As they work with HIV-infected patients, however, their fears diminish. They begin to see the patient, and not the disease.

Stage 5: Caring Concern. This stage is a natural consequence of stage 4: seeing the patient as a person with fears, concerns, and desires like those of any other patient with a life-threatening disease. They express the caring concern that is natural to persons who have chosen one of the caring professions.

People responsible for educational programs for HCWs have discovered these stages by observation and experience in the areas hardest hit by the epidemic. Several educational programs include a hands-on, touching experience with a person with AIDS (PWA). Such programs report an almost immediate positive change in feelings on the part of HCWs. Video or film presentations of such interactions, Although they lack the immediacy of touching, may serve a similar purpose.

Health Care Workers' Feelings and Attitudes

An HCW's feelings and attitudes are communicated to the patient. Fear of infection may be revealed in the way the worker touches—or refuses to touch—a patient. It may be revealed by excessive precautions on the part of the HCW. An HIV-infected person already lives with enough fear without facing feelings of fear or rejection on the part of HCWs. Whether learning of the HIV infection for the first time, or experiencing symptoms and wondering, "Is this it?" the patient is searching for answers, for support. The responses of HCWs, in whatever professional capacity they serve are important to the patient.

As you read the following case studies, consider these questions:

- What types of responses are being given by the health professional(s) involved?
- What effect do these responses have on the patient?
- To what extent do you identify with the patient? With one of the health professionals?
- What would you do differently if you were one of the health professionals involved?
- What difference in the practice of your profession will reading these case studies make to you?
- How many persons do you know personally who have experienced receiving the news that they are HIV-infected? Have symptomatic HIV infection?
- What difference has knowing such persons made in your feelings and attitudes?

CASE STUDY NUMBER 1: A VOLUNTEER WORKER WITH AIDS

As a white gay male, I have been concerned about the AIDS epidemic since its beginning, but I never imagined it would become a personal struggle. Because I am gay, I realized even then that my chances of contracting the disease were increased. In 1982, I volunteered for a health study that was tracking and researching the natural history of AIDS. Samples of my urine, blood, and semen were collected and frozen. In 1985, a blood test was developed to detect antibodies to the HIV. As soon as it became available, I took the test. The test results showed that I was seropositive. The specimens collected earlier were thawed and tested. They were also HIV positive.

By 1986, my immune system had been compromised by the virus. My physician diagnosed AIDS-related complex, or ARC, as it was then called. My health worsened. In 1987, I was diagnosed as having full-blown AIDS. My body had become unable to mount an effective immune response to opportunistic infections, and I contracted *Pneumocystis carinii* pneumonia (PCP). In 1988, as I write this, I am alive and fighting AIDS—and sometimes health care workers as well.

Positive Tests Results. I was determined to be HIV positive at an alternative testing site. After giving me the results, the counselor advised me to "go home and wrap up my affairs." I was afraid of dying. Figuring I did not have very long to live, I managed the situation by indiscriminately overextending my credit limit at several banks and department stores. Eventually, I was forced to face not only the debts I had incurred, but also the disease I had contracted.

If good pretest and post-test counseling had been available, I might have been more objective about my life expectancy and less emotional about my choices. Unfortunately, in the early years of the AIDS epidemic, there were few mental health programs to guide persons who had tested positive.

Once I learned I was antibody positive, I became paranoid. Every time I was ill, I thought I had developed AIDS. Between learning of my positive test result and learning I had full-blown AIDS, I went to a doctor at least 50 times. AIDS was my first and foremost conclusion each time I was not feeling well.

I believed that if I were ever diagnosed as having full-blown AIDS, I could accept it because I had been expecting it. It did not happen that way. I was overwhelmed by my diagnosis of AIDS. I did not feel like doing anything. I felt as if my life were over at the moment, although I was not dead. I felt there was nothing I could do. I felt powerless. I knew I could not return to work. I would not be able to move from my apartment. I could no longer take care of myself. I felt completely overcome.

The media presents people with AIDS as persons experiencing tremendous suffering. I wanted to avoid as much suffering as possible. I often thought that it would be better to contract an opportunistic infection and die rather than experience weight loss, night sweats, fatigue, diarrhea, brain infections, and all the other disorders connected with the disease.

I thought of committing suicide. It seemed the only viable alternative. Mental health professionals, especially my psychiatrist, helped me overcome my desperation. Mental health workers have consistently reminded me there is hope. I've learned that people with AIDS are more likely to commit suicide than persons with other terminal illnesses. Now there are mental health programs and support groups to help. I've learned to employ coping skills as I manage my disease and my life one day at a time.

Once I was diagnosed with full-blown AIDS, I was determined to be disabled and become eligible for benefits through the Social Security Administration. That enabled me to obtain professional psychiatric care I could not have afforded before the diagnosis. During regular sessions with my psychiatrist, I have confided personal concerns too sensitive for group counseling. My trust in my psychiatrist and his concern for my well being have developed our doctor–patient relationship into a lasting friendship.

The Emergency Room. Having a compromised immune system has created several medical emergencies for me requiring treatment in an emergency room. From the time I learned of my initial HIV-positive test results until now, I have been alarmed at the lack of AIDS education on the part of many of the staff in the emergency room, ranging from admitting clerks to physicians. I have been admitted for serious illnesses, and I have been admitted for reactions to treatments I have been receiving. Upon each admission I identified myself as HIV positive—and it has been a mistake every time!

In 1985, after my positive antibody test, I went to an emergency room because I was not feeling well. I had been having flu-like symptoms. Having disclosed that

I was HIV positive, I was quickly moved into isolation. The physician immediately suspected the diagnosis was AIDS. He ordered all the standard tests: blood tests and x-rays.

When the technician arrived to escort me to the radiology clinic, she was fully suited in mask, gloves, and gown; the only thing missing was eye goggles. I realize that not much was known then about transmission of the virus, but no one else had used such extreme precautions. This technician was only going to transport me to the x-ray clinic; she was not going to perform an invasive procedure on me!

I felt like a leper or an alien from Mars. I didn't even feel like a human being. That kind of treatment was very offensive. I thought, "Next time I won't tell them . . . then they can't discriminate against me." On the other hand, if I didn't tell them I woud be jeopardizing my health because I might not receive an accurate assessment.

That technician angered me for another reason. She was protecting herself for fear of contracting the AIDS virus. In reality, I was more at risk of contracting an infection from her because of my suppressed immune system. She had adequate T-helper cells; she could fight off an infection. I couldn't. If I were exposed to any bacteria or virus she was carrying, it could aggravate my condition. Because she worked in a hospital, she came into contact with organisms to which I might not otherwise be exposed. It was—and is—far easier for me to contract a nosocomial infection from her than for her to contract AIDS from me.

I've seen that type of attitude and behavior many times. If it persists, HIV-positive people will go underground. It is impossible to tell HIV status from a person's appearance. People don't have to tell their HIV status. They will hide it. They will be afraid to tell anyone, and they have plenty of reason to feel that way.

In 1988, I returned to the same emergency room. I should have learned from my first experience 3 years earlier. This time I told them I had full-blown AIDS. I thought that in 3 years more information would have made a difference. Instead, the staff was reluctant to believe my diagnosis because I did not fit the stereotype of a person with AIDS. I carry a paunch and am slightly overweight. The staff questioned my diagnosis. I referred the doubters to my primary care physician for confirmation. I had endured 2 months in another hospital with PCP; I told them I was certain of my diagnosis.

A careless phlebotomist came to draw my blood. Across my chart I could see printed clearly the word "AIDS." I watched her ready the needle to draw my blood. She took no precautions as she prepared to insert the needle into my vein. I warned her that she should be wearing gloves and taking precautions in drawing my blood because I was HIV positive. Startled, she dropped the syringe.

I explained to her that she should always use preventive measures when drawing blood. I told her it was not persons like myself she had to fear, but those who do not know, or do not disclose, their HIV status. I advised her always to use precautions with every patient to reduce her chances of infection.

If health care workers only use precautions with persons they know to be seropositive, then they are putting themselves at risk. It is foolish to use precautions only with persons known to be infected, but this is the practice I have observed repeatedly. I have seen my lab work labeled "infectious." To me, it makes more sense to label all specimens "infectious" to ensure proper handling.

Securing Dental Care. With a diagnosis of AIDS, I found that obtaining dental care was more difficult than obtaining treatment for rare infections. For diseases uncommon except among AIDS patients I received experimental drugs and treatments, but for a simple tooth cavity not associated with AIDS, I had trouble securing dental care.

After enduring a few days of an excruciating toothache, I sought care. I hoped my only obstacle would be finding a dentist who would accept my dental coverage through public assistance. Instead, several local dentists refused to treat me when I revealed my AIDS diagnosis. I told them about my infection so they could take precautions while rendering service; instead, their "preventive behavior" was avoidance. They refused to treat me.

Finally, the local AIDS project referred me to a more compassionate dentist. At my appointment, I told the dentist of my conversations with other area dentists. He assured me that it was not ethical behavior in dentistry to discriminate against persons with AIDS. He also shared his belief that all dentists should be using universal precautions, treating patients as though each one were infected with the HIV.

My Respiratory Therapist. I have as much faith in my respiratory therapist as I have in my physicians. Because of my suppressed immune system, I am at greater risk of contracting the frequently fatal PCP than of contracting any other opportunistic infection. My respiratory therapist knows this and always expresses his concern for prevention. I rely on the aerosolized pentamidine treatments he administers as the greatest prophylactic against a recurrence of infection. He has reviewed with me in great detail my lung volume and oxygen diffusion test results. He also updates me on current drug therapies and the latest in AIDS research. It makes me feel a part of my own health care when he includes me in the diagnostic tests and therapy. I am fortunate to have such an AIDS-literate therapist. He maintains a practice of treating only patients with HIV infection and symptomatic AIDS, which keeps him sensitive to their concerns and needs.

My experience with drugs has not always been the greatest. During my bout with PCP, the physician ordered intravenous trimethoprim/sulfamethoxazole (Bactrim), an antibacterial agent used in treating PCP. The drug caused skin rashes covering my entire body, liver and kidney disorders, and heart fluttering. The Bactrim was immediately discontinued, and the doctor prescribed intravenous pentamidine, which eventually resolved the PCP.

During that hospitalization for PCP, the doctors did not think I was going to survive. My attending physician approached my mother, explaining to her that it was difficult for me to breathe, and that I was becoming incapable of diffusing oxygen through my lungs. He informed her I should be moved to an intensive care unit, but he thought it best not to move me. He told my mother he thought it best to "shut me down" because he did not expect me to make it through the night.

I was very upset by the physician's prognosis and recommendations about continuing my life support. I warned my mother that if she let that happen, I would come back from the dead and haunt her! I demanded that the machines be left on for as long as it would take for my recovery. My mother concurred that it was neither her nor the physician's decision to "pull the plug"; as long as I could think, it was my decision.

Obviously, my physician believed I was incapable of making my own choices. At the time, I was taking lorazepam (Ativan), oxycodone HCl (Perdocan), and other pain medications. He thought I was unaware of the conversation and anything else happening around me. But I could—and did—hear their discussion. And I intended to be part of that decision!

A commonly held stereotype about persons with AIDS is that they do not want aggressive life-saving measures exercised because they are terminally ill, and because they are suffering. In my experience, most health care workers seem willing to let AIDS patients die. I want people to know that it is not all suffering. Eventually, I stabilized and recovered. I have been living a quality life. I have had a few minor illnesses, but I have not had another opportunistic infection. I have not had difficulty breathing. And I shouldn't have had to suffer because of someone's insensitivity while I was critically ill in the hospital.

Currently I am under the care of not 1, but 2, primary care physicians as well as several specialists. One of my primary care physicians is a resident at a university hospital. He was the doctor who initially diagnosed my full-blown AIDS. He had not worked with AIDS patients before, nor was he familiar with gays. He has shown me great compassion in my health care. Together we have learned much about the disease and our life experiences. My second primary care physician is an AIDS specialist. He is aggressive in his treatments and current on AIDS therapies. He is constantly in demand but has always made time for my medical needs. I believe a team of doctors is better than a single physician. I also believe it is important to treat AIDS aggressively. I take an active role in my health care management and believe that all AIDS patients should do the same.

Just as there are many persons with AIDS, however, there are many different perspectives on living with AIDS. There are people who do not want to fight the disease. There are people who do not want treatment. I've met them. But there are also people who live a quality life every day waiting for a cure. Not everyone approves of "dignified death" legislation and wishes to be eased into death by a titrated morphine drip!

I view AIDS with optimism. I serve as a member of the board for an AIDS project and I continually share my hope with others. I share my belief with people currently infected with the HIV that chronic infections are manageable through drug therapy. Lives can continue as they once did. I believe a vaccine will be developed for health care workers and others not already infected, alleviating the fear that has resulted in discrimination. I believe there is hope. I have to.

CASE STUDY NUMBER 2:
A HEALTH PROFESSIONAL WITH AIDS

They went to sea in a Sieve, they did,
In a Sieve they went to sea:
In spite of all their friends could say,
On a winter's morn, on a storm day,
In a Sieve they went to sea!*

How do I begin this? I've spent so much energy trying to live in the present and forget what went before that this is not going to be easy. I was active, probably too active. I'd been a physical therapist since 1978, and had settled into a nice home care position as an independent contractor. I loved it. I went to the gym 3 nights a week and I looked good. I went to rehearsal for an ethnic music and dance company 3 more nights a week. We had regular performances and occasionally toured nationally. My significant other and I had purchased a home and recently been to Italy (the word *lover* does not encompass the nuances and complexities of our relationship, and for this reason, I prefer the term *significant other*). My spare time was spent body surfing, carousing, and generally enjoying life. I'd had a rough childhood, but had learned that with some hard work I could make myself a good life and really appreciate the moment.

In the summer of '85 I had a sudden and noticeable decrease in endurance. I couldn't stay up all night anymore, and a day at the beach surfing required another 2 days in bed resting. About 3 weeks later, while lifting a patient, with help and in the proper position, I injured my back. It made no sense. I'd been doing this for years and was very cautious. It seemed like a typical lumbar injury and though activity was painful, I toughed it out and the symptoms gradually disappeared. However, the decreased endurance worsened.

That fall at a dance rehearsal, going over material I'd performed comfortably for years, I felt a ripping sensation at my left sacroiliac (SI) joint. It was frightening but it didn't really hurt at the time. Two days later there was a change. Activity— almost any activity—resulted in severe intermittent pain radiating to my pelvis and both legs. I'm amazed now, remembering that I continued to work for the next 3 months. I had a minimal patient load, finished as quickly as possible every day, and was a sorry excuse as a therapist. All my spare time was spent in bed. I lost weight and became increasingly depressed.

Hunting for the Best Treatment. I went from one doctor to another for 3 months. Regardless of the treatment—or lack of it—nothing improved. I felt totally

---

*From *The Jumblies*, by Edward Lear. Adama Books, New York, with permission.

disoriented and confused. Depression became anxiety, and anxiety became desperation. I've found that I can't properly communicate and describe severe anxiety to persons who have not experienced it. I made an appointment with a counselor at the local gay community center. The man recommended a psychiatrist, but was oblivious to what I was trying to tell him, that I was ready for suicide *now!* I went home and prepared to use a knife on myself. Rance, my significant other, realized what was going on, and we paid an emergency visit to the recommended psychiatrist. My only viable option was admitting myself to an open-door psych unit. Rance and I were left alone for a few minutes, 2 adult men crying. We'd both worked so hard to be independent and in control, and now we had no idea what was going to happen next.

The Psych Unit. As a physical therapist, I had worked with patients in psych units on occasion, and recalled that there often seemed to be a nurse or psych technician that should not have been there because of personality quirks. I found this to be true for the unit to which I was admitted. I remember dealing with an overly controlling and manipulative occupational therapist, but I was confused and found it hard to be objective at the time. By and large, the counselors and attendants were very kind and generous.

I was there only 3 days. A nonaddictive antidepressant temporarily did the trick. But the rest of 1986 was a continuing hell. I was unable to return to work because of the growing severity of my back pain. I was assured I could return to my old position anytime when my condition improved, and I still appreciate that.

My symptoms indicated to me that I had a hypermobile left SI joint—an unusual condition. I went from doctor to doctor, university teaching hospital to hospital, specialist to specialist. Physicians would take me for a short while, then drop me. I was terrified to think I would be without income; I had a house payment to make. I had various tests and nothing turned up. My immunologist didn't recommend the HIV test because I didn't fit the AIDS pattern with which he was familiar. If such a test did turn up positive results, it still wouldn't be conclusive, and he felt it might mark me, preventing my return to work.

Analysing the Symptoms. Over a long period of time, because of my own clinical experience, I was able to analyze what specific activities and positions aggravated my back symptoms. This took a long time because an activity seldom caused immediate pain. Ten to 30 minutes after certain activities, however, I would be howling with pain and would have to stay in bed the rest of the day. For example, I was unable to sit on a hard seat, leaning forward was impossible. I could use the toilet only in the standing position. Putting on pants, shoes, and socks all had to be accomplished in the supine position. If I dropped something, which happened frequently, I had to use a mechanical reacher to pick it up. By strictly avoiding aggravating activities, I didn't have to spend as much time in bed. I could wash the dishes, cook, water the lawn, and sometimes even drive.

Eventually, I contacted another physical therapist who had had experience treating a hypermobile SI joint. He instructed me in some self-mobilization techniques, and they worked! During periods of acute pain, I would perform these exercises. I'd feel a shift and a pop, and immediately my pain would lessen. This didn't prevent it all from happening again, but now I could temporarily relieve the worst of the pain. Hallelujah!

Kaposi's Sarcoma.   In the fall of '87 I became aware of a small patch of what looked like scar tissue over my right patella. My immunologist and dermatologist requested that I be patient and watch for any changes. Eventually, I demanded a biopsy and, the results showed I had Kaposi's sarcoma (KS). It was a sad thing to discover, but on the other hand, it was a possible explanation for the things that had been happening. I wasn't necessarily a clinical hysteric. It had all been real; I hadn't made it up.

This past year (1988) has been very different. I've been able to face problems with less self-doubt. I receive a disability income regularly through private insurance. This has freed my mind so I can solve problems better. I have been denied Social Security because I turned in a form 5 days late. I explained that I was caring for my own needs and those of my significant other who also has AIDS. We'd both been ill, but my appeal was still denied. I'm finally feeling confident enough to fight this, and have recently done research to find out which agencies might help. One of the AIDS projects has been the most helpful. They gave me the name of their liaison with the Social Security Administration and a legal aid counsel. The project also set up an appointment for me with a local dentist. In the dental office, masks and gloves were used while I was being treated, but I had expected that. The receptionist, hygienist, and dentist all treated me kindly and professionally, which I really appreciated.

I have wondered how I would be treated by others in the health care field. My primary physician, who is also an immunologist, is involved with AIDS research and treatment. Aside from being tardy with his paperwork, he and his receptionist are magnificent. I couldn't ask for anyone more professional, compassionate, knowledgeable, or devoted.

In May of '88, I came down with *Shigella,* a severe case of dysentery. Up until this time I'd had a series of minor problems, infections that were manageable with medication. When I entered the hospital with *Shigella,* I feared I might be treated poorly, but this was not at all what happened. Even the cleaning crew took time to visit and give me a few kind words. After discharge, it took about 3 more weeks at Mom's for me to recover. During that time I discovered a new problem: the explosive diarrhea had caused a tear in my lower colon. It still doesn't want to heal, but at least it doesn't seem to be worsening. The gastroenterologists involved and their staff have been kind and helpful.

Reiter's Syndrome.   Next I found I had developed arthritis in my right knee. This has now affected my right leg and ribcage. A rheumatologist diagnosed this as Reiter's syndrome, an inherited rheumatic disease often aggravated by dysentery. Most likely Reiter's is also the cause of my weakened and arthritic left SI joint. My physicians say there isn't necessarily a connection between this and AIDS, but AIDS hospice workers have told me that they see this frequently. I've talked to other AIDS patients who also have arthritic symptoms and I am convinced that there is a connection. I believe I've had the active disease for the past 3 years.

I have had some very good things happen. I'd hate to have you think that all I think about is pain and suffering. I'm sad to say that I have an aunt who won't let me in her home, and my father will have nothing to do with me now. My mother, sister, and brother, my partner's family, and my friends have been an army of support. I learned that I could tolerate periods of time standing in front of an easel and started to learn to paint. I have art work in a couple of galleries, and am having my second solo exhibition in a few months at a local community center.

I went through 4 psychiatric counselors before I found one that I thought didn't have problems worse than mine. With the tools he provides and his continuing friendship, I've coped well, I think. With this progress I felt recently that I just might have enough time to focus on spiritual matters. I wasn't happy with the fundamentalist religion in which I'd been raised. I tried others that didn't seem much better. Now I've started attending a Unitarian church and from the first visit it has felt like home. They asked me to give an informational presentation on AIDS. I did, and it seemed to be well received.

I had worked with hospice patients as a physical therapist, so this has helped me to quickly deal with any fear of death. It's physical pain I don't deal well with; I'm a big baby. Often I don't feel well physically, and sometimes this puts me in a very bad mood. Also, my significant other is confused and physically abusive. Today I had a full glass of water thrown at me. I just found out one of our friends died of AIDS; he isolated himself so that most of his friends didn't know. He didn't give us an opportunity to show him that we loved him. I'm angry about that, but it feels good to be angry. I used to feel depressed, but now I use anger to energize me to do positive things. Anger is not a bad thing; it depends on what you do with it.

It's hard to breathe, I have a new Kaposi's spot, and I haven't been able to paint for a month. When I paint, the only problems I have are the ones I've set for myself on canvas—and those I can solve.

> And in twenty years, they all came back,
> In twenty years or more,
> And every one said, "How tall they've grown!
> For they've been to the Lakes, and the Torrible Zone,
> And the hills of the Chankly Bore";
>
> And they drank their health, and gave them a feast
> Of dumplings made of beautiful yeast;
> And every one said, "If we only live,
> We, too, will go to the sea in a Sieve,
> To the hills of the Chankly Bore!"*

---

*From *The Jumblies,* by Edward Lear. Adama Books, New York, with permission.

GLOSSARY

AIDSophobia. Fear of catching AIDS.

Airborne spread. Spread by air, for instance of dust and droplet nuclei.

Antigen. Any foreign substance that causes the formation of antibodies as protective substances in the body. These substances react only with the specific antibody produced.

Arthralgia. Joint pain.

Aspergillosis. Infection caused by species of *Aspergillus* and causing inflammatory lesions or tumors.

Bisexual. Pertaining to sexual, emotional, and/or physical attraction to persons of both genders.

Candidiasis. Infection caused by the *Candida* organism.

Capsid. The shell of protein that protects the nucleic acid of a virus; it is composed of structural units, or *capsomeres*.

Cerebral toxic plasmosis. Inflammation of the brain caused by protozoa.

Colonization. Organisms multiplying on the body's surface (skin or mucosa) without immunologic or physiologic evidence that the host responded (*e.g.*, bacteria growing in the axilla).

Common-vehicle spread. A mode of infectious disease spread in which a contaminated object, usually inanimate, transmits the infectious agent to a person or persons.

Contact spread. A mode of infectious disease spread by which an association between a person and an infected source (animal, environmental contamination, or another person) provides an opportunity for the person to acquire an infection. Contact may be direct or indirect.

Contamination exposure. Exposure by splash to mucous membrane, open wound, or broken skin.

CSF. Cerebral spinal fluid.

CT. Computed tomography.

Countertransference. Behavioral, cognitive, or emotional reaction to another person's circumstances, emotions, or behaviors.

Cytomegalovirus (CMV). A common member of the herpes family of viruses causing an infectious mononucleosis-like illness. Commonly present in blood and urine.

Detoxification. Ridding the body of poison or the effect of poison.

Deoxyribonucleic acid (DNA). A nucleic acid that on hydrolysis yields adenine, guanine, cytosine, thymine, deoxyribose, and phosphoric acid; it is the carrier of genetic information for all organisms except RNA viruses.

Direct contact. The infection transmission mode occurring when the victim actively and directly contacts the infection source.

Distal axonopathy. Disease of the neurons farthest from the cell body (the neurons that conduct impulses).

Droplet. Fluid particle large enough to fall rapidly, before it dehydrates.

Dysphagia. Difficulty swallowing.

Dysphoria. Exaggerated feeling of depression and unrest without an apparent cause.

Dystonia. Impaired or disordered tonicity, especially muscle tone.

Electrophoresis. An electrochemical technique for separating chemical compounds.

Encephalopathy. Any abnormality (disease) of the brain and spinal cord.

Endoscope. An instrument by which one can look directly into a body cavity (lungs, stomach, colon, *etc.*).

Endoscopic retrograde cholangiopancreatography (ERCP). An endoscopic means of directly viewing the biliary and pancreatic ducts and injecting them with dye for radiologic visualization.

Enzyme-linked immunosorbent assay (ELISA). A laboratory testing method using an enzyme substrate reaction for identifying organisms.

Epidemiology. The study of incidence, distribution, environmental causes, and control of a disease in a population.

Epstein-Barr virus (EBV). The viral cause of infectious mononucleosis.

Etiologic agent. The agent that causes a disease.

Etiology. The cause of a disease.

Gallium scan. A nuclear medicine scan that detects infection, other inflammation and malignancy.

Ganglioneuronitis. Inflammation or degenerative inflammation of a mass of nervous tissue composed principally of nerve cell bodies and lying outside the brain or spinal cord.

Gene. A segment of DNA that codes for a functional product.

Genome. The complete set of hereditary factors contained in the haploid set of chromosomes.

Glycoprotein. A protein bound (conjugated) to a carbohydrate group. There are many types of glycoprotein.

Guillain-Barré Syndrome. Inflammation of 2 or more nerves accompanied by progressive muscular weakness of extremities and potentially leading to paralysis.

Hemophiliac. A person with an inherited condition in which normal blood clotting is not possible. Hemophiliacs take a blood product called Factor VIII to assist in clotting. A minor subgroup of hemophiliacs require Factor IX, not Factor VIII. These concentrates are made of the pooled blood of many individuals. Previously, Factor VIII often contained the AIDS virus, but since 1985 in the United States, both Factors VIII and IX are heat-treated to kill the virus. A few cases of AIDs have been diagnosed in patients lacking Factor IX. Because of the high rate of previous infection, hemophiliacs remain a high-risk group for AIDS.

Hemiplegia. Paralysis of only one side of the body.

Heterosexual. Pertaining to sexual, emotional, and/or physical attraction to persons of the opposite sex; or a person who is attracted to persons of the opposite sex.

Homophobia. Fear, dislike, or hatred of homosexuals and homosexuality.

Homosexual. Pertaining to sexual, emotional, and/or physical attraction to persons of the same sex; or a person who is attracted to persons of the same sex.

Host. Person, animal, or other animate site of infection.

Human immunodeficiency virus (HIV). The name chosen by a scientific panel of virologists and other researchers for the AIDS virus.

Human T-cell lymphotropic virus (HTLV). Viruses that infect a population of lymphocytes called T lymphocytes. The name first given to the AIDS virus by American researchers.

Immunosuppressive. Pertaining to or inducing immunosuppression; an agent that induces immunosuppression (by artificially preventing the immune response). Radiation treatment and treatment with antimetabolites are both immunosuppressive.

Indirect contact. The transmission mode involving intermediate objects in the passive transmission from source to victim.

Infection. Invasion of a host by a virus or other organism or by its toxin and manifested by immunologic, physiologic, and/or anatomic changes.

Infectious disease. Symptoms or abnormal physical findings caused by infection.

Infectious mononucleosis. A common infection of late adolescence and young adulthood caused by Epstein-Barr virus, or EBV. Symptoms include sore throat, swollen lymph nodes, fever, and profound weakness lasting several weeks.

Interstitial lung disease. A classification of lung diseases that includes *P. carinii* and other opportunistic infections common in AIDS.

Kaposi's sarcoma. A tumor of the walls of blood vessels. Usually appears as pink or purple painless spots on the skin but may also occur internally. Death occurs from major organic involvement. Originally seen in elderly men of Mediterranean or Ashkenazi Jewish descent and young men from equatorial Africa as a slow-growing, benign lesion, it is now occurring in young men, 80% of whom are gay or bisexual. It is frequently fatal.

Lentivirus. A subfamily of retroviruses that includes the visna viruses (of sheep), the equine infectious anemia virus, and the caprine arthritis–encephalitis virus (of goats). The HIV also belongs to this subfamily.

Leptomeninges. Membranes of the internal spinal cord and brain.

Lymphadenopathy. Enlarged lymph nodes. The diagnosis of generalized lymphadenopathy requires that lymph nodes be more than 1 cm in diameter; that the enlargement cannot be otherwise explained; and that the enlargement be bilaterally symmetric and affect at least 2 extrainguinal sites for at least 3 months. Generalized lymphadenopathy usually involves the neck and axilla and lasts for several years.

Lymphoma. A group of cancers that usually affect the lymph nodes. In HIV infections they often affect other tissues also.

Lymphotropic. Having an affinity for lymphocytes.

Lysogenic. Pertaining to a host cell carrying a provirus.

Lytic. A sequence of replication of viruses that results in host cell lysis, or death.

Macrophage. Any of the large, mononuclear, highly phagocytic cells derived from monocytes that occur in the walls of blood vessels (adventitial cells) and in loose connective tissue (histiocytes, phagocytic reticular cells). They are components of the reticuloendothelial system. Macrophages are usually immobile but become mobile when stimulated by inflammation; they also interact with lymphocytes to facilitate antibody production.

Meningitis. An acute inflammation of the membranes of the spinal cord or brain.

MRI. Magnetic resonance imaging.

Monocyte. A mononuclear, phagocytic leukocyte, $13–25\mu$ in diameter, with an ovoid or kidney-shaped nucleus, and azurophilic cytoplasmic granules. Formed in the bone marrow from promonocytes, monocytes are transported to tissues, such as the lung and liver, where they develop into macrophages.

Myelopathy. Any pathological condition of the spinal cord.

Neuropathy. Nervous system abnormalities or disease.

Neutropenia. Severe decrease in the number of white blood cells.

Nocardida asteroides. Star-shaped abscesses in the brain.

No identified risk (NIR). A technical term used to identify persons with HIV infection who do not acknowledge the practice of high-risk behaviors.

Nonmaleficence. Not causing harm to another.

Nucleocapsid. A unit of viral structure, consisting of a capsid with the enclosed nucleic acid.

Obligate intracellular parasite (OIP). A parasite that requires a living cell in order to grow and reproduce.

Opportunistic infections. Infections caused by opportunistic organisms. Opportunistic organisms require an opportunity to cause disease. They are omnipresent and frequently enter healthy people without causing disease but when they enter people with damaged immune defenses (*e.g.*, people with AIDS), they cause serious diseases.

Organism. A nonspecific word that identifies any type of living thing. Usually the prefix *micro-* is used when referring to the universe of unicellular organisms and smaller organisms.

Palliative. Serving to relieve or alleviate, without curing.

Paraparesis. Partial paralysis affecting the lower limbs.

Parenteral. Denoting any route other than the alimentary canal.

Parenteral exposure. Exposure by means of a needle-stick injury or cut with other sharp instrument.

Paresthesia. Sensation of numbness, prickling, or tingling; heightened sensitivity.

Pandemic. A widespread epidemic disease. A disease of worldwide occurrence. Influenza is an example of such a disease.

PCR. Polymerase chain reaction. (*See entry below*).

Perinatal. Occurring in the period around, during, or just after birth.

Peripheral neuropathy. Disease of the peripheral nerves.

Plasmapheresis. Removing blood from the body and centrifuging it in order to separate the cellular elements from the plasma.

Pneumocystis carini *pneumonia* (PCP). A lung infection usually occurring in immunocompromised people. It is caused by a protozoan that is present almost everywhere but that is normally destroyed by healthy immune systems. By the age of 4 years, 70% of healthy children have evidence of past exposure. The protozoan is air-borne, but cannot be transmitted this way to nonsusceptible individuals. Once a person develops PCP, they are susceptible to recurrence of the disease, which can be fatal.

Polymerase chain reaction (PCR). A laboratory test that can be used to diagnose HIV infection in its early stages.

Polymyositis. Disease of the connective tissue characterized by edema, inflammation, and degeneration of the muscles, and by dermatitis.

Polyneuropathy. Disorder of the peripheral nerves.

Polyradiculopathy. Inflammatory disease of the nerve roots.

Portal of entry. The site where an infectious agent enters a person's body.

Portal of exit. The site by which an infectious agent exits the infected host.

Prophylactic. Something that prevents.

Progressive multifocal leukoencephalopathy (PML). A generally fatal disease of viral origin in which the demyelination is usually found in the white matter of the brain and can be seen in the brain stem or cerebellum.

Prospective studies. Studies that follow cases of a disease in a specified population. Each member is defined, studied, and characterized at the beginning of the study. A prospective study of HIV infection in a population of health care workers might identify all the workers with occupational needle-stick injuries associated with treating HIV-infected patients at the time the injuries occur and follow the cases for an adequate period of time with adequate testing to determine if HIV infection occurred. Then, and only then, will it be possible to define the risk of HIV infection associated with needle stick-injuries caused by treating HIV-infected persons.

Provirus. The genome of an animal virus integrated or incorporated into the chromosome of the host cell, and thus replicated in all of its daughter cells.

Psychopathology. The branch of science that deals with the essential nature of mental disease, its causes, the structural and functional changes associated with it, and the ways in which it manifests itself.

Purulent. Pus-like.

Reiter's syndrome. An inherited rheumatic disease often aggravated by dysentery.

Reservoir. The usual location for an organism. The source for spread under natural conditions. Humans are the reservoir for the HIV. Though chimpanzees can become infected, and a person could get infected from a chimp, the chimp was only an accidental host and thus not the reservoir.

Retrovirus. A class of viruses that contain the genetic material RNA and that have the capability to copy this RNA into DNA inside an infected cell. The HIV is a retrovirus.

Reverse transcriptase. RNA-directed DNA polymerase; an enzyme of RNA viruses that catalyzes the transcription of RNA to DNA, which is then incorporated into the genome of the host cell.

Ribonucleic acid (RNA). A nucleic acid found in all living cells, which on hydrolysis yields adenine, guanine, cytosine, uracil, ribose, and phosphoric acid.

Sedimentation rate. A nonspecific laboratory test useful in monitoring the progress of HIV infection.

Self-actualization. Developing one's greatest potential.

Sensitivity. The ratio between the number of positive test results and the true number of positives in the group tested. A ratio of 1:1 is a perfect test, but a perfect test is never achieved.

Sharps. Needles, scalpels, and other sharp objects that can cause punctures or other injuries.

Simian immunodeficiency virus (SIV). A retrovirus shown to cause an immunodeficiency in a variety of monkey species.

Somatic. Of the body, as distinguished from the mind.

Source. Where organisms come from before being transmitted to a host.

Specificity. The ratio between the number of negative test results and the true number of negatives in the group tested. A ratio of 1:1 is a perfect test, but a perfect test is never achieved.

Syndrome. A set of signs and symptoms that occur together.

Transmission. The process by which a microbe gets from its source to a susceptible host (person).

Transplacental. Through the placenta. The organism that causes syphilis is capable of crossing the placental barrier from the mother to the developing fetus.

Tuberculocidal. Something that is lethal to tubercule bacilli. Tubercule bacilli are used as indicator microorganisms for evaluating chemical germicides. Tuberculocidal chemical germicides provide intermediate- and high-level disinfectant, depending upon how the germicide is used.

Universal precautions. A set of guidelines based on the assumption that every hospital patient has a blood-borne infection that can be transmitted by blood, bloody fluids, or genital secretions. Universal precautions say, "Treat every patient as if he or she is infected with a blood-borne infection."

Vector. Any living carrier, usually a mosquito or other biting insect, that transports an infectious agent from a source to a susceptible host.

Viremia. A virus in the blood stream.

Window. The time during which a person is infectious but does not yet test HIV positive. HIV infection occurs within 2–4 weeks of exposure. The patient immediately becomes infectious and capable of spreading the virus. HIV antibody test results become positive 5–10 weeks (and as long as 14 months) after the patient becomes infectious. During the window period, a person who is infectious has a true-negative test.

APPENDIX A

AIDS RESOURCES

NATIONAL RESOURCES

American Foundation for AIDS
  Research (AMFAR)
40 West 57th St., Suite 406
New York, NY 10019-4001
212-333-3118
(Publishes annual update on AIDS
  resources)

U.S. Public Health Service
Public Affairs Office
Hubert H. Humphrey Building, Room
  725-H
200 Independence Ave. SW
Washington, DC 20201
202-245-6867

National AIDS Information
  Clearinghouse
P.O. Box 6003
Rockville, MD 20850
1-800-458-5231

National AIDS Network
1012 14th St. NW, Suite 601
Washington, DC 20005
202-347-0390

AIDS Action Council
729 8th St. SE, Suite 200
Washington, DC 20003
202-547-3101

National AIDS Research & Education
  Foundation
54 10th St.
San Francisco, CA 94013
415-626-8784

National AIDS/Pre-AIDS
  Epidemiological Network
2676 N. Halsted Street
Chicago, IL 60614
312-943-6600, ext. 424

Women's AIDS Network
707 San Bruno
San Francisco, CA 94117
415-821-7984

American Red Cross
AIDS Education Office
1730 D. St. NW
Washington, DC 20006
202-737-8300

American Association of Physicians
for Human Rights
P.O. Box 14366
San Francisco, CA 94114
415-558-9353

National Council of Churches/AIDS
Task Force
475 Riverside Dr., Room 572
New York, NY 10115
212-870-2421

Los Angeles AIDS Project
1362 Santa Monica Blvd.
Los Angeles, CA 90046
213-871-AIDS

San Francisco AIDS Foundation
333 Valencia St., 4th Floor
San Francisco, CA 94103
415-863-2437

National Association of People with
AIDS
2025 I St. NW, Suite 415
Washington, DC 20006
202-347-1317

Mothers of AIDS Patients (MAP)
c/o Barbara Peabody
3403 E. St.
San Diego, CA 92102
619-234-3432

National People with AIDS Project
c/o AIDS Atlanta
1801 Piedmont Rd., Suite 208
Atlanta, GA 30325
404-872-0600

Coalition of Hispanic Health and
Human Service Organizations
(COSSMHO)
1030 15th St. NW, Suite 1053
Washington, DC 20005
202-371-2100

Federal Office of Minority Affairs
HHH Building, Room 118F
200 Independence Ave. SW
Washington, DC 20201
202-245-0020

National Council of La Raza
20 F. St. NW, 2nd Floor
Washington, DC 20001
202-628-9600

National Minority AIDS Council
714 G St. SE
P.O. Box 28574
Washington, DC 20038
202-544-1076

U.S. Conference of Mayors
AIDS Program
1620 Eye St. NW, 4th Floor
Washington, DC 20006
202-293-7330

Gay Men's Health Crisis
P.O. Box 274
132 W. 24th St.
New York, NY 10011
212-807-6655

Hispanic AIDS Forum
c/o APRED
853 Broadway, Suite 2007
New York, NY 10003
212-870-1902

National Hemophilia Foundation
Soho Building
110 Greene St., Room 406
New York, NY 10012
212-219-8180

INTERNATIONAL RESOURCES

AIDS Health Promotion Exchange
Special Program on AIDS
World Health Organization
20 aVe. Appi
1211 Geneva 27, SWITZERLAND

National Advisory Committee on
  AIDS
c/o Laboratory Centre for Disease
  Control
Health and Welfare Canada
Ottawa, Ontario, CANADA KIA 0L2
613-990-8964

AIDS Network of Edmonton
11303 102nd Ave.
Edmonton, Alberta, CANADA
  T5K 0P6
403-426-1516

AIDS Committee of Toronto
c/o Hassle Free Clinic
556 Church St., 2nd Floor
Toronto, Ontario, CANADA K2P 1B6

Collective D'Intervention
  Communautaire
Auprès des Gasis C.P. 29
O Succursal Victoria
Montreal, Quebec, CANADA

Comité SIDA du Quebec
3757 rue Prud'Homme
Montreal, Quebec, CANADA
  H4A 3H8

AIDS HOTLINE TELEPHONE NUMBERS

AIDS Hotline
U.S. Public Health Service
Atlanta, GA (24 hours, daily)
800-342-AIDS
800-342-2437

National Gay Task Force (NGTF)
800-221-7044 (3 to 9 PM)

STATE HEALTH DEPARTMENTS

Alabama: 205-261-5131
Alaska: 907-561-4406

Arizona: 602-255-1203
Arkansas: 501-661-2395

California: 916-445-0553
Colorado: 303-331-8320
Connecticut: 203-549-6789
Delaware: 302-995-8422
District of Columbia: 202-332-AIDS
Florida: 904-448-2905
Georgia: 800-342-2437
Hawaii: 808-735-5303
Idaho: 208-334-5944
Illinois: 312-871-5696
Indiana: 317-633-8406
Iowa: 515-281-5424
Kansas: 913-862-9360
Kentucky: 502-564-4478
Louisiana: 504-342-6711
Maine: 207-289-3747
Maryland: 301-945-AIDS
Massachusetts: 617-727-0368
Michigan: 517-335-8371
Minnesota: 612-623-5414
Mississippi: 601-354-6660
Missouri: 816-353-9902
Montana: 406-444-4740
Nebraska: 402-471-2937

Nevada: 702-885-4988
New Hampshire: 603-271-4487
New Jersey: 609-588-3520
New Mexico: 505-984-0911
New York: 518-473-0641
North Carolina: 919-733-3419
North Dakota: 701-224-2378
Ohio: 614-466-4643
Oklahoma: 405-271-4061
Oregon: 503-229-5792
Pennsylvania: 717-787-3350
Rhode Island: 401-277-2362
South Carolina: 803-734-5482
South Dakota: 605-773-5482
Tennessee: 615-741-7247
Texas: 512-458-7504
Utah: 801-538-6191
Vermont: 802-863-7240
Virginia: 804-786-6267
Washington: 206-361-2914
West Virginia: 304-348-5358
Wisconsin: 608-267-3583
Wyoming: 307-777-7953

LIBRARY DATABASES

Available through:
BRS Colleague
BRS Information Technologies
555 E. Lancaster Ave.
St. Davids, PA 19087

AIDS Abstracts from the Bureau of Hygiene and Tropical Diseases	AIDD
AIDS Articles from Colleague's Complete Text Library	AACC
Medical and Psychological Previews	PREV
MEDLINE References on AIDS	MRAI
PDQ Cancer Information	PDQC
PDQ Protocols	PDQP
AIDS Knowledge Base (from San Francisco General Hospital)	BRS

National Library of Medicine & NIH Office of AIDS Research: Access to AIDSLINE by joining NLM network, request user code. *Telephone inquiries:* NLM's

MEDLARS Management Section 301-496-6193, or toll-free 800-638-8480. Uses GRATEFUL MED Software (National Technical Information Service, 5185 Port Royal Rd., Springfield, VA 22161)

The National Library of Medicine also publishes a quarterly AIDS Bibliography listing references by sub-topics. Subscriptions are $12 and may be requested from the Superintendent of Documents, U.S. Government Printing Office, Washington, DC 20402.

AIDS INFORMATION RESOURCES DIRECTORY (ed 1, 1988)
Publication of American Foundation for AIDS Research
40 West 57th St., Suite 406
New York, NY 10019-4001
212-333-3118

DATABASE ACCESS TO REFERENCES

AIDSLINE: Updated twice a month. Clinical and research aspects of AIDS, epidemiology, and health policy issues from 1980 to present. References are drawn from MEDLINE, CANCERLIT, Health Planning and Administration databases. Maintained by the National Library of Medicine and the National Institutes of Health Office of AIDS Research.

APPENDIX B

*WHAT YOU SHOULD KNOW ABOUT THE AIDS ANTIBODY TEST**

WHAT IS THE AIDS ANTIBODY TEST?

The AIDS antibody test is a way to find out if you have been infected by the virus that causes AIDS. The test does not show if you have AIDS now or will get sick in the future. Instead, testing detects **antibodies,** chemicals the body makes to fight infection in your blood.

If there are AIDS antibodies in your blood, you are infected with the virus and you can probably pass it on to other people.

The most common test is a simple inexpensive blood test known as the ELISA.

HOW DOES THE TEST WORK?

A technician draws about a tablespoon of blood from your arm. The blood is mixed with chemicals and a dye. If antibodies are present, the fluid will change

---

*Reprinted with permission from *What You Should Know About the AIDS Antibody Test,* 1988, Network Publications, a division of ETR Associates, P.O. Box 1830, Santa Cruz, CA 95061-1830, 1-408-438-4060.

color. This is a positive test. If antibodies are not present, there is no color change. This is a negative test. Test results are usually available in about two weeks.

WHAT DOES A NEGATIVE TEST RESULT MEAN?

A negative test result means no AIDS antibodies have been found in your blood because:

- You have not been exposed to the virus; OR
- You have been exposed to the virus but have not become infected; OR
- You are infected, but your body has not yet produced antibodies. (Some people make antibodies within two weeks after exposure. Others take up to six months or more to respond.)

    A negative test result does NOT mean you can't be infected in the future.

WHAT DOES A POSITIVE TEST RESULT MEAN?

A positive test result means AIDS antibodies have been found in your blood because:

- You have been infected by the AIDS virus and can probably pass the virus to other people during vaginal, anal, or oral sex or while sharing drug needles.

    A positive test result does NOT necessarily mean you are now sick or will get sick with AIDS in the future.

IS THE TEST ALWAYS RIGHT?

The ELISA is a very dependable test, but it does occasionally give false results. You could test negative for AIDS antibodies when you are infected with the virus because:

- You were infected recently and your body hasn't made antibodies yet. On the other hand, you could test positive with the ELISA when you are not infected because:
- Like with any medical test, the technician can make a mistake conducting the test or reading the result.
- Certain medical conditions can sometimes make blood proteins look like AIDS antibodies, which confuses the test.

For these reasons, positive ELISA results should be tested again. If the second test is also positive, one of two other antibody tests (the Western Blot or IFA) should be used to check the result a third time.

If there is any question about your results, you should be retested. This system insures that test results are very accurate.

WHO DOES THE TESTING?

Tests are available in public health clinics, hospitals, doctors' offices and other locations. The test may be free or cost $20–$75. Testing procedures, counseling and the degree to which the results are kept confidential vary from place to place.

- Before deciding to take the test, call locations in your area and ask how the test is done, how results are verified and recorded and if counseling is part of the procedure.

WILL TEST RESULTS BE CONFIDENTIAL?

Medical information is usually confidential, but AIDS antibody testing is sometimes an exception.

In some states, laws require the names of persons with positive test results to be reported to the public health department. Public health records, as well as physician and hospital charts, can sometimes be subpoenaed by the courts.

IS THERE ANY WAY TO KEEP TEST RESULTS CONFIDENTIAL?

Yes. Anonymous test centers are available in many places. You can take the test without giving your name, address, telephone number, social security number or other information that might be used to trace test results to you in the future. You are given a number or code to identify you and your blood sample. To learn the results of your test, you must give this number or code. Counseling may or may not be available at these centers. Some states offer free anonymous testing and counseling. Center offering these free services are called alternate test sites.

Anonymous testing guarantees no one else can know your test results without your permission. Call your local health department for the location of the alternate test site or anonymous test center nearest you.

WHAT ABOUT COUNSELING?

Because AIDS antibody testing has the potential to cause emotional, social and legal problems, counseling is part of the testing procedure in many places. Some centers offer group or individual pretest counseling. The initial counseling session should:

- Help you understand what the test can and can't tell you;
- Explain issues of confidentiality and the procedure used to guarantee your privacy;
- Help you assess your risk of exposure to the AIDS virus by offering information about high risk sexual and drug taking behaviors;
- Help you make a plan to deal with either positive or negative test results;
- Give you names and phone numbers of people you can contact if you have questions or concerns while waiting for your test results.

Individual counseling in private should be provided at the time you learn your test results. No matter what the outcome, the post-test counseling session should:

- Help you understand clearly what your test result means;
- Help you focus on a plan for preventing the spread of the virus.

If your test is positive, counseling should also include:

- Help in coping with emotional stress;
- Information about caring for your health and the health of those around you;
- Referrals for ongoing medical care and emotional support.

WHAT ARE THE ADVANTAGES OF
TAKING THE TEST?

Consider how the test might help you before deciding whether or nt to be tested.

- Testing can reduce your anxiety and uncertainty.
- If you are a woman considering pregnancy or breastfeeding, testing can help you evaluate the risk of transmitting the virus to your child.
- You will know if it is safe to donate blood, organs or sperm to others.
- You might be more likely to protest yourself and others from infection.
- If you learn you do have antibodies to the AIDS virus, you can improve your chances of staying healthy by limiting your use of drugs and alcohol, eating well, getting plenty of rest and reducing stress.

WHAT ARE THE DISADVANTAGES OF TAKING THE TEST?

There are risks that you should carefully consider before deciding to take the test. Being tested may cause:

- Mild to severe emotional reactions, including anxiety, nightmares, depression and fear;
- People to think you have AIDS;
- Problems with sexual desire or arousal, due to stress or anxiety.

If the test is positive:

- Your partner may blame you or refuse to have sex with you.
- You may lose your job or be unable to get insurance if the result is not kept confidential.
- You may experience discrimination in receiving medical care, obtaining housing or attending school.

If the test is negative:

- You may develop a false sense of security. Remember, anyone can get AIDS. Always use condoms if you or your partner have sex with anyone else, and never share needles with anyone.

WHO SHOULD CONSIDER TESTING?

You may want to consider testing if you think you have been exposed to the virus because:

- You have had sex with a gay or bisexual man who has had other partners;
- You have shared needles to use drugs or have had sex with someone who has;
- You have hemophilia, or have had sex with someone who has hemophilia;
- You had blood transfusions between 1979 and March 1985, or have had sex with someone who did;
- You have had sex with a heterosexual man or woman who has had other partners.

You may not want to be tested if your risk of exposure to the AIDS virus is very low or you feel unwilling or unable to cope with a positive test result.

For more information about AIDS antibody testing, call your local health department or the National Public Health Service at the following toll-free number: (800) 342-7514, or the Hotlines listed in Appendix A.

APPENDIX C

*SAFER SEX GUIDELINES**

AIDs, or acquired immunodeficiency syndrome, is caused by a virus called the human immunodeficiency virus (HIV). This virus lives in white blood cells. It is passed from 1 person to another in only a few ways: by having unsafe sex, by sharing needles, from a pregnant woman to her baby before birth, or in rare cases, by blood or blood products that carry the virus.

The HIV cannot be spread by everyday contact like touching, hugging, or sharing a soda with someone who has the virus.

Many of the people who have the HIV have come down with AIDS. But it can take 5–10 years, or more, before the person gets sick. So at this time, **most people who have the HIV are not sick.** They probably don't know they have it. But they can give it to someone else, who may then get AIDS.

These days, many of us may need to change the way we have sex. But we don't have to stop having sex entirely.

And we don't have to stop enjoying sex, either.

WHO SHOULD FOLLOW THE SAFER SEX RULES?

Anyone who is not 100% sure that they and the person they are having sex with do not have the HIV should follow these rules. **This means:**

**Reprinted courtesy of City of Philadelphia, AIDS Coordinating Office.

- People who have had the HIV antibody test (the "AIDS test") and were told they are positive (they have the HIV).
- Anyone, straight or gay, if they or their partner has had sex with more than 1 person since 1976. This means sex between men and women (straight), between men and men (gay), or between women and women (lesbian). Sex involving semen or blood is most risky.
- People who have shared needles with anyone, even once.
- Hemophiliacs ("bleeders") who were given blood or blood products before 1985.
- People who have had sex with anyone who could be on this list.

If you have any questions, call your community AIDS hotline (see Appendix A). You may want to ask about a free blood test to help you find out if you have been infected with HIV (see Appendix B). You don't have to give your name to take this test. There will be someone to talk to about what the test could mean for you.

GENERAL RULES

The basic rule for safer sex is: Don't let semen, blood, vaginal fluids, or pre-ejaculatory fluid get into your mouth, vagina, tip of the penis, or rectum, or into any cuts or sores on the skin.

- Try to keep to 1 sex partner. It's safest to have sex with only 1 person, who has sex only with you. If you or your partner have had sex with anyone else since 1976, or if either one of you has shared a needle, there is a chance you could have the HIV.
- Talk with your partner. Before you begin, talk about what kind of sex you will and will **not** do. Talk about what safer sex is. Get to know the person, but remember, not everyone has the courage to tell the truth about the past.
- If you are high, you may forget to use condoms, so do not use alcohol or drugs when you may want to have sex.

SAFEST SEX

You don't have to worry if you do only these things:

- Solo masturbation
- Massage, body rubs, hugging, cuddling
- Mutual masturbation (using your hands to please each other). Remember, the AIDS virus can get into cuts or sores on your skin, so do not let semen, vaginal fluids, or blood touch any sores. Thin rubber gloves are a good idea if your hands are cut or chapped.

- Body to body rubbing (may be done to orgasm). Be sure no semen or vaginal fluids enter cuts or sores or mucous membranes (vagina, rectum, mouth, tip of penis).
- Kissing on face, lips, breasts, body. Keep in mind that breast milk or breast discharge from an infected woman may pass on the virus.
- Using sex toys (dildoes, vibrators, feathers, and so forth.) Do not share them in any way that could pass on vaginal fluids, semen, blood, or stool to the other person. Clean toys with alcohol or bleach between uses. Or use condoms on the toy and change condoms between partners.

PROBABLY OR POSSIBLY SAFE SEX

You may want to choose which of these you are willing to do:

- *Deep kissing is probably safe—unless there are any cuts or sores or bleeding gums in your mouth or your partner's mouth.*
- *Use a latex condom for vaginal intercourse or anal (rectal) intercourse. Don't use natural membrane condoms, such as Fourex.*

With the condom, you may also want to use a spermicidal (birth control) foam, jelly, cream or lubricant that contains nonoxynol-9. Examples are Delfen Foam, Koromex or Ortho Contraceptive Gel, Today Sponge. (All are sold in drugstores without prescription, and may help protect against disease and pregnancy.) But they will not kill all HIV. **Always** *use it with a condom.*

- Use a condom only once.
- Put it on before the man enters.
- Hold it on while he pulls out.
- Do not use oil-based lubricants (vaseline, baby oil, Crisco), because they may damage the rubber. Use water-based lubricants, like K-Y jelly, to help keep condoms from breaking.
- For extra safety, consider using condoms **and** pulling out **before** the man comes.

Remember that anal sex is even less safe, because condoms are more likely to break during anal sex. There are "extra strength" condoms available in some stores; or use 2 condoms at once.

Use a condom for oral sex on a man. Oral sex may be less risky than vaginal or anal sex, but it is not 100% safe. The main risk is to the person getting semen in the mouth. The other person is at little to no risk from saliva. Keep semen out of the mouth entirely (spitting it out is not enough). Be aware that pre-ejaculatory fluid (pre-cum) may contain the virus.

For oral sex on a woman, or for oral–anal sex on a woman or man, use a latex barrier to protect the person performing oral sex. Some latex barriers are rubber dental dams, cut-apart surgical gloves, or cut-apart condoms, placed over the vaginal opening and clitoris, or anus.

UNSAFE SEX

Do NOT do these things:

- Vaginal sex without a condom is not safe. Other kinds of birth control or douching will **not** help prevent AIDS.
- Anal sex without a condom is not safe. Even with a rubber, this is a very risky kind of sex. Douching or enemas do **not** help, and may even make anal sex **less** safe.
- Oral sex on a man without a condom is not safe.
- Oral sex on a woman is not safe without a latex barrier.
- Oral–anal sex without a latex barrier is not safe. You can get many diseases besides AIDS if you do this.
- Fisting (hand in the rectum) is not safe. It can tear the rectum and make it easy for the AIDS virus to get into the body.

Be well informed about AIDS. If you have any questions, don't be afraid to ask! Call your local community AIDS hotline (see Appendix A).

Index

An "*f*" following a page number indicates a figure. A "*t*" following a page number indicates a table.